PUBLIC HEALTH IN THE 21ST CENTURY

THE DIFFERENT FACES OF BEING OVERWEIGHT

RISK FACTORS FOR THE EVOLUTION TOWARDS OBESITY

PUBLIC HEALTH IN THE 21ST CENTURY

Additional books in this series can be found on Nova's website
under the Series tab.

Additional e-books in this series can be found on Nova's website
under the e-book tab.

PUBLIC HEALTH IN THE 21ST CENTURY

THE DIFFERENT FACES OF BEING OVERWEIGHT

RISK FACTORS FOR THE EVOLUTION TOWARDS OBESITY

EMILIA MANZATO
EDITOR

New York

Library of Congress Cataloging-in-Publication Data

ISBN: 978-1-63483-099-7

Library of Congress Control Number: 2015941528

Published by Nova Science Publishers, Inc. † New York

CONTENTS

FOREWORD

Obesity is considered as a serious and complex condition that heavy interferes with the patients quality of life.

It is increased worldwide, and up to now its treatment remains a challenge.

Yet it is well known that obesity is a chronic condition difficult to treat.

Furthermore actually it is controversial whether a treatment focused only on weight loss can be really effective in promoting health since in most cases a consistent weight loss is not maintained for a long term.

Therefore it is important to give attention to the stages preceding the obesity onset, considering the treatment of overweight patients as the real secondary prevention, and concentrating the research efforts toward the clear identification of risk factors for the weight gain.

So how much important is overweight in the development of obesity? And, furthermore, may overweight be considered itself as a health problem? And yet could a better knowledge of physical and psychological aspects of overweight subjects help in identifying individuals with high risk for developing obesity?

In this book we try to consider overweight not as a single condition, but as a set of clinical conditions very different from each other.

Furthermore, overweight should not be regarded as a stable condition.

Therefore overweight individuals should be assessed in all the factors characterizing their clinical history to decide when, whether and how to operate.

Currently there are no protocols to diagnose every aspect of overweight with a multidisciplinary approach so there is no proper path of care for the overweight patient with high risk factors for developing obesity. We try to affront the overweight problems from different points of view so that to reach a better understanding about this complex problem.

This book is aimed at raising awareness that overweight can be a crucial point in order to prevent obesity progression and it is addressed to therapists who are willing to better understand overweight and accordingly treat overweight patients properly.

PREFACE

The term "obesity epidemic" refers to the rapid increase of obesity prevalence in the Western World. All obese people had previously been overweight.

Because being overweight is a fluctuating condition and it is impossible to treat all overweight individuals, it is crucial to understand specific features of overweight subjects to pinpoint the factors that cause obesity.

Obesity as a medical condition represents an intriguing area of study from both clinical and speculative points of view.

In this book, a general overview concerning epidemiological data of overweight individuals and theories about eating behavior in obese subjects will be discussed thoroughly.

One chapter will be dedicated to dietary restraint as a risk factor for the loss of dietary control.

Epidemiological data and features of overweight individuals throughout life stages will also be discussed.

One chapter will be dedicated to overweight children and adolescents, and how the condition possibly leads to obesity in adulthood.

Eating Disorders as a risk factor for weight gain in overweight people will be discussed, particularly Binge Eating Disorders, Bulimia Nervosa and Night Eating Syndrome.

Furthermore, in the same chapter, other biased eating behaviors leading to weight gain will be widely described.

The characteristics of body dissatisfaction and negative body image in overweight people will also be considered.

Afterwards, the book will focus on sedentary lifestyles and unbalanced diets as a risk factor for obesity.

In the last chapter, the multidimensional approach to overcoming obesity will be discussed.

List of Abbreviations

ACTH	acetylcholine
AN	Anoressia Nervosa
APA	American Psychiatric Association
BN	Bulimia Nervosa
BED	Binge Eating Disorder
BMI	Body Mass Index
BPA	plasticizer bisphenol
CVD	Cardiovascular Disease
DA	dopamine
DR	Dietary Restraint
DSM	Diagnostic and Statistical Manual of Mental Disorders
END	endorphins
ED	Eating Disorders
EDCs	Endocrine Disrupting Chemicals
EDNOS	eating disorders not otherwise specified
FA	Food Addiction
FFM	fat free mass
FM	fat mass
GB	gaba
GWG	Gestional Weight Gain
HFSS	High fat salt sugar (food)
HSME	Homeostasis System of Metabolism and Energy
HSHR	Homeostasis System of Hedonic Reward
LMR	low metabolic rate
NE	norepinephrine
NES	Night Eating Syndrome
NAc	Nucleus accumbens
NCAR	Neural Circuitry of Addiction and Reward
N.E.A.T	Non Exercise Activity Thermogenesis
NES	Night Eating Syndrome
PBDE	polybrominated diphenylether
PIR	prevalence income ratio.
PET	positron emission tomography

REE	resting energy expenditure
RMR	resting metabolic rate
SGA	Small Gestional Age
SUD	Substance Use Disorders
SES	Socio-Economic Status
VTA	Ventral Tegmental Area
COSI	WHO's Childhood Obesity Surveillance Initiative
WHR	Waist/Hip Ratio

In: The Different Faces of Being Overweight
Editor: Emilia Manzato

ISBN: 978-1-63483-099-7

Chapter 1

OVERWEIGHT DURING THE CENTURIES

Emilia Manzato*

Psychiatrist, University of Ferrara, Italy
National Council Member,
Italian Society for the Study of Eating Disorder (SISDCA), Italy

ABSTRACT

There is a growing concern about obesity and overweight worldwide perceived as "epidemic problem".

In this chapter the results of the main surveys regarding the spread of obesity and overweight will be briefly reported.

Most studies have been focused on obesity so far and only recently overweight has gained importance.

Data on overweight give a complex and unclear view: could overweight be considered as a high risk factor to obesity? Or, vice versa, could overweight be the best condition for a longer life expectancy? The results of literature data are contradictory.

In this chapter a broad view about the features of overweight in childhood and adolescence and in women, particularly in the menopausal age will be also given.

Data about health's risks due to overweight condition will be provided in the last part of the chapter.

Keywords: obesity epidemic, obesity in childhood, gender, life expectancy

INTRODUCTION

Despite Hippocrates (460 b.c-377b.c.) many centuries ago had already defined corpulence as "not only an illness itself but also the premonition of other diseases" nevertheless for a long time the excess of body weight has not been considered as a real problem.

* emilia.manzato@gmail.com.

It was only in the second half of last century that obesity started to be considered as a risk condition for health.

Quite recently, at the beginning of XXI century, the World Health Organization (WHO) highlighted the spreading and risks of overweight by using the word "obesity epidemic" to emphasize the rapid increase in the number of subjects suffering from obesity in the Western World [1].

Actually, studies on population show-for the first time in history-a great prevalence of overweight and obese subjects in comparison with normal weight ones in the Western World.

In addition, the perception of overweight and obesity has been changing in the history of mankind in relation with a different social and cultural development in the various geographical areas. In the Western World, in fact, nowadays these conditions are considered as much more negative than in the past concurrently with the development of a different idea of female beauty strictly related to thinness.

Actually, thinness up to emaciation, as in some models, is increasingly exalted as the ability to control hunger, whereas overweight is more and more considered as a negative aspect of the individual, unable to control hunger impulses.

Both conditions may have a negative impact on health.

At present, the World Health Organization defines overweight and obesity as conditions due to abnormal or excessive accumulation of body fat linked to a higher risk of morbidity and mortality.

Obesity in particular, is considered as a serious and complex condition. Two main aspects are examined in details: the need for a multidisciplinary diagnostic/therapeutic approach and the difficulty to achieve a stable weight decrease-which can be reached only in a small percentage of subjects.

Actually it is controversial whether a treatment focused only on weight loss can be really worthy since in most cases a sustained long term weight decrease is not obtained.

In this context, is it so fundamental to focus on overweight? How important is overweight in the development of obesity? And furthermore, may overweight be considered itself a health problem? And yet could a better knowledge of physical and psychological aspects of overweight subjects help us identify individuals at risk of obesity, as well as caregivers find an effective strategy?

Let's consider some main points: first, is overweight a real health problem?

While researches agree that obesity has a real impact on morbility and mortality, on the other hand the debate about a possible impact of overweight on health is still pending.

Recent scientific articles [2] reported an even increased life expectancy in slightly overweight subjects.

Overweight should not be considered as a single condition, but as a set of different clinical conditions varying on the presence or absence of medical or psychiatric complications as well as on genetic, social and family background.

Therefore obesity and overweight should be approached in a similar way.

Furthermore, overweight should not be regarded as a stable condition in most cases but rather as a phase of transition towards a possible further weight gain.

Therefore overweight individuals should be assessed in all the factors characterizing their clinical history to decide when, whether and how to operate.

Normal weight should be restored in patients whenever possible but, if clear obesity risk factors are evident, then a simple stabilization of weight should be achieved.

In this case medical and psychological aspects should be carefully monitored.

Another question still remains unanswered: why is obesity in our industrialized countries societies becoming an epidemic? Does it deal only with wealth, food abundance connected with a decrease in physical activity and contemporary an increase in sedentary jobs?

Furthermore, looking back at the history of human feeding, we can observe a radical change in food consumption in the twentieth century all over the industrialized countries: after the Second World War and especially since the fifties the dietary protein and fat intake has been considerably increasing. In two decades the consumption overcame suggested quantity.

Actually at the end of the nineteenth century the main surveys reported as main causes of death the diseases of gastrointestinal and respiratory tract such as pneumonia, tuberculosis, diseases of infancy and diseases of the circulatory system, while since the 1960's surveys have been showing that cardiovascular diseases were the first cause of death [3,4,5]. These changes may partly be the result of different eating habits.

In addition, changes in the lifestyle as well as the achievement of a better life standard have played an important role as co-factors of obesity in industrialized populations living in developing areas.

Another socio-cultural element that might have contributed to obesity could, paradoxically be represented by a radical change in feminine beauty ideal: since the end of 19'th century it shifted toward a more and more extreme concept of thinness getting to that typical emaciation condition, of some 1970's top models .

Such a challenging goal, so difficult to reach, could lead to unhealthy eating behaviors ranging from restriction to starvation and possible trigger a subsequent loss of control and weight gain.

Finally, it is important to consider the role of psychological problems, such as an altered self-perception of body image, possibly leading unhealthy eating attitudes to real eating disorders. It is well known in fact, that the presence lifetime of any eating disorder represents a risk factor for weight increase.

GLOBAL TREND OF OVERWEIGHT

An impressive amount of studies concerning the trend of obesity and overweight have been published so far: the reports were often conflicting and-especially in recent times- have shown a controversial trend.

The percentage of overweight and obesity has been increasing over a long period from the end of XXth century until recent years when it seemed to level off.

In fact, the prevalence of obesity, relatively constant from 1960 to 1980, increased of about 8% between the 1976-1980 survey and the 1988-1994, as reported by the Third NHANES (National Health and Nutritional Examination Survey) [6].

Also the World Health Organization Consultation on Obesity reported that the incidence of obesity has been increasing rapidly worldwide since 1990: until 1990 the prevalence of obesity in adults was 10–25% in most countries of western Europe and 20–25% in some US countries.

Some years after this percentage increased by 40% in women in eastern European and Mediterranean countries as well as among US Afro-American women [7].

During the 2009-2010 period, obesity prevalence in the US was 35.5 % among men and 35.8% among women [8].

The prevalence of overweight in the USA has continued to increase in children and adolescents between 1999-2004 and the overweight prevalence tripled in the period 1980-2002 in children and adolescents [9].

Similar trends have been observed in many countries throughout the world, for example in Great Britain [10].

Particular news appeared in June 2014: a London newspaper reported figures, provided by the Ministry of Defense, showing how even the royal army had been hit by obesity epidemic.

In fact, over the last three years 22,000 soldiers were found to be overweight and, in addition, 32,419 soldiers (men and women) were no longer able to pass the basic physical tests (according to the UK standards a 30- year- old solder must be able to do 50 flexings on the legs within 120 seconds and 44 flexings on the arms in the same time).

According to World Health Organization estimates for 2003, overweight adults (considering as a threshold body mass index or BMI $\geq$ 25) were more than a billion, of which at least 300 million were obese.

Currently the situation has worsened, the World Health Organization Consultation on Obesity, a worldwide federation of organizations addressing this problem clinically and politically, estimates that approximately 475 million adults are obese and 1.5 billion are overweight. The prevalence of overweight and obesity varies depending on the racial and ethnic groups.

The worldwide prevalence of overweight in 2004 has been found to range from less than 15% in Eritrea to more than 50% in the USA [11].

In low and middle income countries the prevalence of overweight among adults ranges from 18% to 59%. This trend is the result of many factors such as the decline in underweight, the more sedentary lifestyles and the trends in labor force participation [12].

In developing countries overweight trends have been analyzed in relation to the type of working activity: according to the present research women working in agricultural occupations resulted to have a lower overweight prevalence than women working in higher occupational classes [13].

Even in China, where the prevalence of obesity in subjects >20 years old was lower in comparison with other countries, approximately one-third of the subjects were overweight and had an abnormal body fat distribution (abdominal obesity) [14]. In India, which accounts for nearly half of the malnourished population all over the world, 55% of women aged 20 to 69 years are overweight [15].

It is interesting to note that ethnic groups, originating from developing countries, once moved towards industrialized countries will be exposed, within one generation or two, to the same significant weight gain as native subjects, associated with the same or even superior disease risk.

Nonetheless, in the beginning of 2007, Mitchell et al. reported a levelling off in the prevalence of obesity in Scottish schoolchildren [16].

Since then, results from many studies around the world have suggested that the obesity epidemic has levelled off since the early 2000s.

Rokolm et al. [17] systematically reviewed all available data to investigate if there was a real stability or a seeming levelling off in the prevalence of obesity.

Overall results from the 52 studies (44 articles, 4 reports and 4 publicly available database) included in this review indicate a clear tendency towards a stabilization of the obesity epidemic in children and adolescents from Australia, Europe, Russia and the USA.

The leveling off was less evident in the lower socioeconomic status groups.

The tendency in European adults is, however, more ambiguous, as a growth in prevalence was still reported in limited data from Austria, Denmark and Sweden. No obvious differences between genders were detected.

At the end of this brief review of the available data concerning overweight and obesity it is interesting to mention a recent study published in the International Journal of Obesity " A break in the obesity epidemic? Explained by biases or misinterpretation of the data"[18].

The authors underline, somewhat controversially, that the studies concerning the trends of obesity are highly heterogeneous with respect to the quality and comparability of available data. Before concluding that the obesity epidemic is not increasing anymore, the validity of the reports addressing this item should be carefully analyzed.

The authors highlight that most studies suggesting a break or a decrease of obesity were of short duration, in addition studies reporting data on both BMI and waist circumference generally suggest that waist circumference changes were less favorable than BMI variations.

Finally authors conclude that the recent reported break in the obesity epidemic needs to be interpreted with caution.

When Have Overweight and Obesity Become a Problem?

The artistic representation of the human body represents the ideal of beauty expressed by the culture in a definite historical period.

Since the earliest representations of the human body a fair amount of fat was considered a sign of good health and high socio-economic status, as the history of mankind has always been characterized by long periods of famine and undernourishment.

Only in the Middle Ages the body was represented as emaciated and skeletal because a florid body was considered as a source of sin.

Since the 16TH century until the last century overweight and obesity were closely related to the ideal of beauty- it has usually been referred mainly to the female beauty- as well as to good health and fertility as represented, for example, by the women portrayed by Rubens or Renoir.

On the contrary, in recent years, an increasing discrepancy between a new ideal of beauty represented by emaciated models and the real life condition, marked by problems of overweight and obesity, could be observed.

In an old study Wiseman [19] analyzed the weights of Miss USA pageant' finalists and the weights of Playboy models from 1959 to 1987: the results showed a progressive decrease of Misses' and Playboy models 'weight in the last years of the study while on the opposite young women living in Western countries had progressively increased their weight in the same period. For the first time a sizeable gap between the actual physical appearance of females and the current ideal of beauty was evident: in this context, body dissatisfaction and consequent attempts to become as thin as suggested by media have likely contributed to the spreading of unhealthy dietary practices.

At the same time incidence and prevalence of eating disorders such as anorexia and bulimia on one side, overweight up to obesity on the other side did increase.

Furthermore other eating disorders, typically associated to weight gain, such as binge eating disorder, the night eating syndrome and grazing, have been progressively increasing.

These topics, i.e. the change of body image and body dissatisfaction mediated by cultural models, have been specifically discussed in the chapter 7.

It is worth noting that a more accurate assessment of individual's weight has started only in the fifties of last century, when the Metropolitan Life Insurance Company Life, USA, in 1943, introduced for the first time standard height-weight tables for men and women. These tables were based on the hypothesis that a body weight increase above the average value-resulting from statistical analysis- was the main cause of early death due to cardiovascular disease. The "desirable" weight was the one associated with the lowest mortality rates according to insurance longevity statistics of the company.

Afterwards these tables became a guideline for establishing the insurance premium, related to the individual risk of mortality.

Until 50 years ago, more or less, a common way to determine the approximate weight of a person was Bernhardt's formula: (body height in cm x chest circumference) divided by 240. Bernhardt's formula was then replaced by the simpler formula of Broca: body height - 100 ± 10% or 20%.

Nowadays Body Mass Index (BMI) has universally replaced these previous formulas in determining “normal” or “standard” weights. BMI is calculated using the Quetelet formula, developed by a Belgian mathematician for the first time in the 19th century: according to this scientist, individual's BMI [kg / m²] is derives from the ratio of body weight to the square of height.

Since 1972 when it was first applied this index has been more and more extensively used [20].

Nevertheless BMI has also been criticized because, since it doesn’t take into account important factors such as gender, age, percentage of lean or fat body mass and basic morphological characteristics in the formula above.

According to BMI index World Health Organization defined weight standards (26 BMI) beyond which the term "overweight" generally indicates an excess of weight.

A review of the BMI cut-off was made several years ago and resulted into a lowering of the minimum value to define overweight (from 26 to 25).

Currently the almost exclusive use of BMI in epidemiological studies or in scientific research is controversial, due to two main reasons: firstly the terms of comparison are not the same in the different countries of the world, secondly BMI does not seem to be the sole reliable index of severity in a clinical situation related to overweight.

Actually BMI is an inaccurate measurement unit of adiposity since high levels of body fat rather than high body mass could better represent the real health risk. Furthermore, being the relation between body fat and disease occurrence not yet clearly established, a new parameter, the waist circumference, has been included in the assessment of disease risk.

Finally, some authors have criticized the status of alarm created by overweight and obesity epidemic. The term “epidemic” itself has been challenged as it implies an exponential pattern of growth typical of epidemics, not supported by recent data.

Furthermore between 1980 and 2004 media attention to obesity and overweight increased exponentially from 62 articles published in the Lexis-Nexis US News Sources with " obesity" in the headings, lead paragraphs, or key terms in 1980, to over 6500 in 2004.

Pharmaceutical companies could have further contributed to creating a widespread state of alarm about obesity to increase their business.

A different and somewhat revolutionary point of view about obesity epidemic is expressed by Campos [21] in his "point-counterpoint article" (2006) where the author suggests that alarmist claims about obesity are more induced by "moral panic " rather than by a real "health crisis". Campos defines moral panic as the attitude - typical when rapid social changes occur- towards an exaggeration or creation of unmotivated risks: to support this claim the authors report the significant use of alarming terms such as, for instance " time bomb" [22] in as many as 221 newspaper articles concerning obesity.

Campos considers moral panic as a broad concept including also the anxieties about the new gender roles: in this regard he reports that feminist careerism, for example, has been blamed to be a cause of obesity epidemic : "if the mothers work too, few adults and children risk eating balanced meals"!!!!

Finally, he concludes, concerns about obesity epidemic could reflect not only the interests for individuals' health but also political and economic interests of certain groups, while doing immense damage to those whom it blames and stigmatizes.

Overweight in Children and Adolescent

The gradual spreading of overweight in children and adolescents has been extensively studied.

In this book this issue has been specifically deepened in a devoted chapter where the different aspects will be treated in a comprehensive manner (see chapter 5).

We'll mention only some significant data concerning this topic with the purpose to give an overview of the problem "overweight" in childhood and adolescence.

It is to point out that defining obesity and overweight in children and adolescents is quite difficult, both due to the different methods of measuring (weight ? BMI ?) across the survey and to BMI dramatic changes with age.

Until a few years ago, overweight in children was regarded as a sign of well-being and accepted without any concern; nowadays, on the contrary, overweight in childhood is seen as a dangerous condition, even considered as the major risk factor for the development of obesity in adulthood.

Furthermore overweight and obesity in childhood have dramatically increased as well as in adults since 1990. These findings confirm the need for early effective interventions to reverse anticipated trends [23].

A research [24] focused on overweight trend between 1988 and 1994 in children and 16-17 years old adolescents reported a percentage of 11% overweight subjects: the prevalence of overweight was not significantly related to race, ethnicity and income or education status. Over the subsequent years the group of overweight children underwent a further increase of their weight.

In 2010 the prevalence of childhood overweight and obesity was estimated to be 11.7% in developed countries and 6.1% in developing countries, but the majority of affected children -35 million- lived in developing countries [25].

In 2008 The National Center for Epidemiology, Surveillance and Health Promotion of Italian Ministry of Health performed an epidemiologic study named "Okkio alla Salute", subsequently repeated in 2010. This research, focused on weight status and risk behaviors in primary school children, confirmed the high frequency of overweight and obesity, respectively 24% and 12%, in children with 8-9 years. According to the research, overweight and obesity showed an increasing trend from North to South of Italy [26].

The reasons of this phenomenon are still under investigation.

Also for childhood obesity, after decades of rapid increase it appears that the prevalence in developed countries is gradually stabilizing. The data show that the prevalence of obesity and overweight is stabilizing in the US, Australia, Japan and in some European countries such as France and the UK. The levelling of obesity and overweight prevalence is less apparent for more disadvantaged socioeconomics groups [27, 28].

Many studies emphasize the role of family environment in the onset of overweight: actually, parents' feeding practices favouring overweight could be transmitted to their children.

An experiment carried out in a laboratory with children in their pre-school age has documented a relation between maternal consumption of food for mood regulation and children's feeding behaviour when facing negative mood [29].

Furthermore overt parental restriction of some selected food was reported to be related to an increased consumption of such foods when they freely available [30].

It is estimated that approximately 25–40% of infants and toddlers experience feeding problems, often linked with the development of otherwise preventable diseases, such as overweight and obesity as reported by their caregivers.

Indeed, the relationships and interactions around feeding have a crucial role in the development and maintenance of eating difficulties [31].

Furthermore most parents have a job and need grandparents' help for childcare.

In Great Britain approximately 36% of parents ask grandparents to care for their children so that grandparents' attitudes while feeding children may have a great impact upon their eating and weight.

A study [32] comparing parents' and grandparents' feeding practices showed that grandparents might provide even a healthier food for children, but putting in practise maladaptive feeding methods.

According to this research grandparents' eating habits differed from parent's ones in many aspects such as a greater use of emotional food, less encouragement of energy balance and poor model of healthy eating and more dieting for weight reasons.

These feeding practices could have negative effects on adult eating behaviour, by increasing food assumption for emotional regulation and could predict compulsive eating with consequent weight gain over time

Finally, some aspects concerning the tendency toward weight gain in childhood and adolescence are still unclear: weight gain in adolescents suggests an increased calories intake, but actually an increase in calories intake is reported only in late adolescence.

Therefore their weight gain could be mainly due to a change in their lifestyle, much more sedentary than ever before. In fact, despite the lack of studies specifically focusing on the adolescents' attitude toward physical activity, a decline in youth participation to projects of physical education was reported in the period 1984 -1990 [33].

The research study "Health Behavior in School-aged Children" (HBSC) was launched in 1982 to investigate and monitor the health behaviour of teenagers aged 11, 13 and 15 years, as well as to provide more information aimed at promoting health policies [34].

HBSC is an international study providing repeated surveys on these issues every four years, in collaboration with the Regional Office for Europe of the World Health Organization (WHO). Initially promoted by England, Finland and Norway, it now has 43 participating countries. Italy joined in 2000 and three national surveys, in 2001, in 2006 and 2010 have been carried out up to now.

While international guidelines recommended children with developmental age to make a moderate or vigorous physical activity every day for at least 60 minutes, data from the last Italian survey in 2010 show that only 5.2% of eleven-year-old, 6.7% of thirteen-year old and 12.4% of fifteen-year-old never engaged in physical activity.

Still, according to the HBSC study, the acquisition of behavior models during childhood and adolescence would be crucial to maintain a healthy behavior in adulthood.

The lack of adequate space and time, as well as safety in going outdoor shows how children are increasingly confined in an enclosed and more protective space, especially at home watching TV or playing video games [35]. Computers and television reduce needs and opportunities for physical activity [36].

The time spent in front of a screen is considered as one of the main factors responsible for overweight in this age group, since it is often associated with intake of high calorie foods contributing to a daily caloric energy imbalance [37, 38].

The increase in the percentage of overweight is then attributed to several variables that act regardless of age, gender and country of origin.

The early recognition of excessive weight gain relative to linear grow is essential. Routine assessment of all children needs to become a standard practice from infancy.

The guidelines [39] encourage a universal prevention and early treatment: intrauterine, infant and preschool periods are considered as hot periods to possible program a long-term energy-balance regulation.

Overweight on Women

Overweight trends as well as weight related complications could be influenced by genders [40].

Some specific periods in the life of a woman such as menarche, menstruations, pregnancy, postpartum, lactation, menopause are risk conditions for weight gain since the associated neuro-hormonal changes may significantly affect psycho-physical balance. In this context the hormone estradiol plays an important role- well known for 40 years-in the regulation of body weight, fat distribution and the central mechanisms of food intake. All these modifications should be evaluated in relation to the personal history.

In women each biological passage represents a moment of fragility that, whenever enhanced by genetic and environmental risk factors, could lead to changes in weight and development of real eating disorders.

Furthermore, women may suffer from overweight related complications in a differently depending on the stage of their life: e.g. after menopause they become much more vulnerable to cardiovascular events since estrogen levels are no longer enough to prevent protective cardiac complications.

As a matter of fact, the menopausal transition is still a particularly neglected issue whose features have only been delved into by gender medicine.

Sex gender -based medicine proposes an interesting approach to "femininity" and "masculinity" that considers their double biological and historical dimension as not interchangeable but deeply integrated in a reciprocal relationship. This branch of medicine aims at improving prevention, diagnosis and treatment of various pathological conditions in both genders but at the same time to take into account the different expressions of the disease in males and in females. Within this scope new gender-specific biomarkers, risk factors for morbidity, have been studied as well as gender-specific clinical features of a given disease: symptoms, experience of pain, different impact of the disease on psychological, social and cultural status. Another important field of research concerns the different effects of some drugs in men and women; indeed, gender plays a crucial role in pharmacokinetics, pharmacodynamics and drug toxicity. During last decade gender medicine has particularly focused on the cardiovascular vulnerability occurring in post-menopausal women and a gender-specific approach to clinical complications of this period is increasingly accepted.

Several studies showed that the relative risk of health complications due to obesity, particularly cardiovascular disease, have a worse prognosis in women than in men [41, 42, 43]. Furthermore, it has been reported that women with obesity suffer more from stress, headache, fatigue and depression than men with obesity [44]. The higher relative morbidity in obese women compared to obese men suggests that overweight and obesity in female should require a greater attention by health professionals. A Danish study [45] showed that general practitioners (GPs) give different advice and treatment recommendations to overweight male and female patients. Overweight women receive suboptimal cardiovascular disease preventive care and GPs screen and treat them less aggressively than men. In addition, the GPs treat the medical complications due to overweight more rigorously in male than in female patients. The prevalence of overweight in women has been studied in some developing countries where, as previously reported, it has a different distribution depending on the geographic areas, the level of employment etc. A research conducted in 2005 examined the distribution of overweight and underweight among women by using data collected between 1992 and 2000 in 36 developing countries. This study showed that the prevalence of overweight in young women living in both urban and rural areas is higher than the prevalence of underweight. In half of the country surveyed overweight had a prevalence higher or similar to 20% and female overweight exceeded 50% in urban and 40% in rural than female normal weight [46].

Overweight Life Expectancy and Disability

Obesity and its complications are themselves responsible of a Health expenses ranging from 5.5 to 7 per cent in the United States and the percentage drops only slightly (between 2 and 3.5 per cent) in other countries, such as Canada and Japan. The economic burden is mainly linked to two types of costs, the direct costs, resulting from interventions performed to reduce body weight and the indirect ones, attributable to overweight and obesity-related diseases. According to the European Charter on Counteracting Obesity, the impact of overweight and obesity on Health Care expenses is considerable in Europe; its direct costs are amount to a fee up to 8%, while the indirect ones are, at least, twice as much. Substantial differences of mortality by weight categories are still controversial. While the obesity class 2 and 3 are both associated with a significantly higher all-cause mortality, in some studies overweight and obesity class 1 are not. Actually, it has been reported in a metanalysis by Flegal that overweight was even associated with decreased mortality, obesity class 1 was not significantly associated with increased mortality while the main contribution to mortality in obesity was due to higher levels of BMI. These findings were consistent with some other previous studies [47, 48, 49]. The main criticism on meta-analysis by Flegal, concerned the wide-ranging normal weight reference group including a heterogeneous group of people [50].

Another study evaluating mortality in relation to BMI but gender based, found that overweight women compared with normal weight women showed a similar mortality rate, while overweight men showed slightly lower rate than normal weight men [51]. In the same study, the overweight people had longer life expectancy than normal weight participants, results that are consistent with some previous studies [52, 53]. In any case, even if overweight and obesity class 1 subjects in some studies do not seem to be associated with an increased mortality risk, still this does not mean they don't have a serious health problem. In fact, obese and overweight people have higher needs and demands for medical care than normal weight people [54]. Furthermore in a recent review and metanalysis Kramer et al. studied the effect of metabolic status on all cause of mortality in normal weight, overweight and obese subjects. Metabolic status was defined according to Adult Treatment Panel III as healthy or unhealthy depending on the presence or absence of components of the Metabolic Syndrome. Three findings resulted from the review by Kramer: firstly, metabolically healthy obese individuals run a higher risk for all-cause mortality and CV events over the long term (10 years) in comparison with metabolically healthy normal-weight people; secondly, all subjects with unhealthy metabolic status show a higher risk, regardless of BMI; thirdly, blood pressure, waist circumference, insulin resistance increased as well as the BMI, increase such risk independently from baseline metabolic status [55]. In many case overweight is preferred to be maintained rather encouraging weight gain by means wrong treatments: in fact, while major behavioral changes are required to lose weight and maintain such a weight, smaller changes behaviors are required to prevent weight gain. Different results were reported in another wide research on 59.531 women selected from the Breast Cancer Detection Demonstration Project investigating the association between their previous BMI and mortality: underweight, overweight and obese women in comparison with normal weight groups had a shorter average life expectancy even after taking in consideration their education, race / ethnicity, income, etc. [56].

CONCLUSION

In conclusion, the condition of overweight and its impact on individual health is still controversial.

Therefore, it would be necessary to identify the needs and characteristics of different subgroups to organize targeted prevention or therapeutic interventions.

Treatments targeted to weight loss could be harmful in overweight patients showing eating disorders, psychiatric comorbidity and low motivation.

Actually, in such individuals maintenance treatments to prevent possible medical complications are to be preferred since tough weight loss treatments could result totally unsuccessful or even dangerous.

In addition, it would be useful to implement a prevention strategy primarily based on lifestyle in overweight sub-groups with the highest risk of obesity.

Obesity and overweight contribute to worsening the quality of life, and the estimates of years spend with disability vary between 6 and 10 years, depending on age at baseline and sex [57, 58].

Furthermore, women are disproportionally affected by the disability risk induced by excess body weight, whereas men are physically stronger than women and they are more likely to recover from mild disability.

Although it is unclear if overweight is strictly bound to disability risk, as well as obese individuals, the overweight people could develop disability risks in their lower limbs more easily than normal weight people [59].

REFERENCES

[1] World Health Organization. Obesity: preventing and managing the global epidemic Report of a WHO Consultation. *WHO Technical Report Series 894*, 2000.

[2] Flegal, KM; Brian, KK; Orana, H; Graubard, BI. Association of all-cause mortality with overweight and obesity using standard Body mass Index categories. A systematic review and meta-analysis. *JAMA,* 2013 309, 71-82.

[3] Amstrong, GL; Conn, LA; Pinner, RW. Trends in infectious disease mortality in the United States during the 20th century. *JAMA,* 1999 281, 61-66.

[4] Peeters, A; Barendregt, JJ; Willekens; F; Mackenbach, JP; Mamun, AA; Bonneux, L. Obesity in adulthood and its consequences for life expectancy: a life table analysis. *Am. Intern. Med.*, 2003 138, 24-32.

[5] Olshansky, SJ; Passaro, DJ; Hershow, RC; Layden, J; Carnes, BA; Brody, J. A potential decline in life expectancy in the United States in the 21st century. *N. Engl. J. Med*, 2005 352, 1138-1145.

[6] Flegal, KM; Carroll, MD; Kuczmarski, RJ; Johnson, CL. Overweight and obesity in the United States: prevalence and trends, 1960-1994. *Int. J. Obes. Relat. Metab. Disord*, 1998 22 (1), 39-47.

[7] World Health Organisation. Global database on body mass index. Available at: http://who.int/bmi/index.jsp.

[8] Flegal, K; Carroll, MD; Kit, BK; Odgen, CL. Prevalence of obesity and trends in the distribution of body mass index among US adults 1999-2010. *JAMA*, 2012 307 (5), 491-497.

[9] Ogden, CL; Carroll, MD; Curtin, LR; McDowell, MA; Tabak, CJ; Flegal, KM. Prevalence of Overweight and Obesity in the United States, 1999-2004. *JAMA,* 2006 295 (13), 1549-1555.

[10] Rennie, KL; Jebb, SA. Prevalence of obesity in Great Britain, *Obes Rev*, 2005, 6, 11-12.

[11] Low, S; Chin, MC; Duerenberg-Yap, M. Review on Epidemic of Obesity. *Ann. Acad. Med.*, 2009 138 (1), 57-65.

[12] WHO Global status Report on Non communicable Diseases 2010. World Health Organization, 2011, Geneva.

[13] Lopez-Arana, S; Avendano, M; van Lenthe, FJ; Burdorf, A. Trends in overweight among women differ by occupational class: results from 33 low and middle income countries in the period 1992-2009. *Int. J. Obes.,* 2014 38 (1).doi:10.1038/ijo.2013.50

[14] Jia, WP; Xiang, KS; Chen, L; Lu, Jx; Wu, YM. Epidemiological study on obesity and its comorbidities in urban Chinese older than 20 years of age in Shanghai. *China Obes. Rev.*, 2002 3 (3), 157-165.

[15] Sakar, A; Aronson,KJ; Patil, S; Hugar, LB; van Loon, GW. Emerging health risks associated with modern agriculture practices: a comprehensive study in India. *Environ. Res.*, 2012 115, 37-50.

[16] Mitchell, RT; McDougall, CM; Crum, JE. Decreasing prevalence of obesity in primary schoolchildren. *Arch. Dis. Child,* 2007 92, 153–154.

[17] Rokholm, B; Baker, J L;. Sørensen, TIA. The levelling off of the obesity epidemic since the year 1999: a review of evidence and perspectives. *Obes. Rev.*, 2010 11 (12), 835–846.

[18] Visscher, TL; Heitmann, BL; Rissanen, A; Lathi-Koski, M; Lissner, L. A break in the obesity epidemic? Explained by biases or misinterpretation of the data? *Int. J. Obes,* 2014 doi: 10.1038/ijo.2014.98

[19] Wiseman, CV; Gray, JJ; Mosimann,JE; Ahrens,AH;. Cultural expectations of thinness in women:an update. *Int. J. Eat Disord.*, 1992 11, 85-89.

[20] Keys, A; Fidanza, F; Karvonen, MJ; Kimura, N; Taylor, HL. Indices of relative weight and obesity. *J. Chronic. Dis.,* 1972 25 (6), 329-343.

[21] Campos, P; Saguy, P; Ernsberger, P; Oliver, E; Gaesser, G. The epidemiology of overweight and obesity: public health crisis or moral panic? *Int. J. of Epidemiol.*, 2006 35, 55-60.

[22] Saguy, AC; Riley, KW. Weighting both sides: morality, mortality and framing contests over obesity. *J Health Policy Law*, 2005 30, 869- 921.

[23] de Onis, M; Blossner, M; Borghi, E. Global prevalence and trends of overweight and obesity among preschool children. *Am. J. Clin. Nutr.,* 2010 92, 1257-64.

[24] Troiano, RP; Flegal, KM. Overweight in Children and Adolescent: description, epidemiology, and demographics. *Pediatrics,* 1998 101(3), 497-502.

[25] Centers for Disease Control and Prevention; National center for health Statistics. National health and Nutrition Examination survey. http://www.cdc.gov/ nchs/nhanes_ questionnaires.htm.

[26] OKKIO alla SALUTE. https//www.okkioallasalute.it.

[27] Chung, A; Backholer, K; Wong, E; Palermo, C; Keating, C; Peeters, A. Trends in child and adolescent obesity prevalence according to socioeconomic position: protocol for a sistematic review. *Syst. Rev.*, 2014 3, 52.

[28] Odgen, CL; Carroll, MD, Brian , KK; Flegal, KM. Prevalence of obesity and trends in Body Mass Index among US Children and adolescents 1999-2010. *JAMA,* 2012 307(5), 483-490.

[29] Blissett, J; Haycraft, E; Farrow, C. Inducing preschool children's emotional eating: Relationships with parental feeding practices. *Am. J. Clin. Nutr.*, 2010 92, 359–365.

[30] Ventura, A; Birch, L. Does parenting affect children's eating and weight status? *Int. J. Behav. Nutr. Phys. Act.*, 2008 5, 15.

[31] Reau, NR; Senturia, YD; Lebailly, SA; Christoffel, KK. Infant and toddler feeding patterns and problems. Normative data and a new direction. The Pediatric Research Group. *J. Dev. Behav. Pediatr.*, 1996 17, 149–153.

[32] Farrow, C. A comparison between the feeding practices of parents and grandparents. *Eat. Behav.*, 2014 15, 339–342.

[33] Heat, GW; Pratt, M; Warren, CW; Kann, L. Physical activity patterns in American high school students. *Arch. Pediatr. Adolesc. Med.,* 1994 148, 1131-1136.

[34] Studio HBSC-Italia, rapporto sui dati 2010 a cura di Cavallo F, Giacchi M, Vieno A, Galeone D, Tomba A, Lamberti A, Nardone P ISSN ISTISAN13/5.

[35] Sonneville, KR; La Pelle, N; Taveras, EM; Gillman, MW; Prosser, LA. Economic and other barriers to adopting recommendations to prevent childhood obesity: results of a focus group study with parents. *BMC Pediatr*, 2009 21, 9-81.

[36] Task Force on Community Preventive Services. Increasing physical activity. MMWR *Recomm. Rep*, 2001 50 (18), 1-14.

[37] Powell, LM; Szczypka, G; Chaloupka, FJ. Adolescent exposure to food advertising on television. *Am. J. Prev. Med.*, 2007 33(4), 251-6.

[38] Utter, J; Scragg, R; Schaaf, D. Associations between television viewing and consumption of commonly advertised foods among New Zealand children and young adolescents. *Public Health Nutr.*, 2006 9(5), 606-12.

[39] Berg, F; Buechner, J; Parham, E. Guidelines for childhood obesity prevention programs: promoting healthy weight in children. *J. Nutr. Educ. Behav.*, 2003 35 (1), 1-4.

[40] Manson, JE ; Willett, WC ; Stampfer, MJ ; Colditz, GA ; Hunter, DJ ; Hankinson, SE ; et al. Body weight and mortality among women. *N. Engl. J. Med.*, 1995 333, 677-85.

[41] Mosca, L; Mochari, H; Christian, A; Berra, K; Taubert, K. National study of women's awareness, preventive action, and barriers to cardiovascular health. *Circulation,* 2006 113, 525-534.

[42] Grover, SA; Kaouache, M; Rempel, P; Joseph, L; Dawes, M; Lau, DC; Lowensteyn, I. Years of life lost and healthy life-years lost from diabetes and cardiovascular disease in overweight and obese people: a modelling study. *Lancet Diabetes Endocrinol.* 2015 3(2), 114-122

[43] Khan, UI; Wang, D; Karvonen-Guitierrez, CA; Khalili, N; Ylitalo, KR; Santoro, N. Progression from metabolically benign to at-risk obesity in perimenopausal women: a longitudinal analysis of study of women across the nation (SWAN). *Clin Endocrinol Metab,* 2014 99(7), 2516-25.

[44] Muenning, P; Lubetkin, E; Jia, H; Franks, P. Gender and the burden of disease attributable to obesity. *Am. J. Public Health,* 2006 96, 1662-1668.

[45] Rohde, JF; Hessner MV; Lous, J; Műller, P; Hølund, U; Heitmann, BL. The Importance of Gender of Patients and General Practitioners in Relation to Treatment Practices for overweight. *PloS ONE,* 2014 doi: 10.1371/journal.pone.0095706.

[46] Mendez, MA; Monteriro, CA, Popkins, BM. Overweight exceeds underweight among women in most developing countries. *Am. J. Clin. Nutr.,* 2005 81, 714-721.

[47] Flegal, KM; Kit, BK; Orana, H; Graubard, BI. Association of all-cause mortality with overweight and obesity using standard Body mass Index categories. A systematic review and meta-analysis. *JAMA,* 2013 309, (1)71-82.

[48] McGee, DL. Diverse populations collaboration Body Mass Index and Mortality: a meta-analysis based on person level data from twenty-six observational studies. *Ann. Epidemiol.*, 2005 15 (2), 87-97.

[49] Allison, DB; Fontaine, KR; Manson, JE; Stevens, J; Vanitallie, TB. Annual deaths attributable to obesity in the United States. *J. Am. Med. Ass.*, 1999 282, 1530-1538.

[50] Keith, SW; Fontaine, KR; Allison, DB. Mortality rate and overweight: overblown or understimated? A commentary on a recent meta-analysisi of the associations of BMI and mortality. *Mol. Metab.*, 2013 2, 65-68.

[51] Nagai, M; KuriYama, S; Kakizaki, M et al. Impact of obesity, averweight and underweight on life expectancy and lifetime medical expenditure: the Ohsaki cohort study. *BMJ* Open doi:10.1136/bmjopen-2012-000940.

[52] Reuser, M; Bonneux, LG; Willekens, FJ. Smoking kills, obesity disables: a multistate approach of the US Health and Retirement Survey. *Obesity,* 2009 17, 783-789.

[53] van Baal, PH; Hoogenveen, RT; de Wit, GA; et al. Estimating health-adjusted life expectancy conditional on risk factors: results for smoking and obesity. *Popul. Health Metr.* 2006 3, 4-14.

[54] Kuriyama, S; Tsuji, I; Ohkubo, T; et al. Medical expenditure associated with body mass index in Japan: the Ohsaki Study. *Int. J. Obes. Relat. Metab Disord*, 2002 26, 1069-1074.

[55] Krame, CK; Zinman, B; Retnakaran, R. Are metabolically Healthy overweight and obesity benign conditions? *Ann. Intern. Med.,* 2013 159, 758-769.

[56] More, SC; Mayne, ST; Graubard, BI; Schatzkin, A; Albanes, D; Schairer, C; Hoover, RN; Leitzmann, MF. Past body mass index and risk of mortality among women. *Int. J. Obes.*, 2008 32 (5), 730-739.

[57] Walter, S; Kunst, A; Mackenbach, J; Hofman, A; Tiemeier, H. Mortality and disability: the effect of overweight and obesity. *Int. J. Obes.*, 2009 33, 1410-1418.

[58] Steensma, C; Loukine, L; Orpana, H; Lo, E; Choi, B; Waters, C; Marte, S. Comparing life expectancy and health-adjusted life expectancy by body mass index category in adult canadians: a descriptive study. *Popul. Health Metr.*, 2013 19,1-21.

[59] Ferraro, KF; Su, Y; Gretebeck, RJ; Black, DR; Badylak, SF. Body mass index and disability in adulthood: a 20 year panel study. *Am. J. Pubblic Health*, 2002 92 (5), 834-840.

In: The Different Faces of Being Overweight
Editor: Emilia Manzato
ISBN: 978-1-63483-099-7

Chapter 2

FOOD ADDICTION: BRAIN AND MIND

Gian Luigi Luxardi[12*] ***and Fiorenza Marchiol***[34]

[1]Clinical Psychologist, Chief of Center for Eating Disorders of ASL, "Friuli Occidentale", Italy

[2]President of Triveneto Section of Italian Society for the Study of Eating Disorders (SISDCA), Italy

[3]Clinical Psychologist, Center for Eating Disorders of ASL n.6, "Friuli Occidentale", Italy

[4]Member of Italian Society for the Study of Eating Disorders (SISDCA), Italy

ABSTRACT

There have been various attempts to explain why some people chronically overeat and seem unable to restrain their food intake. One explanation relates directly to the markedly "toxic" food environment in recent years. A growing body of clinical and neurobiological evidence has shown how persistent overeating can lead, in vulnerable individuals, to a pattern of compulsive behaviour similar to that seen in addiction disorders. Evidence in scientific literature argues that food reward, not hunger, could be the main driving force behind eating in the modern obesogenic environment. In this chapter, we consider the assumptions related to neural and molecular adaptations in both homeostatic and non-homeostatic appetite regulation that may underlie the formation of an allostatic, non-resilient state, propelling the individual from a basic preference for palatable diets to food craving and compulsive, addiction-like eating behavior. We consider also the interaction of these systems with stress and mood regulation.

INTRODUCTION

Some people chronically overeat and seem unable to restrain their food intake. Some explanations for this focus on the environment in which we live and the plentiful availability of highly refined food rich in fat, sugar and salt. According to Kelly Brownell [1], this

* gianluigi.luxardi@ass6.sanita.fvg.it.

environment can be defined as "toxic" in respect of the availability of highly processed and hyper-palatable foods compared with previous generations [2]. Binge eating, emotional eating, external eating and eating in response to food cravings have been linked to weight gain and weight regain after successful weight loss. Binge eating is characterized by consumption of large amounts of food and loss of control over eating. Although prevalence estimates for binge eating among obese individuals vary [3], evidence indicates that binge eating is a substantial issue among obese individuals. Emotional eating is characterized by consumption of food in response to emotional arousal [4], and external eating is characterized by eating in response to external food-related cues (i.e. the sight, smell and taste of food) [5]. Although there are no prevalence estimates for emotional and external eating behaviors, there is evidence that they are more common among obese individuals than among normal-weight individuals [6]. Food cravings have been shown to lead to obsessive thoughts about food and impulsive consumption of craved foods in some individuals, which increases the risk for weight gain [7].

Several food addiction hypotheses have been published in the scientific literature [8, 9, 10, 11, 12, 13, 14] and two manuals on food addiction have recently been published [15, 16], but there is currently no standardized definition.

The current scientific evidence is insufficient to definitively answer the question of whether food is indeed addictive. Firstly, there are problems with the actual concept of food addiction [11, 12, 17]. Food is required for daily living and a line must be drawn between normal consumption and overconsumption, which can be highly subjective. Drug dependence, on the other hand, is more easily defined because psychoactive substances are not necessary for survival and any amount could be considered overuse. Secondly, experiments demonstrating physiological dependence are currently limited to animal models [8, 18, 19, 20] and have yet to be reproduced in humans. Thirdly, food addiction is routinely compared with known eating disorders, despite fundamental differences in psychopathology and presentation [9]. For instance, food addiction is most often compared to Binge Eating Disorder (BED), which was recently added as a new diagnosis in the 5th edition of the American Psychiatric Association (APA) Diagnostic and Statistical Manual (DSM-5) [21]. Finally, as pointed out by Pelchat [17], the pattern in which food is consumed or made available may be more important than the nutrient content of the food itself.

Studies in animals focus on physiologic addiction using the classic features of the addictive cycle [22] as defined below:

Bingeing in animals is defined as an escalation of intake. This can be measured by a significant increase in lever presses to self-administer a substance [23], or eating after satiation [20]. In humans, this definition is highly subjective, because what is a large amount to some may not be perceived as unusual by others. Nevertheless, there is a definition of bingeing in the APA's Diagnostic and Statistical Manual (DSM-5). There are clinical accounts of increased food consumption in each binge as the disorder becomes chronic [24], with higher body weight correlated with the frequency and severity of binge-eating episodes [25].

Withdrawal is based on signs and symptoms of opioid deficiency and is characterized by physical signs (such as tremors) [18] anxiety, and depression [8]. Studies of food addiction in humans have focused on negative affect or] dysphoria by self-report: clinical reporting of headaches, irritability, and flu-like symptoms when not overeating [24]; clinical accounts in which self-identified food addicts use food to self-medicate, eating when they feel tired, anxious, depressed or irritable in order to escape a negative mood state [26].

Tolerance is also often included as a criterion for dependence and is defined as need for more substance to get the same effect, or as the same amount of substance producing less effect with continued use [8]. This has been attributed to dopamine D2 receptor down-regulation in the nucleus accumbens (NAc) [27]. In humans, the consumption of larger amounts of food is described in the DSM criteria for BED, even though we have no evidence for a need to increase the quantity of food over time, to get the same result.

Craving or seeking in the addiction literature is described as an intense drive to self-administer drugs. In food addiction research, craving is illustrated by the motivation to seek food. Serotonin and opioids are thought to play key roles in this process; serotonin receptor agonists [28], and opioid and cannabinoid antagonists [29] significantly diminish motivation to eat. Drug craving and seeking have been experimentally described as forms of learning in which dopamine signaling facilitates the consolidation of memory such that past experiences are used to inform future decisions [30]. In other words, rats 'press the lever' for drugs because they have learned that it is rewarding [31]. Food cravings are reported at significantly higher rates in adults with BED than non-bingeing controls [32].

Sensitization is defined as a progressive increase in locomotor response observed with repeated administration of a substance [8, 33]. It is attributed to engrained changes in mesolimbic dopamine signaling [34]. In animals, sensitization is usually measured as increased locomotion in response to the substance [8]. Once sensitized, animals or subjects may demonstrate hyper-responsiveness to a new substance. This is referred to as cross-sensitization [8].

In humans, food addiction is often examined in comparison with established criteria for substance dependence [9, 26, 35]. Human substance dependence was defined by the Diagnostic and Statistical Manual IV-TR [36] as "a maladaptive pattern of substance use leading to clinically significant impairment or distress". Seven criteria for substance dependence were identified. Cassin & von Ronson [37] used a structured telephone interview, with the word "food" substituted for the word "drug" in the DSM-IV-TR criteria for substance dependence, showing that 92% of women with BED met the diagnosis.

Gearhardt et al. [38, 39] developed the Yale food addiction scale (YFAS) as an attempt to operationalize the concept of ''food addiction.'' The YFAS translates the substance dependence diagnostic criteria outlined in the Diagnostic and Statistical Manual IV-TR [36] to apply to eating behavior. The YFAS provides two scoring options, one option that measures food addiction ''symptoms'' and another option that provides a food addiction ''diagnosis'' based on the substance dependence diagnosis in the DSM-IV-TR.

The recently published DSM-5 features a new category entitled "Addiction and Related Disorders" [21], which includes both substance use disorders (SUD) and non-substance addictions. In addition, the list of clinical symptoms indicating substance dependence has increased from seven in the DSM-IV-TR to eleven in the DSM-5, and it includes additional features such as failure to fulfill role obligations, use in physically hazardous situations, continued use despite interpersonal problems, and craving or a strong desire or urge to use the substance.

A recent qualitative study [40] compares two groups of overweight women, with or without a diagnosis of BED. The results of this study suggest that obese women with BED are more likely to meet criteria for a food addiction based on the revised criteria for SUD in the

DMS-5. Findings from this and other studies [41, 42] also demonstrate that addictive tendencies toward food do not only characterize BED but can also occur in other individuals who struggle with overeating. In the cited study [40], all participants (except for one person in the non-BED group) met two or more criteria for a substance-use diagnosis (with food as the substance) as specified in the DSM-5. The APA suggests that the seriousness of the disorder can be determined by the number of symptoms endorsed (for example: two or three symptoms are described as "moderate," while greater than four reflects a "severe" condition). The BED participants appear to be more severely addicted because they endorsed more symptoms than their non-binging counterparts. Both groups of women subjectively endorsed DSM-5 SUD criteria (in relation to food) in their narratives, even if there were visible qualitative differences in the manners in which the women experienced these symptoms. The endorsed criterions in both groups were:

Criterion 6: The substance is often taken in larger amounts or over a longer period of time.

Criterion 7: There is a persistent desire or unsuccessful efforts to cut down or control the substance use.

The BED group also strongly endorsed Criterion 10, unlike their obese counterparts (*Criterion 10: The substance use is continued despite knowledge of having persistent or recurrent physical or psychological problems that are likely to have been caused or exacerbated by the substance*). Also Criterion 11 illustrates a difference between the groups (*Criterion 11: Craving or a strong desire or urge to use a specific substance*). This symptom was frequently endorsed by the BED group, but by fewer non-BED counterparts. Another recent study [43] proposes an online survey of 479 adults, a sample of the general public, from the USA (n = 215) and Australia (n = 264). Almost three quarters (72%) of participants believed that an addiction to certain foods caused obesity. Just over half (54%) agreed that obesity should be treated as an addiction, and 64% were prepared to classify obesity as an eating disorder. Most (86%) participants thought that certain foods are addictive (79% in the case of sugar) and 80% believed that some foods could be as addictive as alcohol, nicotine and cocaine. Support for the view that certain foods could be as addictive as drugs increased with BMI. Obese individuals were significantly more supportive of the concept of food addiction than their overweight and normal weight counterparts. They were also more supportive of treating obesity as a type of food addiction.

We can reasonably argue that in the public view there is strong endorsement for the idea of obesity as a food addiction.

Finally, epidemiological data show that rates of comorbid alcohol or drug dependence are significantly elevated in both clinical and community samples of individuals with eating disorders [44, 45, 46]. Recent research has shown that substance abuse is significantly associated with BED [47]. It is important to note that rates of substance abuse are elevated in many disorders, and that depression is a more common co-occurring disorder than substance abuse in both community and treatment-seeking samples of eating disorders and obesity [48, 49, 50].

STUDIES IN ANIMALS

Avena et al., from the group of Bart Hoebel, [51, 52] developed a line of research to show sugar addiction in rats. Their starting point was that: ''many people claim that they feel compelled to eat sweet foods, similar in some ways to how an alcoholic might feel compelled to drink. Therefore, we developed an animal model to investigate why some people have difficulty moderating their intake of palatable foods'' [51]. In this experimental model, developed in Bart Hoebel's laboratory, rats were given 12-h daily access to an aqueous 10% sucrose solution (25% glucose in some experiments) and lab chow, followed by 12 h of deprivation, for three or more weeks [53]. This feeding schedule induced spontaneous binge eating. These rats were compared with control groups offered *ad libitum* access to sucrose and lab chow, *ad libitum* access to lab chow, or 12-h access to lab chow. The rats maintained on 12-h sucrose and lab chow entered a state that resembled drug dependence in several dimensions. They escalated their sugar intake and increased their intake during the first hour of daily access, as happens in a "binge". In addition to first hour binges, spontaneous binge episodes occurred throughout the access period [51]. Signs of opioid withdrawal have been noted after daily intermittent access to sugar, and are seen when withdrawal is precipitated with an opioid antagonist, or when food and sugar are removed [51, 18]. Rats with 12-h daily access to sucrose also lever press for more sugar compared to a control group following a two week sugar abstinence period indicating an increased motivation to obtain the substance. They also show locomotor cross-sensitization to amphetamine and enhanced intake of alcohol [54, 55]. Other groups replicated these results, showing that rats with limited access to sucrose show signs of aggressive behavior [56], withdrawal [57], and cross-sensitization to cocaine [58]. When offered binge access to fat, rats show increased progressive ratio breakpoints compared with non-binge groups, again indicating enhanced motivation to obtain the food [59]. Binge access to sugar/fat combinations results in stress-induced hyperphagia [60], and rats prone to binge eat will more readily endure shock to obtain a highly palatable food [61].

Thus, there is a body of research that supports the suggestion that rats kept under this behavioral regime manifest physiological and behavioral changes consistent with an addiction to sugar. Hoebel et al. [52] describe this eating pattern as a 'natural addiction'. It was proposed that this animal model potentially offered insight into various human disorders. ''We suggest that sugar, as common as it is, nonetheless meets many of the criteria for a substance of abuse. The rise in obesity, coupled with the emergence of scientific findings of parallels between drugs of abuse and palatable foods has given credibility to this idea''. The feeding regimen of the rats ''shares some aspects of the behavioral pattern in people diagnosed with binge-eating disorder or bulimia. Bulimics often restrict intake early in the day and then binge later in the evening, usually on palatable foods'' [51].

These considerations lead to one important question: is sugar the culprit of food addiction, or is it one's eating behavior, or both? Avena et al. [32] claim that "It is important to note that it is not simply the composition of the diet, but an interaction between diet and availability that leads to these addiction-like alterations. Specifically, in our model free access to the highly palatable food does not result in signs of dependence; a limited access schedule is needed in order to see these behaviors emerge".

Another question to be asked is whether these findings can be generalized to humans? And they can, to what extent? Although animal studies can generate hypotheses, they need to be confirmed in humans who are influenced by a cultural and social environment that adds a complexity not seen with rodents. Moreover, even the conditions of the described experiment cannot be considered to be representative of the everyday lives of rats.

NEUROBIOLOGY OF FOOD ADDICTION

As we have seen, drug addiction and overconsumption of food share similarities both from a physiological and behavioral point of view. This can lead us to assume a commonality of the neuronal mechanisms below. There is an impressive body of studies on brain metabolism in relation to feed-forward mechanisms (for a recent review, see Alsiö et al. [62]). Research on the neurochemistry of reward provide a great deal of evidence for similarity between food and drug cravings. Johnson and Kenny [63] found that the development of obesity and compulsive-like eating in obese rats was associated with deficits in brain reward mechanisms. Specifically, striatal dopamine receptors were downregulated in obese rats as has been reported in humans addicted to drugs. The authors suggested that common hedonic mechanisms may underlie obesity and drug addiction. Consistent with the Johnson and Kenny findings of downregulation of dopamine receptors, Stice et al. [64] demonstrated that individuals with higher BMI showed less activation in the striatum, in response to food consumption relative to those with a lower BMI. Stice et al. also found that this dopamine downregulation can be coupled with greater activation in the gustatory cortex and somatosensory brain regions in response to anticipation and consumption of food. Both biological processes would predispose people to overeating and weight gain. In a similar way, Wang et al. [65] used raclopride binding to measure density of D2 receptors and found an inverse relationship between D2 receptor density and BMI. The key question here is to determine the direction of causality for these differences in sensitivity to dopamine. Is it a result of repeated overstimulation of the system? Or, is it a preexisting risk factor for obesity or drug abuse? Stice et al. [64] cautioned that it is unclear whether these brain abnormalities precede or are caused by overeating.

The mesolimbic dopaminergic system is centrally involved in the acute positive effects of a number of rewarding stimuli, including drugs of abuse [66, 67, 68, 69]. Microdialysis and positron emission tomography (PET) studies show that illicit drugs increase extracellular dopamine (DA) preferentially in the ventral striatum, particularly in the nucleus accumbens (NAc) area, in rats, nonhuman primates, and humans [66, 70]. As such, increased DA release could be a crucial mechanism in the reinforcement of rewarding stimuli [66].

We must take into account, as Benton cautioned [11], that a wide range of pleasant phenomena also activate these mechanisms. Music [71], humour [72], winning [73] or expecting to win a prize [74], attractive [75, 76] or smiling faces [77], a mother recognizing their child [78] or being in love [79] also stimulate these pathways.

This may suggest that rather than seeing the stimulation of these pathways by sugars as something unusual or worrying, it can be viewed as one of a wide range of positive experiences that routinely stimulate a common circuitry. When dopamine is released into the synapse, it stimulates a number of dopamine receptors (D1-D5) that bring about a feeling of well-being and stress reduction. This is the result of the interaction of numerous transmitters: serotonin (5HT), endorphins (END), GABA (GB), dopamine (DA), norepinephrine (NE), and acetycholine (ACH). The process of these interactions in the brain rewarding system is called "the reward cascade" [80].

Nevertheless, when there is a dysfunction in the "reward cascade", causing a low or hypodopaminergic trait, the brain requires dopamine to feel good. Bloom described this condition as Reward Deficiency Syndrome, a disease due in-part to a form of a gene (DRD2A1 allele), which prevents the expression, or the normal laying down, of dopamine receptors in the brain reward site [81]. This high-risk genetic trait predisposes individuals to a high risk for multiple addictive, impulsive, and compulsive behaviors.

However, even outside of the pathology, the subjective perception of pleasure varies among individuals based on the degree of dopaminergic activity. Gjedde et al. [82] showed that healthy Danish men who are more sensation-seeking than other healthy men have significantly fewer available DA receptors in striatum because a greater fraction are occupied by the increased extracellular DA. This greater dopamine, in turn, is thought to be the result of constant dopaminergic stimulation, resulting in the lower binding potential of the receptors. At the same time, the tissue apparently compensates for the DA receptor occupation by generating additional receptors.

The feeling of euphoria seems to depend on the rate at which the extracellular DA concentration rises to abnormally high levels [83]. Thus, we can surmise that drugs, or other equivalent stimuli, produces greater DA release associated with a more euphoric "high" [66, 83]. Volkow et al. [83] show that the intensity of the "high" induced by methylphenidate was significantly correlated with the levels of released DA. Thus, the subjects who reported the most intense ''high'' were those who had the greatest increase of DA release. Food does release DA in the NAc [66, 53, 84]. Palatable food (high-sugar or sugar/fat) in particular causes even greater DA release [85].

A possible difference between drugs of abuse and food is that drugs (i.e., opiates, cocaine, methamphetamine) can increase extracellular DA with every administration [8, 87], whereas food induced increases in DA usually wane with additional intake of the same substance [88, 89]. This aspect leads us to believe that an element of novelty is necessary for the food to be addictive. From this perspective it is probable that the expectation for food in a context of restriction, or in relation to forbidden foods, plays a role of certain relevance.

Besides the importance of dopamine in reinforcement intake of palatable foods, we must consider the contribution of endogenous opioids (endorphins). Release of these transmitters leads to higher levels of striatal dopamine, that is, to what we think is rewarding. Palatable food can activate opioid receptors in the VTA and further stimulate DA-releasing cells in the NAc [90]. Opioid peptides and receptors are expressed throughout the brain: in the brainstem, subregions of the hypothalamus, ventral tegmental area (VTA), and within different striatal compartments. At many sites associated with food intake control, opioid receptor antagonism reduces feeding: these include the arcuate (ARC), paraventricular (PVN) and lateral hypothalamic nuclei, nucleus accumbens (NAc), nucleus accumbens shell (NAcSh), VTA, and amygdala [62]. In the VTA and NacSh, opioid receptors are present on GABAergic neurons, tonically inhibiting dopamine signaling [62].

The rewarding properties of alcoholic beverages [91] and of sweet (or palatable) foods [92] are thought to be mediated by this pathway. One of the specific roles for opioids in overeating seems to be in mediating the hedonic impact of, or the pleasure derived from, palatable food. The effects on consumption of palatable food [93], as well as food-induced DA release in the accumbens, were attenuated by the opioid receptor antagonists, naltrexone and LY255582. Although Naltrexone reduces short-term food intake, it is important to note that this effect may be limited to palatable foods. Naltrexone treatment does lead to reduced pleasantness ratings for foods, but it does not appear to affect hunger (see Yeomans & Gray [94] for a review). Because opioids preferentially stimulate intake of food that is palatable, it has been suggested that these peptides have a role also in chronic overfeeding [62].

The type 1 cannabinoid receptor (CB1) and its endogenous ligands (endocannabinoids such as anandamide) have emerged more recently as important players in hedonic aspects of feeding, although such a role had been expected based on the orexigenic effects associated with marijuana. Such appetite typically favors intake of palatable food and stems from CB1 activation in a number of appetite-related sites including the hypothalamus, brainstem and striatum [62, 95, 96, 97]. As with the opioid system and dopamine pathways, alterations are observed in cannabinoidergic tone in reward areas after extended access to palatable food [98]. Cannabinoidergic activity in the hypothalamus is directly regulated by leptin levels: leptin injections reduce hypothalamic levels of endocannabinoids whereas leptin-deficient strains display elevated endocannabinoid levels in the hypothalamus [99].

Initial hypotheses on the neurophysiology of feeding reward focused on very select molecules (opioids, dopamine and, more recently, cannabinoids) acting within the "reward system", but the picture is more complex. Hypothalamic nuclei also receive and integrate signals, such as leptin and ghrelin, from peripheral tissues and coordinate peripheral metabolic need and food seeking. ''Hunger'' and ''satiety'' centers have been described within the hypothalamus and brainstem, and signals within these structures have been identified, including the first-order neurons (receiving input from circulating hormones and nutrients) of the ARC, which contain either neuropeptide Y (NPY)/agouti-related peptide (AgRP), or cocaine- and amphetamine-regulated transcript (CART)/proopiomelanocortin (POMC). Whereas the functions of these systems are often divided into non-homeostatic and homeostatic food intake regulation, it has been established that reciprocal and functional interactions exist between the reward molecules and neuropeptidergic systems responsible for the regulation of calorie intake [62]. In agreement with this integrative view of appetite regulation, receptors for the anorexigenic hormone leptin are present throughout the hypothalamus and brainstem nuclei, but are also expressed and functional in the hippocampus and on dopamine neurons in the ventral tegmental area [100, 101, 102]. Ghrelin is currently the only described orexigenic hormone from the periphery, which acts centrally to modulate the body's energy homeostasis. Both ghrelin and its receptor are ubiquitously expressed in the periphery and in the central nervous system (CNS) and this abundant expression suggests that it is involved in a plethora of biological functions [103]. The appetite-inducing effects of ghrelin are mainly linked to peripherally produced ghrelin, which exerts its effects centrally. Peripheral ghrelin signals to the brain via the blood circulation, passing the blood–brain barrier and travelling via vagal afferents to the nucleus of the solitary tract (NTS) in the brain stem [103]. Ghrelin infusions directly into the VTA and nucleus accumbens have been found to increased food intake in rats [104]. In agreement with such neural interplay, leptin and ghrelin peripheral infusion alter brain activity in striatal as well as cortical structures in humans [105, 106].

This picture has to be completed with cognitive ''top-down'' control from prefrontal areas and input from both limbic and memory systems. Memory plays a crucial role. Food (and drug) cravings can be learned. Environmental cues, not just nutritional deprivation, are effective triggers for food craving - the sight or smell of food or even food imagery may serve as triggers [107; 108; 109]. Gibson & Desmond [110] reported that craving may be an acquired response based on repeatedly eating the craved food when hungry. The complexity of these phenomena, in which the cognitive aspects are intertwined with the modulation of neurotransmitters, is dealt with in the Incentive Sensitization Theory of addiction [111]. Sensitized incentive salience can manifest in behaviour via either implicit (as unconscious wanting) or explicit (as conscious craving) processes, depending on circumstances. According to Robinson & Berridge [111] this process is established through the learning of strong "automatized" stimulus–response (S–R) habits, where dopamine may act to incentive salience attributions to the neural representations of reward-related stimuli. Incentive salience is a distinct component of motivation and reward, and concerns the power of a stimulus to elicit a response, regardless to the subject's "liking". We are in the neurological field, rather than the psychological learning field, here. In other words, dopamine is necessary to stabilize "wanting" incentives, but not for 'liking' them or for learning new "likes" and "dislikes" [111]. Considering the differences between drug and food (we saw previously that the food needs of an element of novelty to stimulate the dopamine system), we think that in this case the model of Pavlovian learning may be reductive. To paint a more comprehensive picture, we need to consider more widely the symbolic system and the attribution of meaning to food, to control, to ourselves and to our ability to manage difficulties. We think that the interaction between likes, needs and frustrations is an important source of arousal to consider.

So far, we have substantial evidence that neuroadaptations in both ''non-homeostatic'' reward pathways (e.g. dopamine, opioid pathways) and ''homeostatic'' appetite signaling (e.g. grehelin, NPY) occur in animals during extended exposure to palatable food. This phenomenon is not restricted to animal models, as overeating/weight gain in overweight women was, in a recent longitudinal study, shown to affect striatal activity in response to palatable food [112]. Palatable high caloric foods can switch the regulation of food intake from homeostatic to rewarding pathways. This process maintains a close interactive relationship between the different systems, and leads to overeating and obesity [113]. We can thus speculate that these systems are hijacked and used for other purpose. The question is, what function do they assume?

Stress and Nutrition

Considering the links between stress and nutrition can be helpful. The relationship between stress and food has its roots in an evolutionary context with the purpose of surviving in an environment of food scarcity. We can assume that overeating had the function of allowing survival in periods in which food was not available. In modern Western society, with the high availability of food, this function does not appear useful. However, a relationship between stress and nutrition persists. The connection between the gut and the brain regulates appetite and satiety, and it maintains the body's energy homeostasis [103, 114, 115]. Its dysregulation is linked to metabolic imbalances leading to obesity as well as to psychological conditions such as stress, anxiety and depression [103, 116, 117]. Overlapping neuronal circuitries also reinforce the link between stress and feeding behaviour [103, 118].

Circuitries that regulate food intake and circuitries that modulate stress, the hypothalamic-pituitary-adrenal (HPA) axis, both converge on the PVN, which contains neurons producing corticotropin-releasing hormone (CRH). The release of this molecule in turn would cause an increase in the levels of glucocorticoids (cortisol in humans, corticosterone in rats), hormones produced in response to a condition of stress, involved in facilitating the adaptation of the individual to the environment [103]. CRH stimulates the release and synthesis of adrenocorticotropin (ACTH), which, in turn, increases the release of cortisol by the adrenal cortex [119]. In particular, variations in HPA axis activity exert a strong influence on metabolic pathways. During acute stress, the brain focuses on the perceived threat, attention is enhanced, catabolism is initiated, and blood flow is redirected to provide the greatest perfusion of the brain and muscles [120]. These changes are transient and occur to improve the individual's chance of survival. By contrast, chronic stress exposure, and a consecutively persistent HPA axis activation shift the metabolism toward a generalized catabolic state. Endogenous opioids are released in response to HPA axis stimulation and feedback negatively to shut off the stress response. These opioids serve to ameliorate the stress response. Recalling that palatable foods also stimulate opioid release, it has been postulated that people may choose these foods to medicate their stress [121, 122]. Consistent with the substance dependence literature, Adam & Epel [122] proposed a model of stress-induced food addiction, in which they postulate that cortisol and endogenous opioids released in response to stress drive overeating of palatable food. Chronic stress can lead to greater cortisol exposure. In turn, this has direct and indirect effects on the reward system. Greater sensitization of the reward system can lead to excessive intake of highly palatable food. Moreover, the combination of high cortisol, dense calories, and consequently high insulin, contributes to visceral fat distribution. High levels of glucocorticoids are also linked to overeating and obesity through upregulation of NPY and resistance to insulin and leptin. Cortisol is believed to increase the drive for and salience of food, while insulin promotes the seeking of highly palatable food.

Response to stress may help to explain why in some subjects there is a transition from substance use to addiction. As has been reviewed by Koob [123], initial drug administration is associated with the classical stress response, which contributes to the reward associated with drug administration and the motivation to seek more. However, repeated HPA axis stimulation results in high circulating levels of glucocorticoids, which simultaneously feedback negatively to shut off the HPA axis and sensitize other areas of the brain to release CRF. This effect has been shown with chronic use of cocaine, opioids, nicotine, and alcohol. Hyperactivity of these extrahypothalamic stress systems (particularly the amygdala) is believed to be a key contributor to the negative affect experienced during withdrawal (Koob, 2010). Thus, while the stress response is associated with the intoxication phase of early use, it is also contributes to the compulsive drug-seeking behavior that marks the transition from use to addiction.

There is a paradox in the relation between stress and food consumption. Stress affects feeding behaviour in humans in both directions, with some individuals increasing their food intake and others eating less [103, 124, 125]. According to Adam & Epel [122], this effect is partly due to the perception of the stressor, whether as a threat (e.g. social rejection) or a challenge (e.g. achievement). Activation of the HPA axis is enhanced when coping skills are perceived as inadequate. Consequently, increased activation of the HPA axis seems to be related, in humans, with feelings of helplessness and inability to manage a difficult situation.

PSYCHOSOCIAL STRESS, MOOD AND DIETING

A growing body of evidence indicates that chronic psychosocial stress leads to visceral obesity [126, 120, 127, 128, 129] and it has been suggested that psychosocial stress predicts the incidence of metabolic syndrome, i.e. a cluster of obesity, impaired glucose tolerance and lipid metabolism, and arterial hypertension [130].

Mood is closely linked to food consumption and body weight regulation, an interrelation that can be confirmed by most non-obese people [131]. It is well known that typical or melancholic depression is accompanied by a decrease in appetite and body weight loss whereas atypical depression is characterized by increased appetite and weight gain [132]. In any case, the diagnosis of a depressive disorder involves alterations in food intake behavior. A recent meta-analysis including more than 58,700 subjects revealed a bidirectional association between depression and obesity: obese persons had a 55% higher risk of developing depression over time in comparison with normal weight subjects, whereas subjects with depression had a 58% increased risk of becoming obese compared with healthy persons [50]. Patients with major depressive disorder display alterations in glucose metabolism as well as high cortisol values [133, 134]. Therapeutic intervention against depression reverses both elevated cortisol concentrations and disturbed mood [135, 136].

Hirth et al. [137] and Brewerton [138] report data that underline the links between posttraumatic stress disorder (PTSD) symptoms and eating disordered behaviors. They extend those links with PTSD to the ingestion of sugary sodas and fast foods, a finding that persists despite race or ethnicity, marital status, education, income level, and body mass index (BMI). They also suggest that the ingestion, and especially over-ingestion, of fatty or sugary energy sources may be just another strategy that traumatized individuals use to numb themselves from their unpleasant feeling states and memories. In essence, certain foods can act just like other substances that alter brain chemistry and, hence, consciousness.

On the other hand, dietary restriction and stress may work in combination to activate addictive overeating. Boggiano et al. [60, 139] have demonstrated this in rats, that binge eat under the combined conditions of stress and food restriction. In humans, dieting appears to mediate the relationship between stress and overeating [140]. That is, dieters eat more in response to an acute stressor. According to Garber & Lustig [121], this may explain the gender effect of stress-eating, whereby women tend to eat more and men to eat less in response to stress, since women are more likely to be on a diet and eat for emotional reasons [141]. The tendency for women who are dieters to eat more when under stress has also been measured outside of the laboratory in subjects experiencing significant work-related stress [142]. In fact, under stress, women tend to eat the foods that are normally forbidden when they are on a diet [140]. Young children, moreover, have been shown to overindulge in foods that they feel are "forbidden" [143].

Obviously, the phenomena described are to be considered in light of the symbolic activity of human beings. The perception of stressors as a threat or challenge, awareness of skills and limitations, self-evaluation, value attributed to food and food control, and what we think is forbidden or allowed, involve cognitive and affective frameworks built through our experience and education in a social cultural context. The attribution of meaning interacts with our biology, through the way in which we read reality, our expectations, our emotional reactions and our behavior. Finally, which model can we assume for food addiction?

PROPOSED MECHANISM

Jauch-Chara & Oltmanns [131] suggest that obesity is a consequence of a vicious circle built on interrelations between chronically enhanced stress axis activity and reward-related mechanisms within the mesolimbic system. During childhood, food intake is a readily accessible and powerful tool to down-regulate HPA. Schellekens [103] proposes feed-forward and feedback loops between stress and diet that are partly regulated by the neuropeptide ghrelin. According to this model, the gut hormone ghrelin mediates the effect of stress in eating behaviour, anxiety, depression and obesity. Prolonged stress increases the risk of developing psychological disorders such as anxiety and depression. Increases in psychological stress elevate plasma ghrelin levels, which activates the hedonic signalling pathway and stimulates the intake of caloric dense 'comfort' foods. Ghrelin-induced enhanced consumption of palatable foods elicits central reward pathways and increase dopamine signalling, which may act to reduce the deleterious effects of stress and minimize depression-like behaviour. However, this stress-induced food reward behaviour and hyperphagia of palatable caloric dense foods increases body weight, which in itself has been linked to major depressive disorders. While obesity generally decreases plasma ghrelin levels, the dopaminergic reward signalling is down-regulated, following prolonged exposure to palatable foods leading to a desensitization of reward signalling similar as observed in addiction behaviour. Thus, prolonged exposure to stress and 'comfort foods' may lead to a worsening of the reward deficit, further fostering anxiety and depression and co-morbid obesity. In turn, the other way to increase ghrelin level is dieting. Going on and off diets may be the human analogue to the restricted access paradigm of rats [51].

We can consider this interplay among different systems as an activation of an allostatic state, the function of which is to cope with stress exposure. As Goldstein offers, "According to the concept of allostasis, there is no single, ideal set of steady-state conditions in life. Allostasis reflects active, adaptive processes that maintain apparent steady states, via multiple, interacting effectors regulated by homeostatic comparators 'homeostats'. Stress can be defined as a condition or state in which a sensed discrepancy between afferent information and a set point for response leads to activation of effectors, reducing the discrepancy." [144, 145]. The allostatic adjustment represents a state that may momentarily appear quite therapeutic but that, in the long run, may cause suffering to the organism. The key to remaining healthy and adaptive over time is in keeping a dynamic state of equilibrium which implies continuous non-linear adaptations and flexibilities. This is one way to define the resiliency of an organism. In engineering, resilience can be defined as the ability of a material to absorb energy, to modify its structure in an elastic fashion and then return to its original state of energy determined configuration [146]. Elsewhere, physicians, psychologists and other researchers have extensively addressed the concept of resiliency under the framework of organismic adaptation to stress (see Charney [147] for a review).

According to this point of view, we can consider food addiction to be a non-resilient adaptation, in other words a 'skew' allostatic state [145], to cope with psychosocial stress. This state involves the metabolic level as well as the symbolic one, the latter determining what is necessary, attractive, dangerous or forbidden. As Garber & Lustig [121] pointed out, certain individuals are more susceptible to transitioning from the use of comfort food to dependence upon it. Several lines of evidence suggest that individuals who are obese, dieting, and/or under stress, are more likely to eat for reward. In addition, dietary restraint is a cognitive state that may be impossible to maintain under stress or when surrounded by forbidden foods.

BASIC NEED SATISFACTION AND OVEREATING

Shriner [145] has offered that "addictions are always a substitute for the genuine article". In this case, the genuine article has to do with unsatisfied basic emotional needs. Timmerman & Acton [148] examined the relationship between basic need satisfaction as identified by Maslow's hierarchy and emotional eating. Maslow's theory [149] proposed that one's perception of a situation and the status of basic need satisfaction are important determinants of behavior. Maslow stated that all persons have needs (i.e., physiological, safety/security, love/belonging, esteem/self-esteem, and self-actualization) existing in a quasi-hierarchy. People have an inherent drive to meet their needs, and as their needs are met repeatedly, resources are built to assist in dealing with life stressors. When individuals perceive life situations as stressful, they draw upon their self-care resources to aid in buffering or reducing the resultant stress. Self-care resources may be internal or external. External resources are acquired from the environment (e.g., social, financial, and material support). Internal resources, such as self-esteem, are dependent on the satisfaction of basic needs over time. If needs are met repeatedly, a resource asset is created and is available for future use. People can draw upon these assets in times of stress to assist them in coping with stressful events. However, if needs remain unmet over a prolonged period of time, then a resource deficit may exist. This means that a person may experience a decreased ability to handle stressful life situations. This could result in engaging in unhealthy coping behaviors such as emotional eating in response to stress, in order to maintain emotional homeostasis.

Timmerman & Acton [148] investigated these factors in a sample of healthy, educated adults, using the Basic Need Satisfaction Inventory (BNSI) [150] and the Emotional Eating Scale (EES) [151]. The BNSI had a strong, negative correlation to the EES ($r = -.49$). Thus, the lower the level of basic need satisfaction, the more likely an individual was to engage in emotional eating.

A recent study [152] replicated the same methodology with a sample of obese subjects and found a similarly strong negative relationship ($\beta = -0.36$). Self-esteem was considered to be a mediator that significantly predicted emotional eating. In addition, incidences of emotional eating and negative coping have been found to be significantly higher and self-esteem to be significantly lower in individuals with BMIs >40 as compared with individuals with BMIs <40.

The manner in which food can achieve the aim of self-soothing, it is probably more complex than just an action on the HPA axis.

In line with the idea that physiological and psychological processes are related, the literature on embodied cognition highlights the interplay between the body, the environment, and the mind. According to Barsalou [153] experiences are fixed within a situation, such that contextual information is coded in association with perception (sensory information), action (information about spatial properties and movement) and introspection (mental states, affects, and motivation). Using and combining the information from different modalities can facilitate learning and aid in the representation of abstract concepts [154]. For instance, children experience physical warmth when someone takes care of them, which over time creates an interrelationship between social proximity and physical warmth [155, 156]. The ability to associate the grounded experience of physical warmth with the abstract concept of friendship facilitates knowledge representation. Embodied cognition may be particularly relevant in relation to comfort food: "a specific food consumed during a specific situation to obtain psychological comfort" [157]. Troisi and Gabriel [158] reasoned that the appeal of eating comfort food may arise from its association with social proximity, due to a history of frequently consuming these food items in the presence of close relationship partners.

People use food as a substitute for other support behaviors in relation to their ability (or inability) to recognize emotions. Rommel et al. [159] found that the obese were less able to identify their own emotions and the emotional states of others than participants of normal weight. Obese people with decreased emotional awareness rely more on emotional eating as a means to regulate emotion, due to a lack of alternative strategies. Alexithymia is a central feature in this context. The term alexithymia literally means "lacking words for feelings" and it was coined to describe certain clinical characteristics observed among patients with psychosomatic disorders who had difficulty engaging in insight-oriented psychotherapy [160]. Alexithymic patients demonstrate deficiencies in emotional awareness and communication and show little insight into their feelings, symptoms, and motivation. It has been hypothesized that this difficulty is due to a deficit in the referential link between the sub-symbolic (visceral, kinesthetic, emotional, etc.) and the symbolic aspects (words, images) that constitute the emotional patterns of the person [161]. Difficulties relate to identifying and describing feelings, externally oriented thinking, and a limited imaginal capacity. Patients fail to activate images and words that give meaning to the experience. Emotions are experienced through the body in an undifferentiated way [161, 162]. Alexithymic people also tend to engage in unhealthy behaviors, particularly substance abuse, compulsive eating or dieting, and pathological gambling. Such behaviors might be conceptualized, in part, as the person's attempt to regulate a noxious, undifferentiated, physiologically aroused state. It appears that alexithymia is a negative prognostic indicator for many psychological treatments, particularly those focusing on insight, emotional awareness, and a close alliance with a therapist (even if it may not affect more structured cognitive-behavioral treatments) [163]. We must take into account the need to help patients to learn more adaptive strategies for affect regulation.

Negative emotions have been shown to result in overeating in obese individuals [164], in eating-disordered women [165], and in normal-weight dieters [166]. Recently, it has been found that there is a relationship between the use of comfort food as a way to manage stress and high body mass index (BMI range 41.8 to 51) [167].

To explain emotional eating, the *affect regulation model* [168] assumes that emotional eaters overeat in response to a stress or negative emotion, because they have learned that it relieves them from aversive mood state. Similarly, the *escape model* by Heatherton & Baumeister [169], posits that emotional eaters overeat to escape or shift attention from an ego-threatening stimulus (e.g. individuals with high standards may binge as an attempt to escape from negative self-awareness when those standards are not met) that causes aversive self-awareness. Focusing the attention on external stimuli, resulting in overeating, leads to increased salience of these stimuli.

If, as posited by the affect regulation models and the escape theory, emotional eating may occur through a process of emotion regulation and avoidance of aversive mood states, it seems plausible that more correct coping strategies fail in down-regulating negative emotions. Lazarus and Folkman [170] defined coping as the cognitive-behavioral attempts at continuous change made by a subject in order to manage internal and/or external demands which exceed his own personal resources. They distinguished two major coping categories or styles: emotion-focused coping and problem-focused coping. Problem-focused coping is directed at modifying the stressful situation or trying to solve the problem. We can refer to it as the "cool" way to solve problems. Emotion-focused coping focuses on reducing the tension and the physiological and emotional responses which arise from the situation. A third category that has also received considerable attention, avoidance coping, involves behaviour directed at denying or not dealing with the stressor or problem [171]. We propose to consider both of them as "hot" ways.

According to the model, all strategies are adaptive, but the excessive use of one type of strategy, or its use in an inappropriate context or out of control, can make them ineffective in managing stress or may give rise to dysfunctional behaviors. Nevertheless, in a recent study [172], the adolescents who reported binge eating use positive-coping strategies (such as trying to solve the problem, focusing on the positive or asking for help) less frequently than the adolescents who reported not having binges. This confirms the hypothesis regarding the link between "hot" coping strategies and emotional eating. These findings indicate that coping skills programs for adolescents may provide a positive approach for the prevention of future maladaptive eating behaviors. In addition, research shows that coping is an important element to consider in the treatment of eating-disordered individuals. Building adequate coping skills may help in their recovery and in relapse prevention [173, 174]. Therefore, coping is an important variable to take into account when designing effective prevention programs for eating pathology in adolescents and when treating eating-disordered individuals.

Conclusion

The idea that some forms of overeating may represent an addictive behavior and that specific foods may have an addiction potential has been widely discussed in the scientific literature in recent years. In the last decade research has strongly increased with the rise of neuroimaging studies. Nevertheless, despite the growing number of studies on food addiction, there is not yet a common point of view in the scientific community, and a clear and agreed upon definition is yet to come.

Food addiction theory is based on some strong pillars. Firstly, some people act as if they are addicted and recognize themselves in the description of addictive behavior. This similarity between drug abuse and overeating has been formalized in the Yale Food Addiction Scale (YFAS) [39], a measure that represents a cornerstone in the literature on human food addiction. The ease with which people accept this point of view is probably due to the comfort that it offers to individuals struggling with eating and weight. It gives them a counterweight to a prevalent view of obesity as a moral failing on the part of the obese individuals. However, we find that feeling guilty or ashamed is not the best way to increase the necessary self-esteem and self-efficacy to cope with such a challenge.

Secondly, studies in animals [51] show addiction-like consumption of sugar and neurobiological changes after several weeks of intermittent access to sugar. This paradigm is often criticized for being artificial and not replicable in humans. Nevertheless, it matches quite well to the eating styles of some individuals (e.g. individuals with bulimia nervosa or also dieters).

Thirdly, biological models give an account of the interplay among homeostatic system, reward circuitry and regulation of mood and stress. From a neuropsychological point of view, overeating displays a striking number of neurobiological similarities and behavioral analogies to substance dependence. Behavioral studies have revealed that overeating/obesity and addiction both activate identical brain structures related to reward processing, motivation, decision-making, learning, and memory. Reward processing in both overeating and addiction activate the mesencephalic dopaminergic system. Moreover, food intake is not only modulated by pathways of the reward system but also by multiple environmental, endocrine, and neurobiological factors, and the mesencephalic dopaminergic system interacts with peripheral hormones, in particular with ghrelin. Plasma ghrelin levels are enhanced under conditions of physiological stress, and it has recently been suggested that ghrelin plays an important role in stress-induced food reward behaviour [103]. Recent evidence suggests that ghrelin is a critical factor at the interface of homeostatic control of appetite and reward circuitries, modulating the hedonic aspects of food intake. These findings highlight the close interaction between food, mood and stress and the development of obesity. Thus, as Jauch-Chara & Oltmanns [131] suggest, obesity may be viewed as a consequence of a vicious circle built on cross-links between chronically enhanced stress axis activity and reward-related mechanisms within the mesolimbic system. According to this point of view, we can consider food addiction as a non-resilient adaptation, in other words a 'skew' allostatic state [145], to cope with psychosocial stress. Food addiction represents a pervasive and enduring pattern of both food perception (how we view and feel about food) and food related behavior (how we go about procuring and ingesting food) which biases our relationship with food in harmful, non-resilient and unhealthy ways [175]. This construct involves the metabolic level as well as the symbolic one, the latter to determine what is necessary, attractive, dangerous or forbidden. We must be aware of this complexity if we are to build more effective treatments.

As Curtis and Davis [40] suggest, overeating should probably be viewed as a dimensional prototype with several degrees of severity and different factors that lead to overconsumption. Some people may overeat because they are highly sensitive or responsive to rewarding stimuli, others may use food to "self-medicate" in respect to a negative feeling. A smaller proportion of individuals do show signs of disordered or dysregulated overeating associated with a range of psychiatric co-morbidities. It is probable that the subset of BED patients classified as having YFAS "food addiction" represents a more disturbed variant characterized by greater eating disorder psychopathology and associated pathology [42].

Other problems remain to be solved: It is unclear whether certain foods *per se* could determine a state of addiction or whether a specific pattern of consumptions is necessary. There is a tendency to regard food as a drug of abuse, but we can also use the model of behavioral addiction, like pathological gambling, which can help us to shed light on the complex interaction of biological elements with behavioral, cognitive, motivational and emotional factors.

Further studies will help to clarify the real dimension of food addiction, particularly from the neurobiological point of view. However, at the moment, we find that this perspective gives us, at least, a good heuristic hypothesis that can explain part of the continuum of dysregulated eating behavior. Starting from there, we can take an overview of the complex interplay of biological and psycho-social dimensions that underlies overeating and, most important, we can try to tailor a treatment that matches the different facets of the problem.

REFERENCES

[1] Horgen, KB; Brownell, KD. Comparison of price change and health message interventions in promoting healthy food choices. *Health Psychol.* 2002 21(5), 505-12.

[2] Gearhardt, AN; Davis, C; Kuschner, R; Brownell, KD. The addiction potential of hyperpalatable foods. *Curr Drug Abuse Rev.* 2011 4(3),140-5.

[3] Stunkard, AJ; Allison, KC. Two forms of disordered eating in obesity: binge eating and night eating. *Int J Obes Relat Metab Disord.* 2003 Jan;27(1),1-12.

[4] van Strien, T; Herman, CP; Verheijden, MW. Eating style, overeating, and overweight in a representative Dutch sample. Does external eating play a role? *Appetite.* 2009 52(2), 380-7. doi: 10.1016/j.appet. 2008.11.010.

[5] Patel, KA; Schlundt, DG. Impact of moods and social context on eating behavior. *Appetite.* 2001 36(2), 111-8.

[6] May, J; Andrade, J; Batey, H; Berry, LM; Kavanagh, DJ. Less food for thought. Impact of attentional instructions on intrusive thoughts about snack foods. *Appetite.* 2010 55(2), 279-87. doi: 10.1016/j.appet.2010.06.014.

[7] Avena, NM; Rada, P; Hoebel, BG. Evidence for sugar addiction: behavioral and neurochemical effects of intermittent, excessive sugar intake. *Neurosci Biobehav Rev* 2007 32 (1), 20-39.

[8] Corsica, JA; Pelchat, ML. Food addiction: true or false? *Curr Opin Gastroenterol* 2010 26 (2), 165-9.

[9] Wang, GJ; Volkow, ND; Fowler, JS. The role of dopamine in motivation for food in humans: implications for obesity. *Expert Opin Ther Targets* 2002 6 (5), 601-9.

[10] Benton, D. The plausibility of sugar addiction and its role in obesity and eating disorders. *Clin Nutr.* 2010 29(3),288-303. doi: 10.1016 /j.clnu.2009.12.001.

[11] Wilson, GT. Eating disorders, obesity and addiction. *Eur Eat Disord Rev.* 2010 18(5), 341-51. doi: 10.1002/erv.1048.

[12] Ziauddeen, H; Fletcher, PC. Is food addiction a valid and useful concept? *Obes Rev.* 2013 14(1), 19-28. doi: 10.1111/j.1467-789X.2012.01046.x.

[13] Krashes, MJ; Kravitz, AV. Optogenetic and chemogenetic insights into the food addiction hypothesis. *Front Behav Neurosci.* 2014 28, 8, 57. doi: 10.3389/fnbeh.2014.00057. eCollection 2014. Review.

[14] Brownell, KD; Gold, MS. *Food and Addiction*, Oxford University Press. 2012.

[15] Melchionda, N. *Food Addiction.* Modena: Mucchi Editore. 2014.

[16] Pelchat, ML. Food addiction in humans. *J Nutr.* 2009 139 (3), 620-2.

[17] Colantuoni, C; Rada, P; McCarthy, J; Patten, C; Avena, NM; Chadeayne, A; Hoebel, BG. Evidence that intermittent, excessive sugar intake causes endogenous opioid dependence. *Obes Res.* 2002 10(6), 478-88.

[18] Colantuoni, C; Schwenker, J; McCarthy, J; Rada, P; Ladenheim, B; Cadet, JL; Schwartz, GJ; Moran, TH; Hoebel, BG. Excessive sugar intake alters binding to dopamine and mu-opioid receptors in the brain. *Neuroreport.* 2001 12(16), 3549-52.

[19] Boggiano, MM; Dorsey, JR; Thomas, JM; Murdaugh, DL. The Pavlovian power of palatable food: lessons for weight-loss adherence from a new rodent model of cue-induced overeating. *Int J Obes (Lond).* 2009 33(6), 693-701. doi: 10.1038/ijo.2009.57.

[20] American Psychiatric Association. Diagnostic and statistical manual of Mental Disorders (5th ed.). *The American Psychiatric Association*: Washington, DC, 2013

[21] Koob, GF; Le Moal, M. Drug abuse: hedonic homeostatic dysregulation. *Science* 1997 278 (5335), 52-8.

[22] Avena, NM; Long, KA; Hoebel, BG. Sugar-dependent rats show enhanced responding for sugar after abstinence: evidence of a sugar deprivation effect. *Physiol Behav.* 2005 16, 84(3), 359-62.

[23] Davis, C; Carter, JC. Compulsive overeating as an addiction disorder. A review of theory and evidence. *Appetite.* 2009 53(1), 1-8. doi: 10.1016/j.appet.2009.05.018. Review.

[24] Picot, AK; Lilenfeld, LR. The relationship among binge severity, personality psychopathology, and body mass index. *Int J Eat Disord.* 2003 34(1), 98-107.

[25] Ifland, JR; Preuss, HG; Marcus, MT; Rourke, KM; Taylor, WC; Burau, K; Jacobs, WS; Kadish, W; Manso, G. Refined food addiction: a classic substance use disorder. *Med Hypotheses.* 2009 72(5), 518-26. doi: 10.1016/j.mehy.2008.11.035.

[26] Spangler, R; Wittkowski, KM; Goddard, NL; Avena, NM; Hoebel, BG; Leibowitz, SF. Opiate-like effects of sugar on gene expression in reward areas of the rat brain. *Brain Res Mol Brain Res.* 2004 19, 124(2), 134-42.

[27] Acosta, JI; Boynton, FA; Kirschner, KF; Neisewander, JL. Stimulation of 5-HT1B receptors decreases cocaine- and sucrose-seeking behavior. *Pharmacol Biochem Behav.* 2005 80(2), 297-307.

[28] Solinas, M; Goldberg, SR. Motivational effects of cannabinoids and opioids on food reinforcement depend on simultaneous activation of cannabinoid and opioid systems. *Neuropsychopharmacology* 2005 30 (11), 2035-45.

[29] Arias-Carrión, O; Stamelou, M; Murillo-Rodríguez, E; Menéndez-González, M; Pöppel, E. Dopaminergic reward system: a short integrative review. *Int Arch Med.* 2010 6, 3-24. doi: 10.1186/1755-7682-3-24.

[30] Roitman, MF; Stuber, GD; Phillips, PE; Wightman, RM; Carelli, RM. Dopamine operates as a subsecond modulator of food seeking. *J Neurosci.* 2004 11, 24(6), 1265-71.

[31] Avena, NM; Bocarsly, ME; Hoebel, BG; Gold, MS. Overlaps in the nosology of substance abuse and overeating: the translational implications of "food addiction". *Curr Drug Abuse Rev.* 2011 4(3), 133-9.

[32] Richtand, NM. Behavioral sensitization, alternative splicing, and d3 dopamine receptor-mediated inhibitory function. *Neuropsychopharmacology.* 2006 31 (11), 2368-75.

[33] Phillips, TJ; Roberts, AJ; Lessov, CN. Behavioral sensitization to ethanol: genetics and the effects of stress. *Pharmacol Biochem Behav.* 1997 57 (3), 487-93.

[34] Corwin, RL; Grigson, PS. Symposium overview--Food addiction: fact or fiction? *J Nutr* 2009 139 (3), 617-9.

[35] American Psychiatric Association. Diagnostic and Statistical Manual of Mental Disorders (4th ed.). *The American Psychiatric Association*: Washington, DC, 2000.

[36] Cassin, SE; von Ranson, KM. Is binge eating experienced as an addiction? *Appetite.* 2007 49(3), 687-90.

[37] Gearhardt, AN; Corbin, WR; Brownell, KD. Food addiction: An examination of the diagnostic criteria for dependence. *JAMA* 2009 3, 1–7.

[38] Gearhardt, AN; Corbin, WR; Brownell, KD. The preliminary validation of the Yale food addiction scale. *Appetite* 2009 52,430–436.

[39] Curtis, C; Davis, C. A qualitative study of binge eating and obesity from an addiction perspective. *Eat Disord*. 2014 22(1), 19-32. doi: 10.1080/10640266.2014.857515

[40] Davis, C; Curtis, C; Levitan, RD; Carter, JC; Kaplan, AS; Kennedy, JL. Evidence that 'food addiction' is a valid phenotype of obesity. *Appetite*. 2011 57(3), 711-7. doi: 10.1016/j.appet.2011.08.017.

[41] Gearhardt, AN; White, MA; Masheb, RM; Morgan, PT; Crosby, RD; Grilo, CM. An examination of the food addiction construct in obese patients with binge eating disorder. *Int J Eat Disord*. 2012 45(5), 657-63. doi: 10.1002/eat.20957.

[42] Lee, NM; Lucke, J; Hall, WD; Meurk, C; Boyle, FM; Carter, A. Public views on food addiction and obesity: implications for policy and treatment. *PLoS One*. 2013 25, 8(9), e74836. doi: 10.1371/journal.pone.0074836. eCollection 2013.

[43] Garfinkel, PE; Lin, E; Goering, P; Spegg, C; Goldbloom, DS; Kennedy, S; Kaplan, AS; Woodside, DB. Bulimia nervosa in a Canadian community sample: prevalence and comparison of subgroups. *Am J Psychiatry*. 1995 152(7), 1052-8.

[44] Calero-Elvira, A; Krug, I; Davis, K; López, C; Fernández-Aranda, F; Treasure, J. Meta-analysis on drugs in people with eating disorders. *Eur Eat Disord Rev*. 2009 17(4), 243-59. doi: 10.1002/erv.936.

[45] Pozzi, M; Luxardi, GL; Sabbion, R. Disturbi del comportamento alimentare e disturbi da uso di sostanze: una revisione della recente letteratura. *Dipendenze Patologiche Addictive Disorders*. 2010 5 (2), 59-66.

[46] Root, TL; Pisetsky, EM; Thornton, L; Lichtenstein, P; Pedersen, NL; Bulik, CM. Patterns of co-morbidity of eating disorders and substance use in Swedish females. *Psychol Med*. 2010 40(1), 105-15. doi: 10.1017/S0033291709005662.

[47] Keel, PK; Klump, KL; Miller; KB; McGue, M; Iacono, WG. Shared transmission of eating disorders and anxiety disorders. *Int J Eat Disord*. 2005 38(2), 99-105.

[48] Wilson, GT; Wilfley, DE; Agras, WS; Bryson, SW. Psychological treatments of binge eating disorder. *Archives of General Psychiatry*. 2010 67,94–101.

[49] Luppino, FS; de Wit, LM; Bouvy, PF; Stijnen, T; Cuijpers, P; Penninx, BW; Zitman, FG. Overweight, obesity, and depression: a systematic review and meta-analysis of longitudinal studies. *Arch Gen Psychiatry*. 2010 67(3), 220-9. doi: 10.1001/archgenpsychiatry.2010.2. Review.

[50] Avena, NM; Bocarsly, ME; Rada, P; Kim, A; Hoebel, BG. After daily bingeing on a sucrose solution, food deprivation induces anxiety and accumbens dopamine/acetylcholine imbalance. *Physiol Behav*. 2008 (3),309-15. doi: 10.1016/j.physbeh.2008.01.008.

[51] Hoebel, BG; Avena, NM; Bocarsly, ME; Rada, P. Natural addiction: a behavioral and circuit model based on sugar addiction in rats. *J Addict Med*. 2009 3(1), 33-41. doi: 10.1097/ADM.0b013e31819aa621.

[52] Avena, NM; Rada, P; Moise, N; Hoebel, BG. Sucrose sham feeding on a binge schedule releases accumbens dopamine repeatedly and eliminates the acetylcholine satiety response. *Neuroscience*. 2006 139(3), 813-20.

[53] Avena, NM; Carrillo, CA; Needham, L; Leibowitz, SF; Hoebel, BG. Sugar-dependent rats show enhanced intake of unsweetened ethanol. *Alcohol.* 2004 34(2-3),203-9.
[54] Avena, NM; Hoebel, BG. A diet promoting sugar dependency causes behavioral cross-sensitization to a low dose of amphetamine. *Neuroscience.* 2003 122(1), 17-20.
[55] Galic, MA; Persinger, MA. Voluminous sucrose consumption in female rats: increased "nippiness" during periods of sucrose removal and possible oestrus periodicity. *Psychol Rep.* 2002 90(1), 58-60.
[56] Wideman, CH; Nadzam, GR; Murphy, HM. Implications of an animal model of sugar addiction, withdrawal and relapse for human health. *Nutr Neurosci* 2005 8(5-6), 269-76.
[57] Gosnell, BA. Sucrose intake enhances behavioral sensitization produced by cocaine. *Brain Res* 2005 1031(2), 194-201.
[58] Wojnicki, FH; Babbs, RK; Corwin, RL. Reinforcing efficacy of fat, as assessed by progressive ratio responding, depends upon availability not amount consumed. *Physiol Behav.* 2010 16, 100(4), 316-21. doi: 10.1016/j.physbeh.2010.03.004.
[59] Boggiano, MM; Chandler, PC; Viana, JB; Oswald, KD; Maldonado, CR; Wauford, PK. Combined dieting and stress evoke exaggerated responses to opioids in binge-eating rats. *Behav Neurosci.* 2005 119(5), 1207-14.
[60] Oswald, KD; Murdaugh, DL; King, VL; Boggiano, MM. Motivation for palatable food despite consequences in an animal model of binge eating. *Int J Eat Disord.* 2011 44(3), 203-11. doi: 10.1002/eat.20808.
[61] Alsiö, J; Olszewski, PK; Levine, AS; Schiöth, HB. Feed-forward mechanisms: addiction-like behavioral and molecular adaptations in overeating. *Front Neuroendocrinol.* 2012 33(2), 127-39. doi: 10.1016/j.yfrne.2012.01.002.
[62] Johnson, PM; Kenny, PJ. Dopamine D2 receptors in addiction-like reward dysfunction and compulsive eating in obese rats. *Nat Neurosci.* 2010 13(5), 635-41. doi: 10.1038/nn.2519.
[63] Stice, E; Spoor, S; Bohon, C; Veldhuizen, MG; Small, DM. Relation of reward from food intake and anticipated food intake to obesity: A functional magnetic resonance imaging study. *Journal of Abnormal Psychology.* 2008 117, 924–935
[64] Wang, GJ; Volkow, ND; Logan, J; Pappas, NR; Wong, CT; Zhu, W; Netusil, N; Fowler, JS. Brain dopamine and obesity. *Lancet.* 2001 357, 354–7.
[65] Umberg, EN; Shader, RI; Hsu, LKG; Greenblatt, DJ. From Disordered Eating to Addiction. The ''Food Drug'' in Bulimia Nervosa. *J Clin Psychopharmacol.* 2012 32, 376-389
[66] Di Chiara, G. Drug addiction as dopamine-dependent associative learning disorder. *Eur J Pharmacol.* 1999 375, 13-30.
[67] Di Chiara, G; Imperato, A. Drugs abused by humans preferentially increase synaptic dopamine concentrations in the mesolimbic system of freely moving rats. *Proc Natl Acad Sci U S A.* 1988 85, 5274-5278.
[68] Hoebel, BG. Brain neurotransmitters in food and drug reward. *Am J Clin Nutr.* 1985 42, 1133-1150
[69] Di Chiara, G. Nucleus accumbens shell and core dopamine: differential role in behavior and addiction. *Behav Brain Res.* 2002 137, 75-114

[70] Blood, AJ; Zatorre, RJ. Intensely pleasurable responses to music correlate with activity in brain regions implicated in reward and emotion. *Proc Natl Acad Sci U S A*. 2001 25, 98(20), 11818-23.

[71] Mobbs, D; Greicius, MD; Abdel-Azim, E; Menon, V; Reiss, AL. Humor modulates the mesolimbic reward centers. *Neuron*. 2003 4, 40(5), 1041-8.

[72] Breiter, HC; Aharon, I; Kahneman, D; Dale, A; Shizgal, P. Functional imaging of neural responses to expectancy and experience of monetary gains and losses. *Neuron* 2001 30, 619–39

[73] Knutson, B; Adams, CM; Fong, GW; Hommer, D. Anticipation of increasing monetary reward selectively recruits nucleus accumbens. *J Neurosci*. 2001 15, 21-16.

[74] Aharon, I; Etcoff, N; Ariely, D; Chabris, CF; O'Connor, E; Breiter, HC. Beautiful faces have variable reward value: fMRI and behavioral evidence. *Neuron*. 2001 8, 32(3), 537-51.

[75] Ishai, A. Sex, beauty and the orbitofrontal cortex. *Int J Psychophysiol.* 2007 63(2), 181-5.

[76] O'Doherty, J; Winston, J; Critchley, H; Perrett, D; Burt, DM; Dolan, RJ. Beauty in a smile: the role of medial orbitofrontal cortex in facial attractiveness. *Neuropsychologia*. 2003 41(2), 147-55.

[77] Noriuchi, M; Kikuchi, Y; Senoo, A. The functional neuroanatomy of maternal love: mother's response to infant's attachment behaviors. *Biol Psychiatry.* 2008 15, 63(4), 415-23.

[78] Fisher, HE; Aron, A; Brown, LL. Romantic love: a mammalian brain system for mate choice. *Philos Trans R Soc Lond B Biol Sci*. 2006 361(1476), 2173-86.

[79] Blum, K; Liu, Y; Shriner, R; Gold, MS. Reward circuitry dopaminergic activation regulates food and drug craving behavior. *Curr Pharm Des*. 2011 17(12), 1158-67.

[80] Comings, DE; Blum, K. Reward deficiency syndrome: genetic aspects of behavioral disorders. *Prog Brain Res*. 2000 126, 325-41. Review.

[81] Gjedde, A; Kumakura, Y; Cumming, P; Linnet, J; Møller, A. Inverted-U-shaped correlation between dopamine receptor availability in striatum and sensation seeking. *Proc Natl Acad Sci U S A*. 2010 107(8), 3870-5. doi: 10.1073/pnas.0912319107.

[82] Volkow, ND; Wang, GJ; Fowler, JS; Logan, J; Gatley, SJ; Wong, C; Hitzemann, R; Pappas, NR.. Reinforcing effects of psychostimulants in humans are associated with increases in brain dopamine and occupancy of D(2) receptors. *J Pharmacol Exp Ther*. 1999 291, 409-415.

[83] Hajnal, A; Smith, GP; Norgren, R. Oral sucrose stimulation increases accumbens dopamine in the rat. *Am J Physiol Regul Integr Comp Physiol*. 2004 286, R31-R37.

[84] Martel, P; Fantino, M. Mesolimbic dopaminergic system activity as a function of food reward: a microdialysis study. *Pharmacol Biochem Behav*. 1996 53, 221-226.

[85] Pothos, E; Rada, P; Mark, GP; Hoebel, BG. Dopamine microdialysis in the nucleus accumbens during acute and chronic morphine, naloxone-precipitated withdrawal and clonidine treatment. *Brain Res*. 1991 566, 348-350.

[86] Wise, RA; Newton, P; Leeb, K; Burnette, B; Pocock, D; Justice, JB Jr. Fluctuations in nucleus accumbens dopamine concentration during intravenous cocaine self-administration in rats. *Psychopharmacology (Berl).* 1995 120(1), 10-20.

[87] Di Chiara, G; Tanda, G. Blunting of reactivity of dopamine transmission to palatable food: a biochemical marker of anhedonia in the CMS model? *Psychopharmacology (Berl).* 1997 134, 351-353.

[88] Bassareo, V; Di Chiara, G. Modulation of feeding-induced activation of mesolimbic dopamine transmission by appetitive stimuli and its relation to motivational state. *Eur J Neurosci.* 1999 11, 4389-4397.

[89] Tanda, G; Di Chiara, G. A dopamine-mu1 opioid link in the rat ventral tegmentum shared by palatable food (Fonzies) and non-psychostimulant drugs of abuse. *Eur J Neurosci.* 1998 10, 1179-1187.

[90] Ray, LA; Hutchison, KE. Effects of naltrexone on alcohol sensitivity and genetic moderators of medication response. *Arch Gen Psychiatry.* 2007 64, 1069–77.

[91] Pecina, S; Smith, KS; Berridge, KC. Hedonic hot spots in the brain. *Neuroscientist.* 2006 12, 500–11.

[92] Sahr, AE; Sindelar, DK; Alexander-Chacko, JT; Eastwood, BJ; Mitch, CH; Statnick, MA. Activation of mesolimbic dopamine neurons during novel and daily limited access to palatable food is blocked by the opioid antagonist LY255582. *Am J Physiol Regul Integr Comp Physiol.* 2008 295(2), R463-71. doi: 10.1152/ajpregu.00390.2007.

[93] Yeomans, MR; Gray RW. Effects of naltrexone on food intake and changes in subjective appetite after eating: evidence for opioid involvement in the appetizer effect. *Physiol Behav.* 1997 62, 15–21.

[94] Bellocchio, L; Lafenêtre, P; Cannich, A; Cota, D; Puente, N; Grandes, P; Chaouloff, F; Piazza, PV; Marsicano, G. Bimodal control of stimulated food intake by the endocannabinoid system. *Nat Neurosci.* 2010 13(3), 281-3. doi: 10.1038/nn.2494.

[95] Di Marzo, V; Ligresti, A; Cristino, L. The endocannabinoid system as a link between homoeostatic and hedonic pathways involved in energy balance regulation. *Int J Obes (Lond).* 2009 33 (Suppl 2), S18-24. doi: 10.1038/ijo.2009.67. Review.

[96] Quarta, C; Bellocchio, L; Mancini, G; Mazza, R; Cervino, C; Braulke, LJ; Fekete, C: Latorre, R; Nanni, C; Bucci, M; Clemens, LE; Heldmaier, G; Watanabe, M; Leste-Lassere, T; Maitre, M; Tedesco, L; Fanelli, F; Reuss, S; Klaus, S; Srivastava, RK; Monory, K; Valerio, A; Grandis, A; De Giorgio, R; Pasquali, R; Nisoli, E; Cota, D; Lutz, B; Marsicano, G; Pagotto, U. CB(1) signaling in forebrain and sympathetic neurons is a key determinant of endocannabinoid actions on energy balance. *Cell Metab.* 2010 7, 11(4), 273-85. doi: 10.1016/j.cmet.2010.02.015.

[97] Harrold, JA; Elliott, JC; King, PJ; Widdowson, PS; Williams, G. Down-regulation of cannabinoid-1 (CB-1) receptors in specific extrahypothalamic regions of rats with dietary obesity: a role for endogenous cannabinoids in driving appetite for palatable food? *Brain Res.* 2002 18, 952(2), 232-8.

[98] Davis, KW; Wellman, PJ; Clifford, PS. Augmented cocaine conditioned place preference in rats pretreated with systemic ghrelin. *Regul Pept.* 2007 3, 140(3), 148-52.

[99] Hommel, JD; Trinko, R; Sears, RM; Georgescu, D; Liu, ZW; Gao, XB; Thurmon, JJ; Marinelli, M; DiLeone, RJ. Leptin receptor signaling in midbrain dopamine neurons regulates feeding. *Neuron.* 2006 21, 51(6), 801-10.

[100] Kanoski, SE; Hayes, MR; Greenwald, HS; Fortin, SM; Gianessi, CA; Gilbert, JR; Grill, HJ. Hippocampal leptin signaling reduces food intake and modulates food-related memory processing. *Neuropsychopharmacology.* 2011 36, (9), 1859-70. doi:10.1038/npp.2011.70.

[101] Scott, MM; Lachey, JL; Sternson, SM; Lee, CE; Elias, CF; Friedman, JM; Elmquist, JK. Leptin targets in the mouse brain. *J Comp Neurol.* 2009 514(5), 518-32. doi: 10.1002/cne.22025.

[102] Schellekens, H; Finger, BC; Dinan, TG; Cryan, JF. Ghrelin signalling and obesity: at the interface of stress, mood and food reward. *Pharmacol Ther.* 2012 135(3), 316-26. doi: 10.1016/j.pharmthera.2012.06.004.

[103] Skibicka, KP; Hansson, C; Alvarez-Crespo, M; Friberg, PA; Dickson, SL. Ghrelin directly targets the ventral tegmental area to increase food motivation. *Neuroscience.* 2011 180, 129-37. doi: 10.1016/j.neuroscience.2011.02.016.

[104] Farooqi, IS; Bullmore, E; Keogh, J; Gillard, J; O'Rahilly, S; Fletcher, PC. Leptin regulates striatal regions and human eating behavior. *Science.* 2007 317(5843), 1355.

[105] Malik, S; McGlone, F; Bedrossian, D; Dagher, A. Ghrelin modulates brain activity in areas that control appetitive behavior. *Cell Metab.* 2008 7(5), 400-9. doi: 10.1016/j.cmet.2008.03.007.

[106] Pelchat, ML; Johnson, A; Chan, R; Valdez, J; Ragland, JD. Images of desire: food craving activation during fMRI. *Neuroimage.* 2004 23, 1486–93.

[107] Fedoroff, IC Polivy, J; Herman, CP. The effect of pre-exposure to food cues on the eating behavior of restrained and unrestrained eaters. *Appetite.* 1997 28, 33–47.

[108] Tuomisto, T; Hetherington, MM; Morris, MF; Tuomisto, MT; Turjanmaa, V; Lappalainen, R. Psychological and physiological characteristics of sweet food ''addiction''. *Int J Eat Disord.* 1999 25, 169–75.

[109] Gibson, EL; Desmond, E. Chocolate craving and hunger state. *Appetite.*1999 32, 219–40.

[110] Robinson, TE; Berridge, KC. Review. The incentive sensitization theory of addiction: some current issues. *Philos Trans R Soc Lond B Biol Sci.* 2008 363(1507), 3137-46. doi: 10.1098/rstb.2008.0093. Review.

[111] Stice, E; Yokum, S; Blum, K; Bohon, C. Weight gain is associated with reduced striatal response to palatable food. *J Neurosci.* 2010 30(39), 13105-9. doi: 10.1523/JNEUROSCI.2105-10.2010.

[112] Batterham, RL; ffytche, DH; Rosenthal, JM; Zelaya, FO; Barker, GJ; Withers, DJ; Williams, SC. PYY modulation of cortical and hypothalamic brain areas predicts feeding behaviour in humans. *Nature.* 2007 450(7166), 106-9.

[113] Blevins, JE; Baskin, DG. Hypothalamic-brainstem circuits controlling eating. *Forum Nutr.* 2010 63, 133-40. doi: 10.1159/000264401.

[114] Suzuki, K; Simpson, KA; Minnion, JS; Shillito, JC; Bloom, SR. The role of gut hormones and the hypothalamus in appetite regulation. *Endocr J.* 2010 57(5), 359-72.

[115] Gariepy, G; Nitka, D; Schmitz, N. The association between obesity and anxiety disorders in the population: a systematic review and meta-analysis. *Int J Obes (Lond).* 2010 34(3), 407-19. doi: 10.1038/ijo.2009.252.

[116] Marijnissen, RM; Bus, BA; Holewijn, S; Franke, B; Purandare, N; de Graaf ,J; den Heijer, M; Buitelaar, JK; Oude Voshaar, RC. Depressive symptom clusters are differentially associated with general and visceral obesity. *J Am Geriatr Soc.* 2011 59(1), 67-72. doi: 10.1111/j.1532-5415.2010.03228.x.

[117] Maniam, J; Morris, MJ. The link between stress and feeding behaviour. *Neuropharmacology.* 2012 63(1), 97-110. doi: 10.1016/j.neuropharm.2012.04.017.

[118] Nieuwenhuizen, AG; Rutters, F. The hypothalamic-pituitary-adrenal-axis in the regulation of energy balance. *Physiol Behav.* 2008 94(2), 169-77. doi: 10.1016/j.physbeh.2007.12.011.

[119] Kyrou, I; Tsigos, C. Stress mechanisms and metabolic complications. *Horm Metab Res.* 2007 Jun;39(6):430-8.

[120] Garber, AK; Lustig, RH. Is fast food addictive? *Curr Drug Abuse Rev.* 2011 4(3), 146-62.

[121] Adam, TC; Epel, ES. Stress, eating and the reward system. *Physiol Behav.* 2007 Jul 24;91(4):449-58.

[122] Koob, GF. The role of CRF and CRF-related peptides in the dark side of addiction. *Brain Res* 2010 1314, 3-14.

[123] Gibson, EL. Emotional influences on food choice: sensory, physiological and psychological pathways. *Physiol Behav.* 2006 89(1), 53-61.

[124] Dallman, MF. Stress-induced obesity and the emotional nervous system. *Trends Endocrinol Metab.* 2010 21(3), 159-65. doi: 10.1016/j.tem.2009.10.004.

[125] Kyrou, I; Chrousos, GP; Tsigos, C. Stress, visceral obesity, and metabolic complications. *Ann N Y Acad Sci.* 2006 1083, 77-110. Review.

[126] Kyrou, I; Tsigos, C. Chronic stress, visceral obesity and gonadal dysfunction. *Hormones (Athens).* 2008 7(4), 287-93. Review.

[127] Rosmond, R; Dallman, MF; Björntorp, P. Stress-related cortisol secretion in men: relationships with abdominal obesity and endocrine, metabolic and hemodynamic abnormalities. *J Clin Endocrinol Metab.* 1998 83(6), 1853-9.

[128] Rosmond, R; Lapidus, L; Mårin, P; Björntorp, P. Mental distress, obesity and body fat distribution in middle-aged men. *Obes Res.* 1996 4(3), 245-52.

[129] Räikkönen, K; Matthews, KA; Kuller, LH. Depressive symptoms and stressful life events predict metabolic syndrome among middle-aged women: a comparison of World Health Organization, Adult Treatment Panel III, and International Diabetes Foundation definitions. *Diabetes Care.* 2007 30(4), 872-7.

[130] Jauch-Chara, K; Oltmanns, KM. Obesity--a neuropsychological disease? Systematic review and neuropsychological model. *Prog Neurobiol.* 2014 114, 84-101. doi: 10.1016/j.pneurobio.2013.12.001.

[131] Schweiger, U; Greggersen, W; Rudolf, S; Pusch, M; Menzel, T; Winn, S; Hassfurth, J; Fassbinder, E; Kahl, KG; Oltmanns, KM; Hohagen, F; Peters, A. Disturbed glucose disposal in patients with major depression; application of the glucose clamp technique. *Psychosom Med.* 2008 70(2), 170-6. doi: 10.1097/PSY.0b013e318164231d.

[132] Nathan, RS; Sachar, EJ; Asnis, GM; Halbreich, U; Halpern, FS. Relative insulin insensitivity and cortisol secretion in depressed patients. *Psychiatry Res.* 1981 4(3), 291-300.

[133] Amsterdam, JD; Maislin, G. Hormonal responses during insulin-induced hypoglycemia in manic-depressed, unipolar depressed, and healthy control subjects. *J Clin Endocrinol Metab.* 1991 73(3), 541-8.

[134] Lustman, PJ; Clouse, RE. Depression in diabetic patients: the relationship between mood and glycemic control. *J Diabetes Complications.* 2005 19(2), 113-22. Review.

[135] Himmerich, H; Fulda, S; Schaaf, L; Beitinger, PA; Schuld, A; Pollmächer, T. Changes in weight and glucose tolerance during treatment with mirtazapine. *Diabetes Care.* 2006 29(1),170.

[136] Hirth, J; Mahbubur, R; Berenson, AB. The association of posttraumatic stress disorder with fast food and soda consumption and unhealthy weight loss behaviors among young women. *J Womens Health*. 2011 20, 1141–1149.
[137] Brewerton, TD. Posttraumatic Stress Disorder and Disordered Eating: Food Addiction as Self-Medication. *Journal Of Women's Health*; 2011 20(8), 1133-4. doi: 10.1089/jwh.2011.3050.DOI: 10.1089/jwh. 2011.3050
[138] Boggiano, MM; Chandler, PC. Binge eating in rats produced by combining dieting with stress. *Curr Protoc Neurosci* 2006 Chapter 9: Unit9 23A.
[139] Zellner, DA; Loaiza, S; Gonzalez, Z; Pita, J; Morales, J; Pecora, D; Wolf, A. Food selection changes under stress. *Physiol Behav*. 2006 87(4), 789-93.
[140] Oliver, G; Wardle, J; Gibson, EL. Stress and food choice: a laboratory study. *Psychosom Med* 2000 62 (6), 853-65.
[141] Wardle, J; Steptoe, A; Oliver, G; Lipsey, Z. Stress, dietary restraint and food intake. *J Psychosom Res*. 2000 48(2), 195-202.
[142] Fisher, JO; Birch, LL. Restricting access to foods and children's eating. *Appetite* 1999 32(3), 405-19.
[143] Goldstein, DS. Computer models of stress, allostasis, and acute and chronic diseases. *Ann N Y Acad Sci*. 2008 1148, 223-31. doi: 10.1196/annals.1410.061.
[144] Shriner, RL. Food as a bariatric drug. *Curr. Pharm. Des*.2011 17 (12), 1198–1208.
[145] Avallone, E; Baumeister, T; Sadegh, A. *Mark's Standard Handbook for Mechanical Engineers. 11th Ed*. New York: McGraw-Hill Professional. 1996.
[146] Charney, DS. Psychobiological mechanisms of resilience and vulnerability: implications for successful adaptation to extreme stress. *Am J Psychiatry*. 2004 161(2), 195-216. Review.
[147] Timmerman, GM; Acton, GJ. The relationship between basic need satisfaction and emotional eating. *Issues Ment Health Nurs*. 2001 22(7), 691-701.
[148] Maslow, AH. *Toward a psychology of being*. Princeton, NJ: Van Nostrand; 1968
[149] Leidy, NK. Operationalizing Maslow's theory: development and testing of the basic need satisfaction inventory. *Issues Ment Health Nurs*. 1994 15(3), 277-95.
[150] Arnow, B; Kenardy, J; Agras, WS. The Emotional Eating Scale: the development of a measure to assess coping with negative affect by eating. *Int J Eat Disord.* 1995 18(1),79-90.
[151] Andrews, RA; Lowe, R & Clair, A. The relationship between basic need satisfaction and emotional eating in obesity. *Australian Journal of Psychology* 2011 63, 207–213. doi:10.1111/j.1742-9536.2011.00021.x
[152] Barsalou, LW. Perceptual symbol systems. *Behav.BrainSci.* 1999; 22: 577–660.
[153] Schubert, TW. Your highness: vertical positions as perceptual symbols of power. *J Pers Soc Psychol*. 2005 89(1), 1-21.
[154] Williams, LE; Bargh, JA. Experiencing physical warmth promotes interpersonal warmth. *Science*. 2008 322(5901), 606-7. doi: 10.1126/science.1162548.
[155] Ijzerman, H; Semin, GR. The thermometer of social relations: mapping social proximity on temperature. *Psychol Sci*. 2009 20(10), 1214-20. doi: 10.1111/j.1467-9280.2009.02434.x.
[156] Wansink, B; Sangerman, C. The taste of comfort. *Am.Demogr.* 2000 22, 66–67.
[157] Troisi, JD; Gabriel, S. Chicken soup really is good for the soul: "comfort food" fulfills the need to belong. *Psychol Sci*. 2011 22(6), 747-53. doi: 10.1177/0956797611407931.

[158] Rommel, D; Nandrino, JL; Ducro, C; Andrieux, S; Delecourt, F; Antoine, P. Impact of emotional awareness and parental bonding on emotional eating in obese women. *Appetite*. 2012 59(1), 21-6. doi: 10.1016/j.appet.2012.03.006.

[159] Sifneos, PE. Clinical observations on some patients suffering from a variety of psychosomatic diseases. *Acta Medicina Psychosomatica*. 1967 7, 1–10.

[160] Bucci, W. Symptoms and symbols: a multiple code theory of somatization. *Psychoanalitic Inquiry* 1997 17 (2), 151-172.

[161] Ostuzzi, R; Luxardi, GL. Le metafore della Bulimia. In Cavanna, D; Stagi, L (eds.). *Sul fronte del cibo. Corpo, controllo, soggettività*. Torino: Franco Angeli; 2009 pp. 123-141.

[162] Lumley, MA; Neely, LC; Burger, AJ. The assessment of alexithymia in medical settings: implications for understanding and treating health problems. *J Pers Assess.* 2007 89(3), 230-46.

[163] van Strien, T; Ouwens, MA. Counterregulation in female obese emotional eaters: Schachter, Goldman, and Gordon's (1968) test of psychosomatic theory revisited. *Eat Behav*. 2003 3(4), 329-40.

[164] Agras, WS; Telch, CF. The effects of caloric deprivation and negative affect on binge eating in obese binge-eating disordered women. *Behavior Therapy* 1998 29, 491–503.

[165] Polivy, J; Herman, CP; McFarlane, T. Effects of anxiety on eating: does palatability moderate distress-induced overeating in dieters? *J Abnorm Psychol.* 1994 103(3), 505-10.

[166] Burgess, EE; Turan, B; Lokken, KL; Morse, A; Boggiano, MM. Profiling motives behind hedonic eating. Preliminary validation of the Palatable Eating Motives Scale. *Appetite*. 2014 72, 66-72. doi: 10.1016/j.appet.2013.09.016.

[167] Hawkins, RC; Clement, PF. Binge eating: Measurement problems and a conceptual model. In Hawkins, RC; Fremouw, WJ; Clement, PF (Eds.). *The binge purge syndrome: Diagnosis, treatment, and research*. New York: Springer; 1984 pp. 229–251.

[168] Heatherton, TF; Baumeister, R F. Binge eating as an escape from self-awareness. *Psychological Bulletin*. 1991 110(1), 86 –108.

[169] Lazarus, R; Folkman, S. *Stress, appraisal and coping*. NY: Springer; 1984.

[170] Endler, NS; Parker, JD. Multidimensional assessment of coping: a critical evaluation. *J Pers Soc Psychol*. 1990 58(5), 844-54.

[171] Sierra-Baigrie, S; Lemos-Giráldez, S; Paino, M; Fonseca-Pedrero, E. Exploring the relationship between coping strategies and binge eating in nonclinical adolescents. *Eur Eat Disord Rev*. 2012 20(1), e63-9. doi: 10.1002/erv.1103.

[172] Bloks, H; Van Furth, EF; Callewaert, I; Hoek,HW. Coping strategies and recovery in patients with a severe eating disorder. *Eat Disord*. 2004 12(2), 157-69.

[173] Hasking, PA. Reinforcement sensitivity, coping, and delinquent behaviour in adolescents. *J Adolesc*. 2007 30(5),739-49.

[174] Shriner, RL. Food sobriety: surviving the holidays. *Gainesville Today*. 2010 p 69.

In: The Different Faces of Being Overweight
Editor: Emilia Manzato
ISBN: 978-1-63483-099-7

Chapter 3

DIETARY RESTRAINT AS A RISK FACTOR FOR LOSS OF CONTROL

Nazario Melchionda[1,2*] ***and Giulietta Tarrini***[3†]
[1]University of Bologna, Italy
[2]President of Italian Society for the Study of Eating Disorder (SISDCA), Italy
[3]Dietista Coordinatrice, Azienda Ospedaliera di Bologna, Policlinico S.Orsola-Malpighi, Servizio di Malattie del Metabolismo e Dietetica Clinica, Italy

ABSTRACT

The subject of the present chapter is extremely topical and it is interesting not only for research purposes but also to find and examine evidence relevant to therapy in clinical practice. This chapter focuses on the risk of loss of control, using definitions for non-experts, recognizing that eating disorders are multi-disciplinary, involving psychological, psychiatric, endocrinological and nutritional disciplines: Binge eating (BE), Binge Eating Disorder (BED), Dietary Restraint (DR), Food Addiction (FA), HSME: Homeostasis System of Metabolism and Energy, HSHR: Homeostasis System of Hedonic Reward, NAc: Nucleus Accumbens, NCAR: Neural Circuitry of Addiction and Reward, VTA: Ventral Tegmental Area. The major sources of historical data are outlined so as to understand the significance of loss of control – in particular, the 1950 Minnesota Study by Angel Keys, in which the characteristic symptoms of eating disorders were activated in volunteer participants by means of caloric restriction; this is followed by observations in Greek literature, the phenomenon of St Anorexics in the Middle Ages and the effect of caloric restriction on a group of Canadian soldiers during World War II. The historical data concludes with the pioneering publication by Stunkard of his case study of a subject with chronic obesity, in which Binge Eating is described for the first time. In addition, there is reference to human and rodent experimental data: in particular regarding the psychological, psychobiological and neurobiological mechanisms related to BED loss of control. Since 2000 considerable research and numerous studies have been carried out employing neuroimaging techniques to determine the effect brain biology has on both normal and pathological behavior. The result is the current recognition that neural

* melchiondauno@gmail.com.
† gtarrini@gmail.com

systems influence the regulation of normal eating behavior and that they also influence the loss of control that characterizes AN, BN, and BED. The neural systems identified by means of neuroimaging radiological techniques are summarized in the definitions and in the section 'What we can learn from brain biology'. Food Addiction (FA) is the latest chapter in the history of ED research. Three important questions are therefore asked: What are the neurobiological effects of intermittent restriction? What is the level of calorie restriction that results in loss of control? Can we stop eating too much hyper-palatable food? By answering these questions we will be able to make recommendations and suggestions. The final conclusion is that inadequate caloric restriction is not the only risk factor for loss of control but also the cognitive intention to lose weight by means of DR.

Keywords: binge eating, binge eating disorder, dietary restraint, loss of control, food addiction, hedonic reward

ACRONYMS

AN	Anorexia Nervosa
BE	Binge Eating
BED	Binge Eating Disorder
BN	Bulimia Nervosa
DR	Dietary Restraint
ED	Eating Disorders
FA	Food Addiction
HSHR	Homeostatic System of Hedonic Reward
HSME	Homeostatic System of Metabolism and Energy
NCAR	Neural Circuitry of Addiction and Reward
NAc	Nucleus Accumbens
SUD	Substance Use Disorder
VTA	Ventral Tegmental Area

INTRODUCTION

Binge Eating (BE) is a symptom in common with all Eating Disorders Diagnostic Categories: Anorexia Nervosa (AN), Bulimia Nervosa (BN) and Binge Eating Disorder (BED). Most individuals feel a sense of loss of control while bingeing. [4]. Regular Binge eating (BE) is present in adolescent and adult populations (prevalence: 1.8–5%) [27,31,34] and is associated with psychopathology. Thus, it is difficult to understand the etiology of BE. Cross-sectional and longitudinal studies suggest that Dietary Restraint (DR) [32] predicts the onset of BE after 1–2 years. [5,32,60,61] Other longitudinal studies also report that DR is a risk factor for the development of BE and BN. [43,44] Because DR and BE are very prevalent among adolescent girls and young women [21,59] and are associated with functional impairment and psychological distress [24,29,64] it is very important to understand the relationships between dieting (or DR) and the loss of control, which is signal of abnormal eating behaviour. [15] Although many women engage in DR, relatively few develop BE. DR may only increase susceptibility for BE in individuals who are at genetic risk. Specifically, DR may be a behavioural 'exposure factor', that activates genetic predispositions for BE. This hypothesis was investigated in a study on young adolescent and adult same-sex female twins from the Minnesota Twin Family Study and the Michigan State University Twin Registry. Twin moderation models were used to examine whether levels of DR moderate genetic and environmental influences on BE. Results indicated that genetic and non-shared environmental factors for BE increased at higher levels of DR. Importantly, these effects were present after checking age, body mass index, and genetic and environmental overlap among DR and BE. Results suggest that DR may be the most important factor for individuals at genetic risk of BE, and the combination of these factors could enhance individual risk for BE. [53] There are many studies on humans that show the effects of the manipulation of palatability and food availability on its consumption. Even when foods are not palatable more food tends to be consumed if the containers are larger. [76,77] Even if the environmental pressure pushes the consumption of food undoubtedly higher, this simple explanation does not take into account the fact that not all individuals exposed to the same environment gain weight. This suggests that the existing differences (genetic and epigenetic) make some individuals more vulnerable to increased availability and to stimuli associated with food.

DEFINITIONS

Binge Eating Disorder (BED) was included until 2013 in the DSM-IV [2] in the third category of Eating Disorders Not Otherwise Specified (EDNOS). [20,69] A standardized detailed diagnostic grid to define BED was proposed. The amount of food, the feeling of not being able to stop eating, or not being in control of what and how much is eaten are key elements. 'Excessive amount of food' is defined as being greater than that which the majority of people would consume at the same time and in the same circumstances. BED is almost always associated with obesity, although it can also be present in normal weight subjects. [17,38,40] BED is further clarified and proposed for inclusion in the DSM-5 as a nosological category. [67,79] On 13-05-2013 BED was officially included in the DSM-5. [3]

Binge Eating (BE). Episode characterized by a rapid and excessive consumption of food with a feeling of loss of control not followed by compensatory behavior (vomiting, compulsive exercise and laxatives). The term is used when the criteria of the DSM-5 proposal for BED are not met.

Dieting, or Dietary Restraint (DR), refers to intentional and sustained deprivation of caloric intake for the purposes of weight loss or weight maintenance. [28,74] Caloric deprivation is supported by a cognitive attitude concerning the compliance of a medical prescription or a decision independently conceived. Caloric deprivation is a potential risk factor for the development of BE and BN and, although many people engage in the food restriction, relatively few develop BE. The caloric deprivation for individuals at genetic risk of BE combined with environmental factors could enhance individual differences. [53] DR increases the risk of onset and maintenance of BE and BN. *"The main effect of chocolate deprivation on consumption was qualified by an interaction with restraint. Chocolate-deprived restrained eaters consumed more chocolate food than did any other group. Restrained eaters experienced more food cravings than did unrestrained eaters and were* *more likely to eat the craved food. …… Converging measures of craving indicate that deprivation causes craving and overeating, but primarily in restrained eaters".* [48] Prospective risk factor studies indicate that females with high versus low scores on DR scales are at greater risk for future onset of BE, bulimic symptoms, and bulimic pathology. [42] *"The fact that only a small proportion of individuals with elevated dietary restraint scores develop bulimic pathology suggests that some extreme but rare form of dietary restriction may increase risk for this disturbance. The authors tested the hypothesis that fasting …… would be a more potent predictor of binge eating and bulimic pathology onset than dietary restraint scores using data from 496 adolescent girls followed over 5 years. Results confirmed that only 23% of participants with elevated dietary restraint scores reported fasting. Furthermore, fasting generally showed stronger and more consistent predictive relations to future onset of recurrent binge eating and threshold/subthreshold bulimia nervosa over 1- to 5-year follow-up relative to dietary restraint, though the former effects were only significantly stronger than the latter for some comparisons. Results provide preliminary support for the hypothesis that fasting is a stronger risk factor for bulimic pathology than is self-reported dieting."* [63] While many individuals with BN attempt to restrict their food intake, the goal of losing weight fundamentally alters the effect of such restriction on BE, and treatment may benefit from helping patients to establish a healthier approach to achieving long-term weight stability. [33] *"..... Initial pressure to be thin and thin-ideal internalization predicted subsequent growth in body dissatisfaction, initial body dissatisfaction predicted growth in dieting and negative affect, and initial dieting and negative affect predicted growth in bulimic symptoms. ......"* [60] *"The cognitive behavioral model of BN suggests that dieting is central to the maintenance of binge eating. However, correlational and experimental studies suggest that additional clarification is needed about the nature of this relationship."* [39]

Food Addiction (FA). Repeated bouts of food consumption, in some subjects (both humans and animals) can place stress on the cortical inhibitory processes that signal satiety and induce compulsive consumption of food in large quantities, in spite of nutritional overload and also behavioral inconsistencies. This loss of control and compulsive behavior in food consumption is similar to the mode of drug use observed in Substance Use Disorder (SUD) and led to the description of obesity as a possible natural condition of food addiction. [41]

HSME (Homeostasis System of Metabolism and Energy), initially known as 'unger center of lateral hypothalamus' for the regulation of energy balance, maintains energy balance, body weight, and adipose tissue fat.

HSHR (Homeostasis System of Hedonic Reward). The following definition has been proposed: *"Understanding the neurobiological mechanisms of addiction requires an integration of basic neuroscience with social psychology, experimental psychology, and psychiatry. Addiction is presented as a cycle of spiralling dysregulation of brain reward systems that progressively increases, resulting in compulsive drug use and a loss of control over drug-taking. …… This framework provides a realistic approach to identifying the neurobiological factors that produce vulnerability to addiction and to relapse in individuals with a history of addiction."* [37] HSHR regulates the hedonic reward homeostasis. Hoebel was the first to conceptualize the 'core', which is represented by the 'reward', for which food is the main stimulus. *"Hypothalamic sites which control feeding exert a corresponding control over lateral hypothalamic self-stimulation. This was demonstrated in rats bearing* *four, intrahypothalamic electrode-cannulas for electrical stimulation or chemical injection. Self-stimulation of the lateral hypothalamus was inhibited by ventromedial excitation or by excessive feeding. ...... Thus food acts via the ventromedial hypothalamus to inhibit not only feeding, but also lateral hypothalamic self-stimulation."*[30]

NAc (Nucleus Accumbens) is a neuron system in the Ventral Tegmental Area (VTA) that has an important role in the mechanisms of motivational reinforcement of food, causing addiction and the development of feelings of pleasure as a result of the consumption of food (and drugs). Berridge K. has called the NAc the 'hot spot of pleasure', in particular for the pleasure that can be experienced by taste. *"Opioid systems in the medial shell of the nucleus accumbens contribute to hedonic impact ("liking") for sweetness, food, and drug rewards. ...... Our maps indicate that opioid-induced increases in sucrose hedonic impact are generated by a localized cubic millimeter site in a rostrodorsal region of the medial shell. ...... Opioid circuits for stimulating food intake are widely distributed, whereas hedonic "liking" circuits are more tightly localized in the rostromedial shell of the nucleus accumbens."* [45] The NAc system is also the action sites for many drugs such as cocaine and amphetamines that trigger release of dopamine.

NCAR (Neural Circuitry of Addiction and Reward) is a system of meso-limbic structures that act like the interface between HSME and HSHR (NAc and VTA). They regulate and control molecular mechanisms through their cortical pleasure pathways. When NCAR is activated, it exerts a behavior reinforcement through the release of dopamine. The association of ED with SUD is due to the fact the activation of these pathways is common to both abnormal food and drug consumption. Food (in particular glucose), cocaine, opioids, nicotine, caffeine and alcohol activate these same neuro-biological pathways. *"Although cells in many brain regions respond to reward, the cortical-basal ganglia circuit is at the heart of the reward system. The key structures in this network are the anterior cingulate cortex, the orbital prefrontal cortex, the ventral striatum, the ventral pallidum, and the midbrain dopamine neurons. ...... Advances in neuroimaging techniques allow better spatial and temporal resolution. These studies now demonstrate that human functional and structural imaging results map increasingly close to primate anatomy."* [25]

VTA (Ventral Tegmental Area) is a group of neurons in the meso-cortico-limbic system that release dopamine as a reward. The VTA plays an important role in cognition, motivation and addiction.

THE MINNESOTA STUDY: THE LESSONS LEARNED AFTER 60 YEARS

The three phases of the study. The loss of control of food consumption was reported for the first time in 1950, and was called 'bulimic symptom'. In the Minnesota Study this loss of control is caused by caloric restriction. This study is the most important one that has been published which has evaluated the effects of caloric restriction and weight loss in people of normal weight. The study, conducted at the University of Minnesota in 1944 for one year, [36] was designed to evaluate the physiological and psychological effects of a severe and prolonged caloric restriction and the effectiveness of nutritional rehabilitation. The main purpose of the study was to understand how to best assist the victims of the famine in Europe and Asia during and after World War II, using data derived from a laboratory simulation of the famine. More than 100 men were recruited as a voluntary alternative to military service. In this initial sample 36 subjects who had the best state of physical and mental health and high motivation for participation in the study were selected. The participants were all white, aged between 22 and 33, and 25 were members of the Historic Peace Churches. The study was divided into three phases:

1) In the first phase of 12 weeks, the volunteers were fed normally while their behavior and personalities were studied in detail. During this time the participants consumed an average of 3,492 kcal for metabolic homeostasis with weight maintenance.
2) In the second phase of 24 weeks the participants were subjected to caloric deprivation, which corresponded to about half of their caloric intake (on average 1,570 kcal). This was a caloric intake similar to the average intake of the European affected by war famine. This regime caused participants to lose 25% of their initial weight.
3) In the third phase of 12 weeks, participants' food intake was gradually increased to a normal level. Most of the reported results related to only 32 men. All men experienced dramatic physical, psychological and social changes.

Behavioral, psychological and psychiatric effects. Towards the end of the period of caloric restriction, volunteers took two hours to eat a meal which previously took them only a few minutes. Every day they devoted hours to the planning of how to divide up the amount of available food. There was an increase in the consumption of coffee and tea: many drank more than 15 cups of coffee a day. In addition, the participants tried to keep their stomachs full by drinking large amounts of other fluids (water and soup), demanding that the food was served hot and that there was a considerable increase in the use of salt and spices. Consumption of chewing gum for some participants was also 40 packs a day. Both smoking and nail biting increased markedly.

Many of these changes also persisted during the 12 weeks of weight regain. During caloric deprivation all participants reported an increase in hunger and worry. Many participants were not able to adhere to the diet and manifested bulimic episodes, followed by self-reproach, self-deprecation and self-harm shaking. During the weight recovery phase, when a large amount of food was offered, many participants lost appetite control, eating either more or less than was necessary. Even after 12 weeks of rehabilitation increased hunger after a big meal was reported.

The normalization of eating habits occurred in most cases, but in a subgroup the consumption of excess food continued. The discriminating factor between those who normalized eating habits and those who continued to eat huge amounts of food was not identified. However, it is important to emphasize the fact that there were differences in the response to malnutrition. In general, participants responded to caloric restriction with reduced physical activity, fatigue, weakness, carelessness, apathy and lack of energy.

The movements of the participants became significantly slower. Some practiced occasional exercise spontaneously. Some tried to lose more weight by attempting to consume energy in order to be able to get a more plentiful ration of bread or to prevent the reduction of rations. From a psychological point of view, close monitoring occurred for a drop in attention span and concentration, poor insight and critical judgment, thinking focused on food, mood swings, irritability, anxiety, depression and psychotic episodes.

Psychiatric symptoms such as depression and suicidal ideas were constantly present. The frequent hoarding of food stolen from others also occurred. It was noted that anxiety developed as a result of hunger, and mental disorders such as psychosis. At the end of the study, focus was given to the similarity of the symptoms of the fast test with those of AN. [35] Considering that fasting has been a common occurrence in human evolution [19] many of the consequences described are protective, such as amenorrhea. [75] Thinking about food is also a strategy to help rather than a pathological sign. Therefore what happens with AN should be considered a realistic event rather than something inexplicable.

HISTORICAL NOTES: FROM SENOFONTE TO STUNKARD

Senofonte used the term 'boulimos' to describe the feeling of hunger, accompanied by prostration, that occurred with soldiers as a result of the small food rations availiable during the war against Artaxerxes. In greek 'limos' means hunger and 'bou' means great or 'boul' castrated bull. In 1959 Stunkard described BE for the first time in case report of Mr Cohen, who was obese: *"All my good intentions have collapsed ...... a part of me comes in black out ...... I do not feel like ...... the guilt haunts me ...... like I'm all alone with the food ...... until my stomach is full ...... constant fear of being found out ......"* [68]

170 medieval saints were anorexic and bulimic. Teresa D'Avila used an olive branch to induce vomiting; wheras St. Catherine da Siena used a feather for the same purpose; St Maria Maddalena dei Pazzi was seen inducing vomiting by the other sisters; and St Veronica was seen eating before Holy Communion. [9,54] The bulimic symptom was described for the first time in 1874 by William Gull in AN as "occasional bouts of overeaing" and later by other observers in their reports. [23]

Canadian soldiers. A similar tendency to overeat after a period of food deprivation has been observed in human beings. Canadian soldiers captured and held prisoner by the Germans after the abortive raid on Dieppe in France during World War II were questioned 59 years later about theis postwar feelings and behaviours. Not surprisingly, they reported more wae-related emotions than did soldiers who were not prisoners. They also reported that they had had episodes of BE after they were released and returned home to Canada and after their normal weight was restored. [52]

WHAT ANOREXIA TELLS US

Patients with AN starve themselves into emaciation and frequently becoming bulimic. They alternate between uncontrollable binges and starvation, prior deprivation appears to produce a tendency to overeat and even binge *"Bulimia is a poor prognostic sign in anorexia nervosa. This raised the question of whether bulimia represented an "end stage" of chronic anorexia nervosa or whether bulimic patients were a distinct subgroup. ...... Bulimic patients had a history of weighing more and were more commonly premorbidly obese. ......The bulimic group displayed a variety of impulsive behaviors, including use of alcohol and street drugs. ……"* [22] despite the restoration of both food availability and weight to their initial levels. [50]

LOSS OF CONTROL IN THE LABORATORY

From dietary restraint to BE in rodents. FA develops in rodents when there is activation of reward circuitry as a natural response to food intake: glucose causes the release of dopamine and opioids. It has been shown that intermittent access to sweetened food and water triggers behavior in rodents that can be compared to BE. [7] This phenomenon, which can be triggered in humans, occurs with access to food or after caloric deprivation.

Loss of control in BED. The antecedent of 'dieting' whit BED is not always observed in a subset of individuals (35-54%). The explanation can be deduced from the Blomquist's data. *"Patients with BED with a parental history of SUD were significantly more likely to start binge eating before dieting, had a significantly earlier age at BED onset, and reported less time between binge eating onset and meeting diagnostic criteria for BED than did patients without a parental history of SUD. …… Our findings suggest that a parental history of SUD is associated with certain distinct trajectories in the development of binge eating (earlier binge onset predating dieting onset) and with elevated rates of comorbidity with mood disorders in patients with BED",* [11] where it is shown that, in individuals with a family history of SUD, BE appears more readily before so-called 'dieting' compared to subjects without a family history of SUD, in which BE appears after dieting. In addition, people during and after the first BE 'dieting' experience manifest more readily the onset of depression and personality disorders, which can also trigger loss of control. It was observed that in BN without purging (89%), BE is preceded by dieting and weight loss, while with BED, BE is much more variable. Previous episodes of AN are significantly more frequent in BN compared to BED. In the two groups, BN and BED, there are no differences in relation to other psychiatric features. However, for many variables BED appears in a very heterogeneous group. [57]

So a question arises: what is the cause of BED that occur before food restriction? The answer is related to the longstanding question of whether the chicken or the egg came first[80] and is to be found in different psychological mechanisms, both biological and psycho-neuro-biological, which of course are combined in the complexity of the entire system of behavioral ED.

a. Psychological mechanisms are characterized by five phases:

- 1st phase: the desire to be thinner is expressed by the tendency to restrict caloric intake or increase calorie consumption but with far higher levels of physical activity
- 2nd phase: stress stimuli or emotional negativity is expressed by the endevour to seek relief from anxiety or by clearing-up eating
- 3rd phase: psychological factors require continued binging if the second stage does not produce the results required to relieve high levels of anxiety and/or depression

- 4th phase: termination is related to the presence/absence of food, stomach capacity and is linked to the possible onset of involuntary vomiting, to a sense of bloating, nausea, stomach pain or intense fear of gaining weight.
- 5th phase is characterized by the immediate negative thoughts and emotions, which are cancelled during subsequent binge, followed by variable somatic discomforts, including those that relate to increase of weight. [51]

b. Psycho-biological mechanisms: in the 80s and 90s, when modern pathophysiology did not know yet understand what regulates appetite and hunger, Blundell and Hill's psycho-biological model was used. [12] This model was based on our knowledge at that time of the biology of appetite that involves behavior, motivation, diet composition, physiological events, and peripheral and central processes. Hypothetical disorders of this system are related to ED such as disinhibition leading to BE. "*Over the past 30 years, the understanding of eating behaviour has been dominated by the concept of dietary restraint. However, the development of the Three Factor Eating Questionnaire introduced two other factors, disinhibition and hunger, which have not received as much recognition in the literature. …… Disinhibition is an important eating behaviour trait. It is associated not only with a higher body mass index and obesity, but also with mediating variables, such as less healthful food choices, which contribute to overweight/obesity and poorer health.*" [14] This model is explained by a much better knowledge of neuro-biological mechanisms.

c. Neuro-biological mechanisms: The neuro-images obtained of obese subjects using PET show a lack of dopaminergic pathways that regulate neuronal systems associated not only with sensitivity to pleasure and encouragement of motivation, but also to conditioning, to self-control, reactivity to stress and its threshold. *"Both drug addiction and obesity can be defined as disorders in which the saliency value of one type of reward (drugs and food, respectively) becomes abnormally enhanced relative to, and at the expense of others. This model is consistent with the fact that both drugs and food have powerful reinforcing effects-partly mediated by dopamine increases in the limbic system-that, under certain circumstances or in vulnerable individuals, could overwhelm the brain's homeostatic control mechanisms. …… Now, brain imaging discoveries have started to uncover common features between these two conditions and to delineate some of the overlapping brain circuits whose dysfunctions may explain stereotypic and related behavioral deficits in human subjects. These results suggest that both obese and drug-addicted individuals suffer from impairments in dopaminergic pathways that regulate neuronal systems associated not only with reward sensitivity and incentive motivation, but also with conditioning (memory/learning), impulse control (behavioural inhibition), stress reactivity, and interoceptive awareness. ……".* [72,73] These mechanisms bring us to the large field of Food Addiction. [41]

What We Can Learn from Brain Biology

The crucial problem is to know what exactly is the makeup of the differences between those people who are susceptible to have ED and those who are not. We can argue that these differences are responsible for changes in the NCAR function. However, it is equally possible that the differences may be related to the HSME homeostatic systems, which manage access to food. In this scenario, an individual would demonstrate short-term hyperphagic behavior and NCAR should be able to counter this in the long term. This does not happen to all parties and we will not know how to diagnose the most vulnerable if we are not familiar with proper investigation. Probably new phenotypic and genetic markers, already partly known as aspects of the Reward Deficiency Syndrome, will be of help. *"In accord with the new definition of addiction published by American Society of Addiction Medicine (ASAM) it is well-known that individuals who present to a treatment center involved in chemical dependency or other documented reward dependence behaviors have impaired brain reward circuitry. They have hypodopaminergic function due to genetic and/or environmental negative pressures upon the reward neuro-circuitry. This impairment leads to aberrant craving behavior and other behaviors such as SUD. Neurogenetic research in both animal and humans revealed that there is a well-defined cascade in the reward site. The experimental question is whether or not sugar can be a substance of abuse and lead to a natural form of addiction. "Food addiction" seems plausible because brain pathways that evolved to respond to natural rewards are also activated by addictive drugs. …… These behaviors are then related to neurochemical changes in the brain that also occur with addictive drugs. …… The evidence supports the hypothesis that under certain circumstances rats can become sugar dependent. This may translate to some human conditions as suggested by the literature on eating disorders and obesity."*[7] This effect is enhanced as a result of repeated exposures. [8]

The evidence of studies that associate food restriction to loss of control confirm the theory that eating behavior is subject to the functions and interactions between NCAR, HSHR and HSME. The effect of food restriction can help speed up weight gain through loss of control. For example, even binge-resistant rodents consume much more food after a short period of restriction. [13] At the neuro-chemical level, there is an increase in the release of dopamine in the NAc after a short period of restriction compared to rodents treated with unlimited access to sucrose.

The repeated release of dopamine in the NAc is also observed with drugs. [18] In rodents both drugs and sucrose significantly increase the sensitivity of the D2R dopamine receptors [16], contributing to greater dependence on food. Interestingly, following a long period of food restriction, with body weight reduction to 85% of normal, rodents undergo binge-like behavior induced by acute food restriction. [6] These results show that alternate and repeated exposure to food and restriction can alter NCAR, potentially increasing the pleasure derived from the consumption of food and thus making food consumption more difficult to control. In conclusion, there are many human studies that show the effects of the manipulation of palatability and food availability on food consumption. The existing differences make some individuals more vulnerable to the increased availability and stimuli associated with food. We can argue that the above is responsible for NCAR function differences, but it is equally possible that the differences may be related to HSME, which manages access to food, and to HSHR, which manages the perception of reward and action. The evidence of studies combining food restriction to the loss of control confirm the theory that eating behavior is subject to NCAR functions. At a neuro-chemical level, an increase in the release of dopamine in the NAc occurs even after a short period of restriction. Repeated exposure to food and restriction can alter the homeostatic systems, potentially increasing the pleasure derived from the consumption of food and therefore making it more difficult to control.

WHAT WE CAN LEARN FROM TODAY'S KNOWLEDGE

Adolescents with unhealthy weight-control behavior increase their body mass index by about 1 unit more than adolescents without any weight-control behavior and were at approximately three times greater risk for being overweight. Adolescents with unhealthy weight-control behavior were also at increased risk of BE with loss of control and for extreme weight-control behavior such as self-induced vomiting and use of diet pills, laxatives, and diuretics 5 years later, compared with adolescents not without any weight-control behavior. "*Dieting and unhealthful weight-control behaviors predict outcomes related to obesity and eating disorders 5 years later. A shift away from dieting and drastic weight-control measures toward the long-term implementation of healthful eating and physical activity behaviors is needed to prevent obesity and eating disorders in adolescents.*" [42]

THREE VERY IMPORTANT QUESTIONS

1. Can repeated exposure to palatable food change reward mechanisms and lead to FA? What are the neuro-biological effects of intermittent restriction?

When exposure to hyper-palatability is frequent and repeated, hyperphagia becomes habitual because this exposure activates neuro-behavioral adaptations. There is reduced cognitive effort when hyperhagia is habitual. *"Contemporary urge models assume that urges are necessary but not sufficient for the production of drug use in ongoing addicts, are responsible for the initiation of relapse in abstinent addicts, and can be indexed across 3 classes of behavior: verbal report, overt behavior, and somatovisceral response. A review of available data does not provide strong support for these assumptions. An alternative cognitive model of drug use and drug urges is proposed that hypothesizes that drug use in the addict is controlled by automatized action schemata."* [70] This is supported by observations on the effect of caloric restriction that triggers BE when food becomes available under certain psychological conditions and when there is genetic and epigenetic vulnerability. [47]

The study of how drugs and food activate NCAR, HSME and HSHR, well known in animals, offers powerful tools for understanding the behavior of man with fMRI and PET. [71] While food restriction methods may be effective in limiting the intake of calories, with a transient effect in providing weight loss, they really do not stop the vicious cycle of desire and pleasure reward. Foodrestrictions have only the mechanical effect of delaying hyperphagia relapse, whereas neuro-molecular mechanisms are adapted to hyper-palatability, which are always present, to quickly restore previous hedonic habits.

The prevalence of HSHR promotes weight gain and therefore restrictions and relapse alternate. Repeated access to food for both humans and animals can tire the inhibitory processes exercised by satiety and induce compulsive food consumption, notwithstanding the overload nutritional and behavioral inconsistencies in humans. This loss of control and compulsive behavior regarding food consumption recall the consumption of drugs observed in SUD, and led to description of obesity as a possible natural condition of 'dependency', subsequently called FA). [71]

The information available from animal studies suggests that repeated access to sugar can up-regulate the release of dopamine, its carrier [7] and D2R receptor availability in the NAc. [7,10] These changes are responsible for BE escalation, the cross-sensitization to amphetamine-induced locomotor activity, the effectiveness of the reinforcement of regular food, [10] and withdrawal symptoms such as increased anxiety and depression. "*Although certain commonalities exist between eating and drug use (mood effects, external cue-control of appetites, reinforcement, etc.), it is argued that the vast majority of cases of (self-reported) food craving and food "addiction" should not be viewed as addictive behavior. An explanation is proposed that instead gives a prominent role to the psychological processes of ambivalence and attribution, operating together with normal mechanisms of appetite control, the hedonic effects of certain foods, and socially and culturally determined perceptions of appropriate intakes and uses of those foods. ......* [55] For food that is not sweet (typically high-fat food) there is less convincing evidence for the development of addiction, although intermittent access of corn oil can stimulate NAc dopamine release.

2. What is the level of calorie restriction that results in loss of control?

One of the most powerful mechanisms to increase the level of food reinforcement is restriction. This is important because the approach to changing eating behavior requires a reduction in energy consumption. Research is needed to identify the relationship between the level of food restriction and changes in food reinforcement. One hypothesis is that reinforcement increases when there is an energy deficit.

That is to say there is a dose-response relationship between the degree of restriction and the increase of the level of the food reinforcement. Work must be done to assess how many calorie parametric restrictions of food intake there are linked to reinforcement and if there is a window of possibility in which the energy deficit can be lowered without increasing the level of reinforcement. For example, is an energy restriction of 50, 100, 250, or 500 calories sufficient to increase the motivation to eat? Although a reduction of 250 calories per day may represent a small change behavior, this could lead to a weight loss of 13 kg in 1 year, which represents a substantial therapeutic effect. Research suggests that the changes are more moderate than those that occurs in the long term compared to traditional dietary approaches. [58] It is also possible that it is not energy deficit that causes the increase in the level of reinforcement, but rather deprivation of specific food rewarding.

3. Can we stop eating too much hyper-palatable food? The Feed-forward Model

Food palatability and hyper-palatability are important factors that drive the desire to eat a lot and are the main causes of obesity. The fact that hyper-palatable foods, which are high in calories and fats, are more easily consumed is an evolutionary phenomenon that becomes useful in the physiological environment of food shortages. The relatively well defined functions of the mechanisms that push an increase in the intake of palatable food occasionally by an individual are intuitively understandable.

The problem that still puzzles us is why the pleasure gained from an abundance of food can so easily cause loss of control, compromise HSME and cause negative consequences for health, both short and long-term. Why is it so difficult to refrain from consuming hyper-palatable food even if the hazards far outweigh the benefits? Based on a wealth of evidence, the Feed Forward Model developed by Alsiö illustrates how food intake, motivated by palatability, consequently determines an increase in weight that requires restriction and then loss of control similar to that of addiction is established. *"Food reward, not hunger, is the main driving force behind eating in the modern obesogenic environment. …… However, our understanding of long-term neural adaptations to food reward that oftentimes persist during even a prolonged absence of palatable food and contribute to the reinstatement of compulsive overeating of high-fat high-sugar diets, is much more limited. Here we discuss the evidence from animal and human studies for neural and molecular adaptations in both homeostatic and non-homeostatic appetite regulation that may underlie the formation of a "feed-forward" system, sensitive to palatable food and propelling the individual from a basic preference for palatable diets to food craving and compulsive, addiction-like eating behavior."*[1] This pattern suggests a therapeutic strategy for weight loss that consists of periodically interrupting therapeutic restriction periods prior to loss of control, until the hedonic deprivation adaptation is established. It is a strategy to reduce reinforcement of restriction. The hypothesis that neuro-molecular changes occurring initially following experiential learning hyper-palatability that is isolated can be considered as a possible explanation. This hypothesis also explains positive reinforcement of food and hedonic behaviors, with a food consumption that exceeds the energy requirements on certain occasions. This phenomenon concerns HSMS and HSHR.

Curiously, when exposure to hyper-palatability is frequent and repeated, hedonic excess food intake becomes habitual, with very complex consequent neurobehavioral adaptations for a broad range of regulatory processes. Once food consumption becomes habitual, the vicious circle of BE and DR is established. It is of particular interest that the health consequences of overeating loss of control that occur after abstinence from hyper-palatable food are not only in the short term, but also occur long after new healthy eating habits have been established. This indicates that hyper-palatability causes neuro-behavioral and molecular adaptations that determine our attitude and our responses for a long period of time in respect of food consumption behavior rewarding. While caloric restriction methods may be effective for weight loss, these only have a transitory effect, because in reality they do not stop the vicious cycle of desire and compulsive eating. Caloric restriction methods retard only transiently relapse of excessive food consumption, while the neuro-molecular mechanisms, adapted to hyper-palatability, always quickly restore previous habitual overeating, which frequently can become a compulsive disorder.

Recommendations and Suggestions

Behavioral effects that today we can read as Angel Keys' Lesson are fundamental, [36] yet they have not been sufficiently understood by the healthcare community because the phenomenon of caloric deprivation has been applied, and is still applied, indiscriminately in obesity therapy despite evidence of loss-of-control behavioral relapse. The DR present in AN is the cause of the symptoms described by Keys, which should be interpreted as manifestations secondary to energy deficit. This teaches us that refeeding assumes a primary therapeutic role that breaks the vicious cycle of food refusal. Only now, in the light of the knowledge of neural circuits, can we give the evidence-based recommendations that Keys had already highlighted. DR is the most powerful reinforcement that is given to food, with a significant level of saliency. This is important because an effective approach to change eating behavior requires a reduction in energy consumption. Research is needed to identify the relationship between food restriction and changes in food reinforcement.

Diets that require the DR and loss-of-control cycle with calorie restriction are inadequate to induce weight loss. It should be understood that 'deprivation tolerance' is variable: the effect of fasting always generates loss of control while moderate caloric restriction must be assessed case by case. 'Therapeutic' deprivation may be harmful even when weight loss is necessary and it is the most powerful food reinforcement with a significant level of salience.

Conclusion

An eating pattern consisting of gorging, alternating with dieting and purging is identified as a clinical problem in patients of normal weight, in the obese, and in patients with AN. Clinical reports have used a variety of names for this problem, and this has obscured the similarity between the various descriptions. Another perspective on the problem is offered by experimental research on DR and counter-regulation. Counter-regulation, found in subjects from all weight groups who are restricting their food intake, is construed as a laboratory version of BE. Clinical and experimental reports have been combined to provide suggestions for the aetiology and treatment of the problem of BE. DR may lead to BE in numerous ways.

1) Reduced caloric intake leads to BE via physiological deprivation. In support of this, animal research demonstrates that cycles of caloric restriction result in binge-like consumption of palatable food. [46] Dieting and stress are etiological factors in ED, and dieting strongly predicts stress-induced overeating. Animal model with sated rats, BE was evoked by stress, but only in rats with a history of caloric restriction and only if highly palatable food was available after stress. [26] Although adolescent girls with elevated DR scores are at increased risk of future BE and bulimic pathology, they do not eat less than those with lower restraint scores. The fact that only a small proportion of individuals with elevated DR scores develop bulimic pathology suggests that some extreme but rare form of DR may increase risk of this disturbance. Only 23% of study participants with elevated DR scores reported fasting. The hypothesis that fasting is a stronger risk factor for bulimic pathology. [60] Indeed, a recent longitudinal study associated fasting with the onset of BE and eating over a 1–5 year follow-up. [63]
2) Cognitive factors may be important for BE. [50,78] Because dieting is a cognitively mediated activity, dieters can become susceptible to disinhibited eating when their cognitive control is disrupted by the presence of foods. [49,56]
3) Finally, DR may represent an intent to diet' rather than actual caloric restriction. A series of studies suggest scores on self-report measures of DR may not correspond with objectively measured reductions in food intake. [64,62] Thus, individuals who have a desire to diet may be at increased risk of BE even in the absence of decreased caloric intake.

REFERENCES

[1] Alsiö, J; Olszewski, PK; Levine A.S., Schiöth H.B. Feed-forward mechanisms: addiction-like behavioral and molecular adaptations in overeating. *Front. Neuroendocrinol, 2012* 33, 127-139.

[2] American Psychiatric Association (APA). DSM-IV draft criteria, 1993, Washington, DC.

[3] American Psychiatric Association (APA). Diagnostic and Statistical Manual of Mental Disoders: DSM-5. *Am. Psy. Pubbl, 2013 Washington DC.*

[4] American Psychiatric Association (APA). Diagnostic and Statistical Manual of Mental Disorders. Revised 4th ed., Washington, DC, 2000.

[5] Andrés, A; Saldaña, C. Body dissatisfaction and dietary restraint influence binge eating behavior. *Nutr Res,* 2014 34, 944-50.

[6] Avena, NM; Rada, P; Hoebel, BG. Underweight rats have enhanced dopamine release and blunted acetylcholine response in the nucleus accumbens while bingeing on sucrose. *Neuroscience,* 2008 156, 865-71.

[7] Avena, NM; Rada, P; Hoebel, BG. Evidence for sugar addiction: behavioral and neurochemical effects of intermittent, excessive sugar intake. *Neurosci Biobehav Rev,* 2008 32, 20-39.

[8] Bassareo, V; Di Chiara, G. Modulation of feeding-induced activation of mesolimbic dopamine transmission by appetitive stimuli and its relation to motivational state. *Eur J Neurosci,* 1999 11, 4389-97.

[9] Rudolph, M; Bell, RM. Holy Anorexia. Chicago University Press, 1985.

[10] Bello, NT; Lucas, LR; Hajnal, A. Repeated sucrose access influences dopamine D2 receptor density in the striatum. *Neuroreport* 2002 13, 1575-578.

[11] Blomquist, KK; Masheb, RM; White, MA; Grilo, CM. Parental substance use history of overweight men and women with binge eating disorder is associated with distinct developmental trajectories and comorbid mood disorder. *Compr Psychiatry,* 2011 52, 693-00.

[12] Blundell, JE; Hill, AJ. Binge Eating: Psychobiological Mechanisms. In: Fairburn C.G., Wilson G.T. eds. Binge Eating. Nature, Assessment, and Treatment. The Guilford Press, Chapter 2, 208-24, 1993.

[13] Boggiano, MM; Artiga, AI; Pritchett, CE; Chandler-Laney, PC; Smith, ML; Eldridge, AJ. High intake of palatable food predicts binge-eating independent of susceptibility to obesity: an animal model of lean vs obese binge-eating and obesity with and without binge-eating. *Int J Obes,* 2007 31, 1357-67.

[14] Bryant, EJ; King, NA; Blundell, JE. Disinhibition: its effects on appetite and weight regulation. *Obes Rev,* 2008 9, 409-19.

[15] Burger, KS; Stice, E. Relation of Dietary Restraint Scores to Activation of Reward-Related Brain Regions in Response to Food Intake, Anticipated Intake, and Food Pictures. *Neuroimage,* 2011 55, 233–39.

[16] Colantuoni, C; Schwenker, J; McCarthy, J; Rada, P; Ladenheim, B; Cadet, JL; Schwartz, GJ; Moran, TH; Hoebel, BG. Excessive sugar intake alters binding to dopamine and mu-opioid receptors in the brain. *Neuro Report,* 2001 12, 3549-52.

[17] Devlin, MJ; Goldfein, JA; Dobrow, I. What is this thing called BED? Current status of binge eating disorder nosology. *Int J Eat Disord,* 2003 34, 2-18.

[18] Di Chiara, G; Bassareo, V; Fenu, S; De Luca, MA; Spina, L; Cadoni, C; Acquas, E; Carboni, E; Valentini, V; Lecca, D. Dopamine and drug addiction: the nucleus accumbens shell connection. *Neuropharmacology*, 2004 47 (1), 227-41.
[19] Diamond, J. The double puzzle of diabetes. *Nature,* 2003 423, 599-602.
[20] Fairburn, CG; Wilson, GT. Binge Eating: Definition and Classification. In: Fairburn C.G., Wilson G.T. eds. Binge Eating. Nature, Assessment, and Treatment.,The Guilford Press, Chapter 2, 3-14, 1993.
[21] French, SA; Jeffery, RW; Wing, RR. Food intake and physical activity: a comparison of three measures of dieting. *Addict Behav,* 1994 19, 401-09.
[22] Garfinkel, PE; Moldofsky, H; Garner, DM. The heterogeneity of anorexia nervosa. Bulimia as a distinct subgroup. *Arch Gen Psychiatry,* 1980 37, 1036-40.
[23] Garner, DM; Garfinkel, PE. Handbook of Treatment for Eating Disorders, 2nd Edition, The Guilford Press, 1987.
[24] Grilo, CM; Sanislow, CA; Shea, MT; Skodol, AE; Stout, RL; Pagano, ME; Yen, S; McGlashan, TH. The natural course of bulimia nervosa and eating disorder not otherwise specified is not influenced by personality disorders. *Int J Eat Disord,* 2003 34, 319-30.
[25] Haber, SN; Knutson, B. The reward circuit: linking primate anatomy and human imaging. *Neuropsychopharmacology,* 2010 35, 4-26.
[26] Hagan, MM; Chandler, PC; Wauford, PK; Rybak, RJ; Oswald, KD. The role of palatable food and hunger as trigger factors in an animal model of stress induced binge eating. *Int J Eat Disord,* 2003 34, 183-97.
[27] Hay, P.J. Quality of life and bulimic eating disorder behaviors: Findings from a community-based sample. *Int J Eat Disord,* 2007 33, 434-42.
[28] Herman, CP; Polivy, J.(1984). A boundary model for the regulation of eating. In: Stunkard, AJ; Stellar, E. Eating and its disorders. 1984 141-156, Raven Press New York.
[29] Herzog, DB; Greenwood, DN; Dorer, DJ; Flores, AT; Ekeblad, ER; Richards, A; et al. Mortality in eating disorders: A descriptive study. *Int J Eat Disord,* 2000 28, 20-6.
[30] Hoebel, BG; Teitelbaum, P. Hypothalamic control of feeding and self-stimulation. *Science,* 1962 135, 375-7.
[31] Hudson, JI; Hiripi, E; Pope, HG; Kessler, RC. The prevalence and correlates of eating disorders in the National Comorbidity Survey Replication. *Biological Psychiatry,* 2007 61, 348-58.
[32] Jacobi, C; Hayward, C; de Zwaan, M; Kraemer, HC; Agras, WS. Coming to terms with risk factors for eating disorders: Application of risk terminology and suggestions for a general taxonomy. *Psychological Bulletin,* 2004 130, 19-65.
[33] Johnson, F; Wardle, J. Dietary restraint, body dissatisfaction, and psychological distress: a prospective analysis. *J Abnorm Psychol,* 2005 114, 119-25.
[34] Jones, JM; Bennett, S; Olmsted, MP; Lawson, ML; Rodin,G. Disordered eating attitudes and behaviours in teenaged girls: A school-based study. *CMAJ,* 2001 165, 547-52.
[35] Kaye, WH; Barbarich, NC; Putnam, K; Gendall, KA; Fernstrom, J; Fernstrom, M; McConaha, CW; Kishore, A. Anxiolytic effects of acute tryptophan depletion in anorexia nervosa. *Int J Eat Disord,* 2003 33, 257-67.

[36] Keys, A. The biology of human starvation (Vol. 2)., Minneapolis: University of Minnesota Press, 1950.

[37] Koob, G; Le Moal, M. Drug abuse: hedonic homeostatic dysregulation. *Science,* 1997 3, 52-8.

[38] Loro, AD Jr; Orleans, C.S. Binge eating in obesity *Addict Behav,* 1981 6, 155-66.

[39] Lowe, MR; Witt, AA; Grossman, SL. Dieting in bulimia nervosa is associated with increased food restriction and psychopathology but decreased binge eating. *Eat Behav,* 2013 4, 342-7.

[40] Marcus, MD. Binge Eating in Obesity. In: Fairburn, CG; Wilson, GT. Binge Eating. Nature, Assessment, and Treatment. *The Guilford Press,* 77-96, 1993.

[41] Melchionda, N. Food Addiction. Sviluppo dei Disturbi Alimentari e delle Obesità. STEM Mucchi Editore Srl. Modena (IT) 2014. ISBN 978-7000-627-8.

[42] Neumark-Sztainer, D; Wall, M; Guo, J; Story, M; Haines, J; Eisenberg, MJ. Obesity, disordered eating, and eating disorders in a longitudinal study of adolescents: how do dieters fare 5 years later? *J Am Diet Assoc,* 2006 106, 559-68.

[43] Neumark-Sztainer, D; Wall, M; Haines, J; Story, M; Eisenberg, ME. Why does dieting predict weight gain in adolescents? Findings from Project EAT-II: A 5-year longitudinal study. *J Am Diet Assoc,* 2007 107, 448-55.

[44] Patton, GC; Selzer, R; Coffey, C; Carlin, JB; Wolfe, R. Onset of adolescent eating disorders: Population based cohort study over 3 years. *Br Med J,* 1999 318, 765-68.

[45] Peciña, S; Berridge, KC. Hedonic hot spot in nucleus accumbens shell: where do mu-opioids cause increased hedonic impact of sweetness? *J Neurosci,* 2005 25, 11777-86.

[46] Placidi, RJ; Chandler, PC; Oswald, KD; Maldonado,C; Wauford, PK; Boggiano, MM. Stress and hunger alter the anorectic efficacy of fluoxetine in binge-eating rats with a history of caloric restriction. *Int J Eat Disord,* 2004 36. 328-41.

[47] Polivy, J. Psychological consequences of food restriction. *J Am Diet Assoc,* 1996 96, 589-92.

[48] Polivy, J; Coleman, J; Herman, CP. The effect of deprivation on food cravings and eating behavior in restrained and unrestrained eaters. *Int J Eat Disord,* 2005 38, 301-09.

[49] Polivy, J; Herman, CP. Effects of alcohol on eating behavior: Influence of mood and perceived intoxication. *J Abnorm Psychol,* 1976 85, 601-06.

[50] Polivy, J; Herman, CP. Dieting and binging: A causal analysis. *Am Psychol,* 1985 40, 193-01.

[51] Polivy, J; Herman, CP. In: Fairburn, CG; Wilson, GT. Binge Eating. Nature, Assessment, and Treatment. 1993 173-205, The Guilford Press.

[52] Polivy, J; Zeitlin, SB; Heramn, CP; Beal, A.I. Food restriction and binge eating: a study of former prisoners of war. *J Abnorm Psychol,* 1994 103, 409-11.

[53] Racine, SE; Burt, SA; Iacono, WG; McGue, M; Klump, KL. Dietary restraint moderates genetic risk for binge eating. *J Abnorm Psychol,* 2011 120, 119-28.

[54] Reda, M. Anorexia and the Holyness of St Catherine of Siena. *Journal of Criminal Justice and Popular Culture,* 2001 8, 37-47.

[55] Rogers, PJ; Smith, HJ. Food craving and food "addiction": a critical review of the evidence from a biopsychosocial perspective. *Pharmacol Biochem Behav,* 2000 66, 3-14.

[56] Ruderman, AJ; Wilson, GT. Weight, restraint, cognitions and counterregulation. *Behav Res Ther,* 1979 17, 581-90.

[57] Santonastaso, P; Ferrara, S; Favaro A. Differences between binge eating disorder and nonpurging bulimia nervosa. *Int J Eat Disord,* 1999 25, 215-8.

[58] Sbrocco, T; Nedegaard, RC; Stone, JM; Lewis, EL. Behavioral choice treatment promotes continuing weight loss: Preliminary results of a cognitive-behavioral decision-based treatment for obesity. *J Consult Clin Psychol,* 1999 67, 260-66.

[59] Serdula, MK; Collins, ME; Williamson, DF; Anda, RF; Pamuk, E; Byter, TE. Weight control practices of United-States adolescents and adults. *Ann Intern Med,* 1993 119, 667-71.

[60] Stice, EA. Prospective test of the dual-pathway model of bulimic pathology: mediating effects of dieting and negative affect. *J Abnorm Psychol,* 2001 110, 124-35.

[61] Stice, E; Agras, WS. Predicting onset and cessation of bulimic behaviors during adolescence: A longitudinal grouping analysis. *Behav Ther,* 1998 29, 257-76.

[62] Stice, E; Cooper, JA; Schoelle, DA; Tappe, K; Lowe. MR.). Are dietary restraint scales valid measures of moderate-to long-term dietary restriction? Objective biological and behavioral data suggest not. *Psychol Assess*, 2007 19, 449-58.

[63] Stice, E; Davis, K; Miller, NP; Marti, CN. Fasting increases risk for onset of binge eating and bulimic pathology: a 5-year prospective study. *J. Abnorm. Psychol.* 2008 117, 941-46.

[64] Stice,E; Fisher, M; Lowe, MR. Are dietary restraint scales valid measures of acute dietary restriction? Unobstrusive observational data suggest not. *Psychol. Assess* 2004 16, 51-59.

[65] Stice, E; Killen, JD; Hayward, C; Taylor, CB. Age of onset for binge eating and purging during late adolescence: A 4-year survival analysis. *J. Abnorm. Psychol.* 1998 107, 671-75.

[66] Stice, E; Marti, CN; Shaw, H; Jaconis, M. An 8-year longitudinal study of the natural history of threshold, subthreshold, and partial eating disorders from a community sample of adolescents. *J. Abnorm. Psychol.* 2009 118, 587-97.

[67] Striegel-Moore, RH. Development an Evidence Based Classification of Eating Disorders. Scientific Findings for DSM-5, American Psychiatric Association. 2011

[68] Stunkard, AJ. Eating patterns and obesity *Psychiatr. Q.* 1959 33, 284-95.

[69] Stunkard, AJ. A hystory of Binge Eating. In: Fairburn C.G., Wilson G.T. eds. Binge Eating. Nature, Assessment, and Treatment. Guilford Press, 1993 pag 15-34.

[70] Tiffany, ST. A cognitive model of drug urges and drug-use behavior: role of automatic and nonautomatic processes. *Psychol. Rev.* 1990 97, 147-68.

[71] Volkow, ND; O'Brien, CP. Issues for DSM-V: Should obesity be included as a brain disorder? *Am. J. Psychiatry* 2007 164, 708-10.

[72] Volkow, ND; Wang, GJ; Fowler, JS; Tomasi, D; Baler, R. Food and drug reward: overlapping circuits in human obesity and addiction. *Curr. Top. Behav. Neurosci.* 2012 11, 1-24.

[73] Volkow, ND; Wang, GJ; Tomasi, D; Baler, RD. Obesity and addiction: neurobiological overlaps. *Obes. Rev.* 2013 14, 2-18.

[74] Wadden,TA; Brownell, KD; Foster, GD. Obesity: Responding to the global epidemic. *J. Consult. Clin. Psychol.* 2002 70, 510-25.

[75] Wade, GN; Jones, JE. Neuroendocrinology of nutritional infertility. *Am. J. Physiol. Regul. Integr. Comp. Physiol,* 2005 287, R1277-96.

[76] Wansink, B; Kim, J. Bad popcorn in big buckets: portion size can influence intake as much as taste. *J Nutr. Educ. Behav,* 2005 37, 242-45.

[77] Wansink, B; van Ittersum, K; Painter, JE. Ice cream illusions bowls, spoons, and self-served portion sizes. *Am. J. Prev. Med.* 2006 31, 240-43.

[78] Wardle, J. Dietary restraint and binge eating. *Behavioral Analysis and Modification.* 1980 4, 201-09.

[79] Wilfley, DE; Bishop, ME; Wilson, GT; Agras, WS. Classification of eating disorders: toward DSM-5. *Int. J. Eat. Disord.* 2007 40 Suppl, S123-9.

[80] Yanovski, SZ. The chicken or the egg: binge eating disorder and dietary restraint. *Appetite* 1995 24, 258.

In: The Different Faces of Being Overweight
Editor: Emilia Manzato

ISBN: 978-1-63483-099-7

Chapter 4

LIFE STAGES AND OVERWEIGHT/OBESITY RISK

Ottavio Bosello[1]*, MD, and Angiola Vanzo[2]†, MD
[1]Department of Medicine, University of Verona, Italy
[2]Department of Prevention, Food Hygiene and Nutrition Service,
ASL 6 Veneto, Italy

ABSTRACT

Looking at the natural history of obesity, people tend to accumulate fat during all the life span. In recent years, this phenomenon has modified and the age at highest risk is now the childhood. The prevalence of childhood obesity has increased rapidly to high levels over recent decades, particularly in some communities and states at high economic level but also in developing countries. Given such a high prevalence, is now crucial to identify the risk factors best predicting incident obesity in childhood and what are the contributory characteristics resulting in obesity. The environment is the main accused. Furthermore the children at highest risk must be accurately targeted for early intervention.

As a consequence, in the adulthood the main risk factor for obesity is to have been overweight at the younger age.

The prevalence studies show that the peak of obesity is in the younger elderly (60-65 years). Despite the increase in life expectancy, over the years more advanced obesity is becoming less frequent. The phenomenon is due to the increased risk of morbidity and mortality carried by overweight and obesity, with the finding that at older ages the prevalence of obesity is less common.

Last but not least consideration: nowadays, there is a new tendency to redefine obesogenic environments not as environments that make bodies fat, but as environments that make fat bodies problematic and considering alternative theoretical frameworks in order to avoid the pitfalls of environmental determinism.

---

* ottavio.bosello@univr.it. Past president SIO (Italian Society for Obesity) Past president SISDCA (Italian Society for Eating Disorders).
† angiola.vanzo@ulssvicenza.it.

INTRODUCTION

Overweight/obesity is a worldwide epidemic among children, adolescents, and adults and also among the elderly [1, 2]. It has become a major issue for healthcare facilities in both developing and developed countries, with nearly 1 billion adults globally being reported as obese [3, 4, 5] and its prevalence continues to be significantly high within most countries and showing a noticeable tendency to increase [5, 6]. In the USA, the 2009-2010 prevalence of overweight/obesity was 35.5% among adult men and 35.8% among adult women, with no significant change compared to 2003-2008 [7].

Overweight/obesity is a strong growing chronic condition and is associated with significant morbidity and mortality in both men and women [8, 9].

It has also been characterized by the American Heart Association/ American College of Cardiology [9, 10, 11, 12] and the Nutrition Council of the American Heart Association [13, 14], as a major and modifiable risk factor for cardiovascular morbidity and mortality [9].

The Framingham study showed that the excess of body weight is as an independent risk factor for cardiovascular disease [15].

Obesity, particularly severe obesity, affects nearly every organ system of the human body. Most obesity-related medical conditions are caused by the metabolic effects of adipose tissue, but some are caused by the increase of body mass itself. Overweight/obesity is associated with an overall increase in mortality. The relationship between weight and mortality follows a J-shaped curve, with the lowest mortality traditionally believed to occur with a BMI of 20.0-24.9 kg/m^2 (i.e. normal weight) [16].

In a prospective cohort of more than one million American adults, overweight/obesity doubled the risk of death in general and in particular, cardiovascular death [17].

Even though there is ample evidence and widespread agreement that a massive epidemic of overweight/obesity has spread across most countries [5], there is less clarity and still much more debate regarding the consequences this epidemic confers on the public health. Both false and scientifically unsupported beliefs concerning overweight/obesity pervade both scientific literature and the popular press [18]. Overweight/obesity and its impact on health and the healthcare system is one of the most important public health issues facing Western society [19]. Although increases in overweight/obesity over the past 30 years have adversely affected the health of the U.S. population, there have been simultaneous improvements in health because of reductions in smoking. Having a better understanding of the joint effects of these trends on longevity and quality of life will facilitate a more efficient targeting of health care resources. Stewart et al., found that the negative effects of an increase in BMI overwhelmed the positive effects in multiple scenarios of the reduction in smoking. Increases in the remaining life expectancy of a typical 18-year-old are held back by 0.71 years or 0.91 quality-adjusted years between 2005 and 2020. If all U.S. adults became nonsmokers with a normal weight by 2020, they forecast that the life expectancy of an 18-year-old would increase by 3.76 life-years or 5.16 quality-adjusted years. If past overweight/obesity trends continue unchecked, the negative effects on the health of the U.S. population will increasingly outweigh the positive effects gained from decreasing smoking rates. Failure to address continued increases in overweight/obesity could result in an erosion of the pattern of steady gains in health observed since early in the 20th century [20].

Natural History

Looking at the natural history of obesity, people tend to accumulate fat during all their life span. A Swedish study has been able to assess the performance of the weight of a large sample of obese subjects aged 20 to 60 years of age and compared with a sample of the general population [21]. These obese subjects were of an age 60 with BMI> 30, and were considered normal weight those individuals who at age 60 had a normal weight range (BMI between 20 and 25). Obese subjects gradually increase to 1-2 kg per year (over 2 kg in women), while in the general population with normal body weight these increases are of 0,2 to 0,3 kg per year. Virtually all obese subjects report weight loss attempts during their lifetime. Significant correlations were observed between relative weights of obese males, but not females and both of their biological parents. Birth weight was, weakly but significantly associated with the current weight in both males and females; while in the two sexes significant associations with current BMI do not emerge. This phenomenon might suggest that birth weight is a predictor of constitutional configuration, like the height of the individual, but does not seem to connect with the future development of obesity.

Early Stages of Life

Maternal Prepregnancy

In recent years, maternal prepregnancy BMI has increased among the childbearing age women in developed countries. Recent studies reported that prepregnancy BMI was positively associated with infant birth weight [22]. It has also confirmed that maternal prepregnancy overweight/obesity is associated with higher birth weight and birth length, and greater weight gain and length gain of their children in the first year of life [22]. Infants born to mothers with prepregnancy overweight/obesity but adequate gestational weight gain (GWG) did not have a higher risk of childhood overweight/ obesity at 12 months of age, compared with infants born to mothers with prepregnancy normal weight and also with adequate GWG.

Li N et al., [23] found that maternal prepregnancy BMI plays a more important role than GWG in maternal outcomes, especially in pregnancy complications. They also found that pregnancy-induced hypertension, caesarean delivery, and infant size at birth were important outcomes of maternal prepregnancy overweight/obesity.

A very large study examined the effects of prepregnancy BMI and prenatal smoking on SGA risk in over 34,900 term pregnancies [24]. Findings support that prenatal smoking increases risk of small for gestational age (SGA) and decreases birth weight in women who enter pregnancy in the underweight and normal weight BMI categories relative to normal weight non-smoking women in a large, multiethnic cohort of term births. Of course, this does not suggest that women who are overweight or obese prior to pregnancy should smoke or that smokers should gain weight, as overweight and smoking cause numerous other health risks to the mother and her offspring.

The impact of maternal prepregnancy overweight/obesity on fetal brain development is unclear. The brain undergoes rapid development during the fetal period and early childhood. Any insult during this critical period of brain development may be detrimental for individuals' central nervous system development. Animal studies have shown that maternal prepregnancy overweight/obesity induced by high-fat diet consumption is associated with alterations in performance among the offspring. In humans, few studies examining these associations have produced mixed results: some found inconsistent evidence for the intrauterine effects of maternal prepregnancy overweight/obesity on a child's cognitive skill using two European cohorts [25]. In contrast, others [26] have shown the association between maternal prepregnancy overweight/obesity and reduction in child IQ scores among low-income African American population.

Tanda R et al., found that maternal prepregnancy overweight/obesity was associated with a reduction in cognitive test scores among generally healthy children from term birth. The magnitude of the reduction due to prepregnancy overweight/obesity is large compared to the magnitude of the changes in income or education that would be required to produce a comparable effect [27]. Compounded with an adverse childhood environment, a large and long-term impact on a child's future may result.

Maternal Pregnancy

Gestational weight gain (GWG) has also been thoroughly studied as a predictor of adverse pregnancy outcomes, mainly because of the belief that it is potentially modifiable after conception. Low gain is associated with birth of a small-for-gestational age (SGA) infant and preterm birth, whereas high gain is associated with greater risks of macrosomia, cesarean section, and excess postpartum weight retention. Women in the Western world are heavier than ever, and being pregnant contributes further to overweight/obesity [28]. Moreover, many data show that the proportion of women with excessive GWG has increased during the past 15 years.

Maternal and neonatal complications associated with BMI and GWG are of public health importance because they add to the disease burden in women and children and increase medical costs. However, understanding these associations is also complex, because both BMI and GWG are closely linked to lifestyle factors, diseases, and genetic traits that also correlate with the outcome of pregnancy. In addition, pregnancy outcomes (e.g., birth weight) may be in the causal pathway between GWG and other pregnancy outcomes (e.g., cesarean delivery), which also complicates the interpretation of these relations.

What does an adequate weight gain mean? The subject is still widely debated. One of the most authoritative references is the guideline of the Institute of Medicine (IOM) USA [29]. The tables (figure 1) provide increases related to prepregnancy BMI. These ranges are those that, based on the evidence available, have not produced any proven adverse pregnancy outcomes. Of course, these guidelines should be used in combination with a good clinical evaluation.

Since 1990, the last time the IOM released guidelines for weight gain during pregnancy; many key aspects of the health of women of childbearing age have changed. This population now includes a higher proportion of women from racial/ethnic subgroups and prepregnancy body mass index (BMI) and gestational weight gain (GWG) have increased among all population subgroups. Moreover, high rates of overweight and obesity are common in the population subgroups that are at risk for poor maternal and child health outcomes. Finally, women are also becoming pregnant at an older age and, as a result, are entering pregnancy more commonly with chronic conditions such as hypertension or diabetes, which put them at risk for pregnancy complications and may lead to increased morbidity during their post-pregnancy years.

	Total Weight Gain		Rates of Weight Gain* 2nd and 3rd Trimester	
Prepregnancy BMI	Range in kg	Range in lbs	Mean (range) in kg/week	Mean (range) in lbs/week
Underweight (< 18.5 kg/m^2)	12.5–18	28–40	0.51 (0.44–0.58)	1 (1–1.3)
Normal weight (18.5–24.9 kg/m^2)	11.5–16	25–35	0.42 (0.35–0.50)	1 (0.8–1)
Overweight (25.0–29.9 kg/m^2)	7–11.5	15–25	0.28 (0.23–0.33)	0.6 (0.5–0.7)
Obese (≥ 30.0 kg/m^2)	5–9	11–20	0.22 (0.17–0.27)	0.5 (0.4–0.6)

* Calculations assume a 0.5–2 kg (1.1– 4.4 lbs.) weight gain in the first trimester.

Figure 1. New Recommendations for Total and Rate of Weight Gain during Pregnancy, by Prepregnancy BMI [29].

A weight gain during pregnancy greater than the values indicated by the Institute of Medicine is often associated with the risk of maintaining this excess weight and of developing obesity as time goes on. Observations show that women who exceed the 16kg cut-off during pregnancy acquire double the risk of keeping on more than 9kg as long as two years after the termination of the pregnancy. The period during pregnancy when weight gain is associated with greater fetal growth is the second quarter, which is the crucial period during which the weight of the product of conception is strengthened. In general, it has also been observed that, regardless of pre-pregnancy BMI, women with a higher weight gain during the first week of pregnancy are those that have the greatest risk of maintaining the excess weight after pregnancy has been terminated.

Childhood

Individuals can become overweight at any age, but it is more common at certain times. At birth, individuals who will and will not become obese later in life cannot be distinguished by weight, except in the case of infants of diabetic mothers, for whom the likelihood of overweight/obesity is increased. Thus, at birth, there is a large pool of individuals will eventually become overweight, and a smaller group will never become overweight.

In recent years, the overweight/obesity phenomenon has modified and the age at highest risk is now the childhood. The prevalence of childhood overweight/obesity has increased rapidly to high levels over recent decades, particularly in some communities and states at the high economic level but also in developing countries. Because of such high prevalence is now crucial to identify the risk factors best predicting incident overweight/obesity in childhood and what are the contributory characteristics resulting in obesity. The environment is the main accused. Furthermore the children at highest risk must be accurately targeted for early intervention.

According to a study published in the JAMA earlier 2014, the number of severely obese children is growing, even if overweight/obesity rates in the United States have declined among 2- to 5-year-olds and remained stable, at about 17% overall since 2003–2004. [30]

Many studies revealed that socio-economic status (SES) is an important correlate of body weight [31, 32, 33] and found that children from a lower socio-economic background are at higher risk for the development of overweight/obesity [32, 34]. SES needs to be considered as an important factor in the prevention of childhood obesity.

Furthermore, we must keep in mind that specific physical activity, dietary and stress related behaviors are associated with the development of childhood obesity. Physical activity and sedentary behavior are two components of energy expenditure that contribute to the development of childhood overweight/obesity [35, 36]. Several studies demonstrated that higher levels of physical activity during early childhood are protective in developing body fat [37, 38]. A recent literature review from Monasta and colleagues [39] reported that less than 30 minutes of daily physical activity at preschool age is associated with an increased risk for overweight and obesity.

A sedentary behavior consistently associated with the development of childhood overweight/obesity is viewing TV. The reduction of this behavior is suggested to be one of the more successful ways to prevent childhood overweight/obesity [35, 40, 41]. Reilly et al. [41] found that watching more than eight hours TV per week at the age of three is independently related to the risk of obesity. The association between watching TV and childhood overweight/obesity is possibly mediated by an increased energy intake in children [35, 36, 42], underlining the need to target TV viewing as a sedentary risk behavior in the prevention of childhood overweight/obesity [42].

Nowadays there is an increasing interest in overprotective parenting and on the potential role in child development. While some have argued that a trend towards increased parental fear and reduced opportunity for independent mobility may be linked to increasing rates of child overweight and obesity, there is limited empirical information available to support this claim. One possible reason for this shift is that overprotection increasingly represents normative parenting behavior because more parents perceive the world as a dangerous place for children.

There is also an increasing amount of evidence linking parental fear and the level of physical activity in children. As discussed, parental fear is thought to be a key factor in the decline in the amount of free and outdoor play undertaken by children [43].

Physical activity of children has declined over time as rates of child overweight and overweight/obesity have increased. At the same time, there has been a shift in perceptions of safety for children, even though children arguably face the same or fewer risks today than in previous decades. Parents have become more risk averse and protective over time, and as a result children have enjoyed fewer opportunities for active free play and independent mobility. It is possible, therefore, that one of the many factors related to a decline in children's physical activity levels – and perhaps contributing to the increase in overweight/obesity – is the increase in parental fear and protectiveness. These results were observed after controlling for maternal BMI, household income, maternal mental health and sibling position.

We must not forget that the strongest predictor of child overweight and overweight/obesity is maternal BMI. The effect of maternal BMI significantly increases over time. Household income was also associated with the odds of child overweight and obesity.

Childhood weight gain and growth are markedly influenced by nutritional factors, such as type of milk feeding [31]. Many findings show that genetic factors also contribute to early weight gain and growth.

One of the first, and most intimate, experiences of commercial food promotion is television. Therefore, unsurprisingly, the effects of television advertising on children's brand preferences are well established. However, its effect on actual food intake and the food choices in children of various weight statuses has only recently been characterized. Despite regulation, children are often exposed to considerable numbers of food adverts on television. These are predominantly for foods high in fat, salt and sugar (HFSS), which are marketed to children using promotional characters and themes of fun. Such adverts have been shown to cause significant increases in intake, particularly in overweight and obese children, and enhanced preference for high carbohydrate and high fat foods in children who consume the greatest amounts of televisual media.

The survey 2012 of Italian Childhood Overweight/obesity Surveillance System "OKkio alla salute" [44], related to the project of the European Region of WHO "Childhood Overweight/obesity Surveillance Initiative (COSI)", confirm worrying levels of overweight; however, there was a slight decrease with respect to previous surveys: 22.2% of children are overweight and 10.6% obese, with higher rates in the central and southern regions. The 2012 survey has highlighted the prevalence of eating habits that can encourage weight gain among children. In particular, it was found that 9% of children skip breakfast and 31% do not have a proper breakfast (unbalanced in terms of carbohydrates and proteins); 65% have a mid-morning hypercaloric snack while 22% of parents stated that their children do not eat daily fruits and/or vegetables and 44% habitually consume sweetened drinks and/or sodas. Even the values of physical inactivity and sedentary behavior, while showing an improvement, remain high: 18% of children practice sport for no more than one hour a week, 44% have a TV in the room, 36% watch TV and/or playing video games more than 2 hours a day and only 25% go to school on foot or by bicycle.

Parents do not always have an accurate perception of their child's weight status: among mothers of children overweight or obese, most do not believe their children are overweight and only a third thinks excessive the amount of food they eat. In addition, only a part of mothers of children less physically active believe that their sons undergo insufficient physical activity.

Weight status of children is related to weight of parents. Higher educational level of parents relates to lower percentage of overweight/ obesity in children.

Many problems related to overweight/obesity and physical inactivity tends to start in childhood, and often disproportionately affect disadvantaged socio-economic groups [45].

As a result, individuals of lower socio-economic status and children and young people have been identified in the Strategy as priority targets for action.

Eating and physical activity habits are established at an early age: addressing the issue of healthy eating and physical activity in early life can help children and their families to develop and maintain healthy lifestyles. By learning and adopting healthy habits when young, the chance that such habits will be sustained into adulthood is greatly increased.

Appropriate nutrition during pregnancy and lactation is essential for the future wellbeing of both mother and child. In addition, when pregnant and lactating, mothers (and families) are arguably more willing to modify their behavior. They may also engage more frequently with routine medical care services, meaning more opportunities to encourage beneficial lifestyle change. Furthermore, during these periods different socioeconomic groups may be easier to reach through maternal and child health care centers. Effective interventions during pregnancy and lactation do therefore have strong potential to positively affect the health of both mother and child throughout their life spans.

The consumption of sweetened beverages is a known common risk factor for the development of overweight/obesity and dental caries in children and children consume sweet drinks frequently and in large volumes from an early age. Limiting intake of sweet drinks is considered an important step for child general and oral health. However, the choice of drinks for children has influences from social, environmental and behavioral domains, indicating that a multi-strategy approach is required to bring about this change.

Little children do not have the cognitive ability to understand commercial messages, while older children and adults may have: little children are therefore particularly affected by targeted marketing and advertising. Significant correlations between the increase in food advertising directed at children and the increased prevalence of childhood overweight/obesity have been found. The commercials for "hazardous" food and drink are often specifically targeted to the young and are designed to influence the food preference of children [46, 47]. Results of several studies suggest that marketing aimed at women and girls may contribute to body dissatisfaction, eating disorders, low self-esteem and depression.

The Environment

The environmental component that influences overweight/obesity can be explained starting from the ecological model of human development of Bronfenbrenner [48], which studies the interactions of different contextual levels that affect human development, including many environmental situations and various relational mechanisms and institutions that define its function and organization. This model can then be employed to understand all human behavior, including feeding behavior and practice of physical activity that, through multiple levels of interaction, affect the nutritional status of the individual (Figure 2).

The World Health Organization [49] reports data and trends observed that are important to assess the environmental factors that affect the weight of individuals: in 2011 more than 40 million children under five years of age are overweight. Overweight and obesity are no longer, as in the past, a problem exclusive to high-income countries, but also in countries with low and middle incomes, especially in urban areas. More than 30 million overweight children now live in developing countries, while only 10 million are located in developed countries. The low-and middle-income countries are now forced to deal with the "double impact" of deaths from malnutrition and disease on the one hand, and overweight and overweight/obesity on the other hand. This is not difficult to find, not only in the same community, but also within the same four walls.

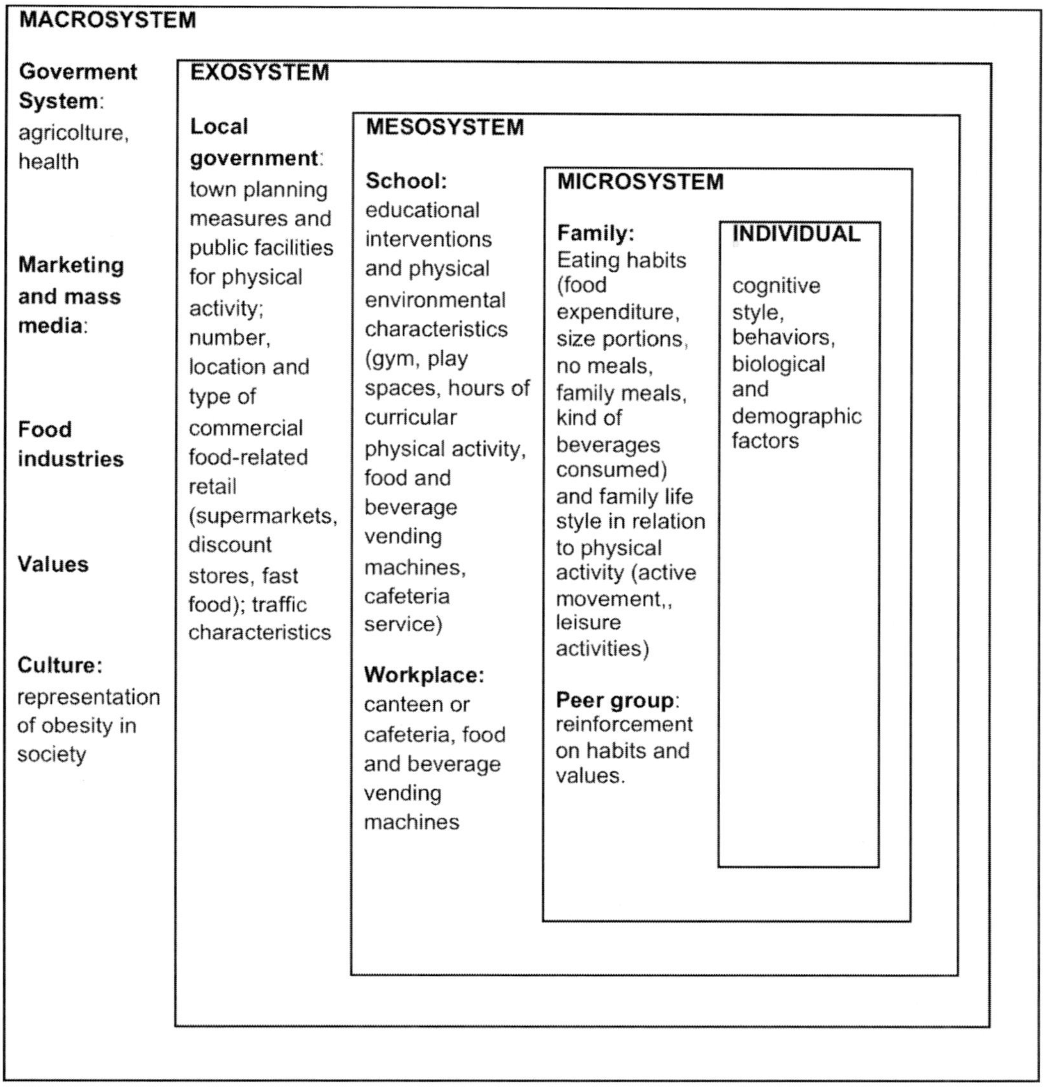

Figure 2. The ecological model of human development. From, Bronfenbrenner U, modified [48].

Researches indicate that in low-income countries there is a positive association between wealth and obesity; this trend evens out in those middle-income countries to become a negative association in the richer countries, where the risk of overweight/obesity is higher in the most disadvantaged socio-economic groups.

Family Environment

The family environment is an important risk factor, since children tend to acquire the lifestyles of parents such as unhealthy diet and sedentary lifestyle [50]. Risk factors related to parenting include having at least one obese parent, the lack of culinary skills, food preferences and beliefs of the parents, the role of modeling and the interactions of the child/parent. Similarly, the physical activity levels of children are strongly influenced by parents' decisions on the use of going by car or on foot, the habits of the family to watch television, and leisure time activities. In addition, parents allow greater access to the computer, television and other sedentary activities and may give greater security to car use and to be reluctant to allow outdoor games.

Children living in single-parent families have increased the number of women working outside the home and consequently decreased the time available for the preparation of meals. Over time, there are fewer family meals and so increasing those outside the home for children who are often cared for by non-family members [51] and for adolescents who become more independent from the family [52].

Epigenetics and Obesity

The nature-versus-nurture debate or the nature versus the environment (or education, learning, behavior) has been solved assuming that both factors have a crucial role and that the phenotypes are the result of actions and interactions of both, which often change over time.

A relatively new area of medicine is epigenetics. The term, which has more than 60 years [53], was coined by Conrad Hal Waddington to describe what is now called developmental biology [54], that is, the idea that the phenotype, or the morphological and functional properties of an organism, develops as part of a program defined by the genome under the influence of the environment in which the organism lives [55]. Early environmental exposures play a significant role in susceptibility to various diseases in adulthood [56]: some of these environmental effects can be transmitted through successive generations. There is evidence that maternal behavior [57] and physical activity [58] may induce "plastic" epigenetic modifications [55].

Epigenetics of Obesity: A Piece of the Puzzle

Epigenetics recently drew the attention of researchers and even the media as an alternative point of view in the etiology of metabolic disorders such as overweight/obesity [59]. A defect in genomic expression is quite often associated with abnormalities during childhood and with physical characteristics often exemplified by excess body weight.

In recent years, epidemiological data have connected the earliest living conditions and poor fetal growth with adult onset of cardiovascular and metabolic diseases, including obesity. This hypothesis, already advanced by David Barker and often referred to as the *Barker hypothesis*, was born from epidemiological observations linking low birth weight with subsequent risk of death from cardiovascular disease [60].

Essential (or polygenic) obesity thus arises when the genetic makeup of an individual is susceptible to an environment that promotes calorie consumption compared to spending energy. Most westernized societies have an environment that promotes weight gain due both to abundance of food and lack of physical activity: thus polygenic overweight/obesity has become the most widespread epidemic of the modern era. Overweight/obesity is, therefore, the result of interactions between environmental and genetic factors.

A matter of debate it's now whether epigenetic modifications introduced during the early stages of development may increase the risk of obesity. Many studies have focused on the hypothesis that early environmental influences induce epigenetic changes, so as to permanently affect the metabolism and the risk of chronic diseases. As for obesity, it has been shown that obese mothers tend to have obese children [61, 62]; it has also been shown that the correction of the maternal weight can have positive effects on reducing the risk of overweight/obesity in children [63].

The current epidemic of overweight/obesity seems not of close genetic origin, but resulting from adverse changes in lifestyle and the environment (the environment 'obesogenic'). The obesogenic environment has different effects on different people, but in the same environment, highlighting an underlying inherited susceptibility to overweight/obesity and body fat distribution.

The role of genetics underlying the common forms of overweight/obesity has been rather vague. The contribution of epigenetics to common forms of overweight/obesity is still largely unknown, but the study of rare syndromes and animal models can support the hypothesis that the effects of both genetic effects and those environmental factors on epigenetics are themselves associated with obesity. New models suggest that a component of the individual response to an obesogenic environment is even partially driven by neurobehavioral pathways [63].

In summary, considering the great changes that have affected the physical and social environment in recent decades, and noting that the prevalence of overweight and overweight/obesity in the population has been gradually increasing, it can be assumed that the environmental component plays a crucial role in pathogenesis obesity. It seems inappropriate, however, to restrict one's attention to the environmental determinants of overweight/obesity as a cause as if they could affect individuals indiscriminately. It seems more logical to look at the problem using the ecological model described above and to consider the continuous interaction and mutual influence between the individual and the higher levels of the environment (social, physical and macro-level).

With the same social pressures and environmental components, differences in lifestyle and the nutritional status of the people can be observed; this is due to the fact that the individual does not suffer the environment in a passive way, but is located in connection to it and should also use coping skills to cope with the obesogenic situations.

The most fascinating idea concerning medical epigenetics is now that it would give the possibility to intervene at the level of the connection between the genome and the environment, to modify the effects of deleterious genes and influence the impact of the environment on phenotypic plasticity, on aging and metabolic diseases and on age-related ones.

The forms of interaction with which you compare personal identity and the environment provide a multivariate explanation of the same: for example, the individual characteristics of genetic, cultural, which give the ability to counteract obesogenic environmental characteristics, introduce us to a situation where every action is multidimensional, every event, every emotion is read at the micro level (family and friends), meso (school, work, city), exo-social (institutions that govern life contexts) and macro (culture and laws).

This ecological approach is crucial for interventions targeted on environmental determinants: food availability, quality and price, opportunities for physical activity and socialization, non-misleading advertising can change lifestyles and reduce health inequalities. Of course, next to the interventions in the health setting with investments in social systems in which people live, is the fundamental approach to prevention and direct mechanisms of information and empowerment of individuals (empowerment and motivational counseling) [64].

Last consideration, but not least: nowadays, there is a new tendency to redefine obesogenic environments not as environments that make bodies fat, but as environments that make fat bodies problematic and considering alternative theoretical frameworks in order to avoid the pitfalls of environmental determinism.

ADULTHOOD

In the adulthood the main risk factor for overweight/obesity is to be overweight in the younger age (Figure 3) [65].

Unfortunately, it seems difficult to reverse this situation that poses complex problems of management and care.

George Bray proposed many items responsible of overweight/obesity at any age [66].

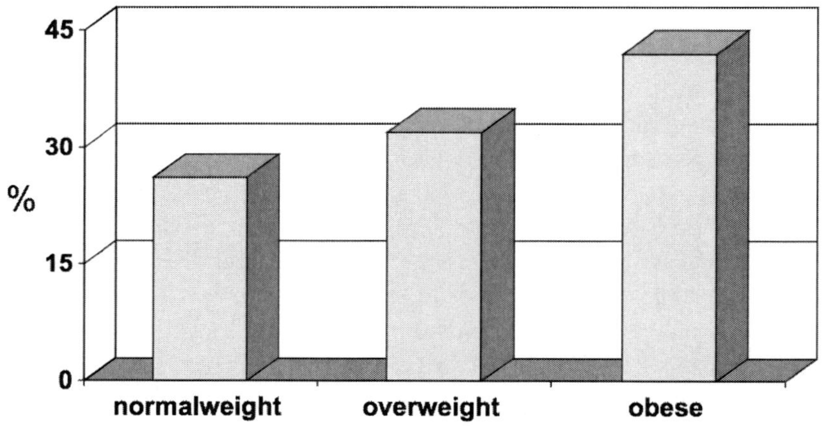

Figure 3. Persistence of overweight/obesity from childhood to adulthood (from 65, modified).

Table 1. Predictors of weight gain for adulthood age (from, 66, modified)

To be overweight at the childhood
Low socioeconomic status
Recent marriage
Multiple pregnancies
Low metabolic rate
Low level of physical activity
Smoking cessation
Frequently dieting
Menopause

McAllister [67] proposed another set of possible risk factors of obesity: below will be considered those who have had the greatest evidence in the literature (Table 2). Of course, many others have been described, but probably of less significance from a point of view statistical and clinical.

Table 2. Ten Putative Contributors to the Overweight/obesity Epidemic (from, 67, modified)

Infections
Epigenetics
Maternal Age
Assortative Mating
Reproductive Fitness
Sleep Debt
Endocrine Disruptors
Pharmaceutical Iatrogenesis
Ambient Temperature
Intrauterine and Intergenerational Effects

Young Adults Born Large

There is some evidence that people born with high birth weight may be at increased risk of cardiovascular disease in adulthood. Young adults born large for gestational age are more likely to be obese: they have increased carotid intima-media thickness, a marker of subclinical atherosclerosis, consistent with an increased risk of cardiovascular disease [68].

Familiar Overweight

The presence of many obese people in the same family environment is quite undisputed. Genetic liability may be invoked: it is estimated that genetics play a 30% risk of obesity. But in the same family environment, there are other factors that can be taken into account, first and foremost lifestyle, including diet and physical activity. It is quite clear that if the parents are sedentary big eaters it is difficult for children to have healthy eating habits and to play an active life. In addition, it will be discussed of socioeconomic and cultural status. Anyway, familiar environment is crucial for the risk of overweight/ obesity at any age of man.

Socioeconomic Status

Socioeconomic status is an important risk factor in childhood, but it becomes even clearer in adulthood. Some studies have shown a relationship between overweight/obesity prevalence and socioeconomic status measured as education level or income [69, 70]. This data briefly presents the recent national observations on overweight/obesity in United States adults and its association with the poverty income ratio (PIR) and education level. The relationship between overweight/obesity and income in men varies by race and ethnicity. Among non-Hispanic black and Mexican-American men, overweight/obesity prevalence decreases as income decreases. There is no significant difference in overweight/obesity prevalence by poverty level among non-Hispanic white men. The trends are similar for non-Hispanic white, non-Hispanic black, and Mexican-American women, but they are only significant for non-Hispanic white women. Among non-Hispanic white women with income at or above of the poverty level, 27.5% are obese, less than the 39.2% of those with income below the poverty level.

In the USA, there is no significant trend between education level and overweight/obesity prevalence among men. Among women, on the contrary, overweight/obesity prevalence increases as education decreases [71]. Between 1988–1994 and 2007–2008 the prevalence of overweight/obesity among adults increased at all income levels. Between 1988–1994 and 2007–2008 the prevalence of overweight/obesity among adults at all levels of education increased. (Figure 4).

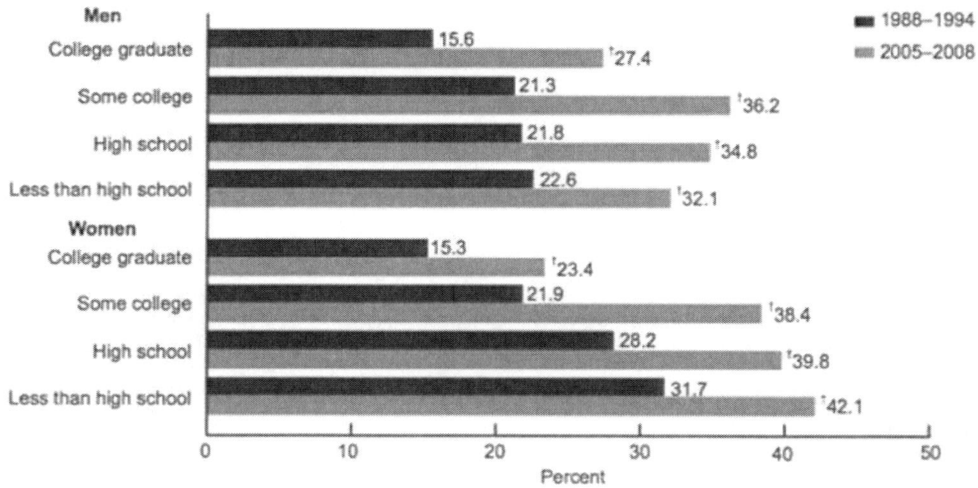

Figure 4. Prevalence of overweight/obesity among adults by education level [71].

In conclusion, in the USA the relationship between overweight/obesity and socioeconomic status differs by sex and race and ethnicity group. Among women, and specifically non-Hispanic white women, overweight/obesity prevalence increases as income decreases, while among non-Hispanic black and Mexican-American men overweight/obesity prevalence decreases as income decreases. Although the prevalence of overweight/obesity among women with income below of the poverty level is higher than among those with higher incomes, most obese women do not have incomes below of the poverty level. Among men and women with a college degree, the prevalence of overweight/obesity is lower than among those with some college education. Moreover, college educated women are less likely to be obese compared with those with less than a high school diploma. Between 1988–1994 and 2005–2008 the prevalence of overweight/obesity increased in adults at all levels of income and education [71, 72].

Evidence also suggests that the differences observed in the different socio-economic classes are becoming more and more widely apparent.

The socio-economic components of low income and low education levels influence overweight/obesity in both countries at high and medium-low income, both for adults and for children and adolescents, and shows important regional variations even within the individual countries.

For adults, however, in Italy, the study *2012 Passi* [73] notes that overweight increases significantly with age and is more common in men, in people with low levels of education and those with major economic difficulties. Also a clear North-South gradient in the comparison between the regions, to the detriment of the southern regions.

Recent Marriage

Marriage increases overweight/obesity rates [66]. Getting married raises the risk of a woman becoming overweight compared to peers who did not marry [74]. The effect is more pronounced for men [75]. The nature of the connection between marriage and weight gain is a matter of conjecture [76, 77]. One possible explanation is the "marriage market hypothesis": single people remain thin for no other reason than to attract a mate ([6, 76]. If people quit smoking, wear sunscreen, and eschew suicide for the sake of their families, why would they allow themselves to become obese? It's important to note that mere age is not the explanation for the link between overweight/obesity and marriage. The researchers control for our tendency to gain weight, as we get older, and the correlation is still easily detectable. Someone suggests that there may be a simple explanation: people eat more when they're together [78]. A study that asked participants to record their food consumption for a week found that eating with one companion increased meal size by 41 percent compared with eating alone, while breaking bread with six or more people increased an individual's caloric intake by a whopping 76 percent. Other studies have found somewhat more modest increases, but the effect is remarkably consistent [67, 76].

Somebody asks why we do eat more when we eat with others. It may be a result of social norms. Communal meals tend to last longer than eating solo, and people who sit in front of food can't resist eating it. The habit may, alternatively, lie deep in evolutionary history. Chimpanzees and marmosets spontaneously share food, probably to help form social bonds. From the innocent, altruistic act grew a regrettable human custom. Perhaps you feed (and feed, and feed) your spouse to strengthen your marital bond, even if you're ultimately shortening its duration.

Adult Women

Multiple Pregnancies

Most overweight women gain their excess weight after puberty. This weight gain may be precipitated by a number of events, including pregnancy, oral contraceptive therapy, and menopause.

Pregnancy

Weight gain during pregnancy and the effect of pregnancy on subsequent weight gain are important events in the weight gain history of women. A few women gain considerable weight during pregnancy, occasionally the gain is more than 50 kg. The pregnancy itself may leave a legacy of increased weight. This was suggested by one study that evaluated women prospectively between the ages of 18 and 30 years [79].

Women who remained nulliparous (n = 925) were compared with women who had a single pregnancy of 28 weeks' duration during that period and who were at least 12 months postpartum. The primiparas gained 2-3 kg more weight and had a greater increase in waist/hip ratio (WHR) compared with the nulliparas during this period. Overweight at each decade increased with increasing parity [80]. The overall risk of weight gain associated with childbearing after age 25, however, is quite modest for American women [80].

Oral Contraceptives

In some women oral contraceptive use may initiate weight gain, although this effect is diminished with currently used low-dose contraceptives. One study evaluated 49 healthy women, initiating treatment with low-dose oral contraceptives (30 mg ethinyl estradiol plus 75 mg gestodene) [79]. Anthropometric measurements before and after the initiation of this formulation were used to compare 31 age- and weight-matched women. Baseline BMI, percent fat, percent water, and WHR did not change significantly after 6 cycles among women who used birth control pills. A similar number of women gained weight in both groups (30.6% of users, 35.4% of controls). The typical weight gain in the group taking pills was only 0.5 kg, attributable to the accumulation of fat, not body water. It is interesting to note that approximately 20% of women in both groups lost weight [76].

Menopause

Weight gain and changes in fat distribution occur after menopause. The decline in circulating levels of estrogen and progesterone alters the fat cell biology so that central fat deposition increases. Central or abdominal fat deposition (as estimated clinically from waist circumference or WHR) is an important determinant of cardiovascular risk. Estrogen replacement therapy does not prevent weight gain, although it may minimize fat redistribution [81]. A prospective study of 63 early postmenopausal women compared 34 who initiated continuous estrogen and progesterone therapy with women who did not. Body weight and fat mass increased significantly in both the treatment (73.2-75.6 kg) and control groups (71.5-73.5 kg). However, WHR increased significantly only in the control group (0.80-0.85). Caloric and macronutrient intake did not change in either group. Similarly, a 2-year trial examining the effects of supplemental estrogen in postmenopausal women showed an increase in body fat [82].

Physical Inactivity

The transition from an active lifestyle during the young years to a more sedentary lifestyle is often associated with weight gain. A rise in body weight continues through the adult years until about the sixth decade. After ages 55 to 64 years, relative weight remains stable and then begins to decline. Evidence from the Framingham Study and studies of men in the armed services suggests that men have become progressively heavier for height during the last decades [67].

Overweight/obesity and sedentary behavior coexist and that both are associated with cardiovascular disease (CVD) in women. Data from the Centers for Disease Control (CDC) show that in areas of the United States where rates of overweight/obesity are higher than 30%, the prevalence of adults who report no leisure-time physical activity is also higher than 30%. Likewise, the prevalence of overweight/obesity and physical inactivity predicts the presence of CVD death [83].

Few studies, however, have examined the association between sedentary behaviors such as prolonged television (TV) watching and obesity. Using data from a large prospective cohort study, the Health Professionals' Follow-up Study, it has been demonstrated that increasing TV watching is strongly associated with overweight/obesity and weight gain, independent of diet and exercise [84].

Men who watched TV more than 40 h per week had a nearly threefold increase in the risk of overweight/obesity and type 2 diabetes compared with those who spent less than 1 h per week watching TV. The increased risk was not entirely explained by the decreased physical activity and unhealthy eating patterns associated with TV watching. Thus, public health campaigns to reduce the risk of overweight/obesity and type 2 diabetes should promote not only increasing exercise levels but also decreasing sedentary behaviors, especially prolonged TV watching.

An observational study on Canadian men and women, the odds of being obese increased as weekly hours of television viewing rose. Furthermore, associations between time spent watching television and overweight/obesity were independent of leisure-time physical activity and diet. When the effects of age and other potential confounding variables were controlled, a modest association was observed between frequent computer use and overweight/obesity among men and women. Reading was not associated with overweight/obesity for either sex [85].

Low Metabolic Rate

There is no significant evidence that overweight/obesity is associated with lower RMR; on the contrary, experience shows that obese persons reveal a higher RMR because it relates to body mass. However, different is the case with easy to gain weight after a diet with relative weight loss. There are evidences that weight loss leads to a reduction in resting energy expenditure (REE) beyond that explained by losses in fat free mass (FFM) and fat mass (FM) [86, 87]. Decreases in specific REE (i.e., the decrease in REE beyond what could be predicted from the changes in FM and FFM) have been described as "adaptive thermogenesis" [88]. Some authors considered adaptive thermogenesis a transient phenomenon that is at least partly explained by a weight loss–induced reduction in serum triiodothyronine concentrations (T3) [89], whereas others suggest a persistence of reduced specific REE after weight loss [90]. Because a decline in specific metabolic rate may predispose to regain of lost weight [91], the metabolic response may be maladaptive in the case of intended weight loss. After weight loss, almost 50% of the decrease in REE can be explained by losses of FFM and FM. The variability in REE explained by body composition increased to 60% after the weight of individual organs was considered. However, adaptive thermogenesis after weight loss remained significant after the decrease in individual organ masses was accounted for. High adaptive thermogenesis is associated with lower weight loss and a conservation of visceral organ mass. [92].

Smoking Cessation

It has been suggested that to give up smoking can be a contributing factor to the increase of excess body weight. There exists a considerable rise in prevalent overweight people among smokers who have given up during the previous 10 years. However, since this group represents a relatively small percentage of the population, the net effect of giving up smoking on the prevalent overweight segment of the population is on the whole rather small. Only about a quarter of the increase in overweight people (2.3 of 9.6%) among men, and about one sixth (1.3 of 8.0%) among women can be attributed to having given up smoking [76].

These results suggest that smoking cessation accounts for a small part of the recent increase in the prevalence of overweight in the U.S. population.

Boyle et al. [93] similarly concluded that increasing weight among Australians could not be explained by decreases in the prevalence of cigarette smoking. To the extent that weight gain is a physiologic process reflecting nicotine withdrawal. Weight gain follows promptly on smoking cessation; relapse or initiation of smoking is followed by weight loss.

Reducing concern about weight gain after the cessation of smoking may be preferable to trying to prevent weight gain [94].

The 1990 report of the Surgeon General concluded that the health benefits of smoking cessation far exceeded the risks associated with weight gain and that smoking cessation had major and immediate health benefits for men and women of all ages [95]. This conclusion is supported by epidemiologic studies that examined the association between weight and mortality separately for smokers and nonsmokers [96].

At present, efforts to prevent weight gain immediately after smoking cessation appear relatively unsuccessful. Despite its long-term health benefits, stopping smoking may involve a gain of 4 to 5 kg or more.

The health benefits of smoking cessation are undeniable. Public health efforts to discourage the initiation of smoking and to promote its cessation must continue. To the extent these efforts are successful, they are likely to lead to further increases in the proportion of the population that is overweight. Nonetheless, it is important to discourage the use of smoking as a means of weight control and to encourage the cessation of smoking, while continuing research aimed at understanding and moderating the degree of weight gain among former smokers.

Frequently Dieting

As above reported in the natural history of obesity, people tend to accumulate fat during all the life span. In a Swedish study on a large sample of obese subjects, normal weight at 20 and obese at 60, retrospectively followed from 20 to 60 years of age, obese subjects gradually increases to 1-2 kg per year, and virtually all reported many weight loss attempts during the lifetime [21].

The mechanism that maintains the responsibility of dieting is a complex psychological, neuroendocrine and metabolic system, among others. The most accepted explanation is the psychobiological one: a person subjected to caloric restriction tends to force all homeostatic mechanisms designed to maintain a certain weight. A sort of adipostatus which tends to resist the weight loss. After a variable period of time, the subject on diet undergoes cognitive disinhibition, breaks the rules of the restriction, increases caloric intake, and recovers the lost weight. It is the rule that retrieves in favor of body fat and reaching values higher than those before the diet: the more are attempts to diet, the greater the weight gain.

Endocrine Disrupters

Endocrine disrupting chemicals (EDCs), such as the flame retardant polybrominated diphenyl ether (PBDE), and the plasticizer bisphenol A (BPA), are very stable in the environment and many have been steadily increasing in levels in humans. PBDE, BPA, and other EDCs exposure have been implicated as contributing to overweight/obesity in both humans and model animals, possibly by interfering with estrogen and androgen signaling [68].

Weight Gain Inducing Pharmaceuticals

The contribution of commonly prescribed medications to the growing overweight/obesity epidemic is stressed by the fact that several million people take the above-mentioned drugs on a chronic basis. Furthermore, weight, once gained, is not easily lost, accumulating an even larger group of people who have taken the drugs for shorter periods of time. This source of weight gain is preventable, and highlights the need for increased education among clinicians.

In many cases, there are alternative medications with little or no potential for weight gain. A lack of acceptable alternatives warrants prescribing the minimal dose to produce clinical efficacy and careful monitoring of weight, with early institution of a program of diet and lifestyle that may minimize drug-induced weight gain.

Intrauterine and Intergenerational Effects

The intrauterine environment is crucial for normal growth and for its physiological development. The reduced or excessive intrauterine growth induced by environmental factors and low or great birth weight is associated with increased susceptibility to future successive multiple diseases, such as obesity, type 2 diabetes and cardiovascular disease.

The 'developmental origins of adult disease' hypothesis, often called the 'Barker hypothesis' after one of its leading proponents, states that adverse influences early in development, and particularly during intrauterine life, can result in permanent changes in physiology and metabolism, which result in increased disease risk in adulthood. This hypothesis originally evolved from observations by Barker and colleagues that the regions in England that had the highest rates of infant mortality in the early twentieth century also had the highest rates of mortality from coronary heart disease decades later [60]. As the most commonly registered cause of infant death at the start of the twentieth century was low birthweight, these observations led to the hypothesis that low birthweight babies who survived infancy and childhood might be at increased risk of coronary heart disease later in life.

Adverse events during pregnancy can affect not only the offspring of that pregnancy, but also the next generation. It has long been recognized that the birthweight of the mother is related to the birthweight of her children [97]. A colony of rats fed a low-protein diet for several generations and then re-fed took three generations for fetal growth and development to return to [98]. A similar effect was seen during the Dutch hunger winter of 1944– 1945; a 5-month period of severe famine at the end of the Second World War. Women who were severely undernourished during the first trimester of pregnancy gave birth to babies who were on average of normal birthweight, but those babies themselves then went on to give birth to smaller babies in the next generation [99]. Many are possible explanations for these inter-generational effects on birthweight. Hormonal environment of the uterus of undernourished mothers may affect the developing reproductive tract of the fetus. Mothers who were small at birth have reduced uterine and ovarian size. It is proposed that smaller uterine size may impose a greater 'maternal constraint' on the fetus, thereby reducing its growth, although there is not yet any direct evidence for such an effect [100]. Furthermore, any epigenetic changes to the genome may be passed on to the second generation [101].

There are also intergenerational effects on risk factors for cardiovascular disease. Lower maternal birthweight is associated with an increased risk of hypertension during pregnancy [102], which in turn is associated with lower birthweight of the offspring. Furthermore, maternal birthweight is negatively related to blood pressure in the offspring, regardless of maternal blood pressure during adult life [103]. This effect may be mediated by exposure to excess glucocorticoids [100].

ELDERLY

Effect of Aging

The prevalence studies show that the peak of overweight/obesity is in the young elderly (60-65 years). Despite the increase in life expectancy, over the years more advanced overweight/obesity is becoming less frequent. The phenomenon is due to the increased risk of morbidity and mortality carried by overweight and obesity, with the finding that at older ages the prevalence of overweight/obesity is less common.

Notwithstanding, it must be stressed that overweight/obesity prevalence is growing progressively even among older age groups. Currently, more than 35% of these individuals are obese and if the current trend continues, nearly half of the elderly population will be obese by 2030 [104].

Controversy exists about the potential harms of overweight/obesity in the elderly. Some studies have suggested that the association between overweight/obesity and mortality risk weakens with age [105, 106, 107].

Bender R et al., made a large study (6193 obese patients) with a long mortality follow-up (median follow-up time of 14.8 years) of a cohort of obese patients, including a considerable number of grossly obese (BMI of 32 to <40 kg/m2) and morbidly obese (BMI ≥40 kg/m2) subjects. They tried to assess the effect of age on the excess mortality associated with all degrees of obesity. They found that the excess mortality associated with overweight/obesity declined considerably with age for both sexes in all degrees of overweight/ obesity [106].

It is possible to argue that these results were derived from biased estimates of the obesity-mortality relationship because models failed to account for confounding influences from ages of respondents at survey and/or cohort membership.

Debate persists about the relation between overweight/obesity in old age and total or disease-specific mortality, the definition of overweight/obesity in the elderly, its clinical relevance, and about the need for its treatment. Knowledge of age-related body composition and fat distribution changes will help us to better understand the relationships between obesity, morbidity and mortality in the elderly. Review of the literature supports that central fat and relative loss of fat-free mass may become relatively more important than BMI in determining the health risk associated with overweight/obesity in older ages. Weight gain or fat redistribution in older age may still confer adverse health risks (for earlier mortality, comorbidities conferring independent adverse health risks, or for functional decline). Evaluation of comorbidity and weight history should be performed in the elderly in order to generate a comprehensive assessment of the potential adverse health effects of overweight or obesity. The risks of overweight/obesity in the elderly have been underestimated by a number of confounders such as survival effect, competing mortalities, relatively shortened life expectancy in older persons, smoking, weight change and unintentional weight loss. Identification of elderly subjects with sarcopenic overweight/obesity is probably clinically relevant, but the definition of sarcopenic obesity, the benefits of its clinical identification, as well as its relation to clinical consequences requires further study. Studies on the effect of voluntary weight loss in the elderly are scarce, but they suggest that even small amounts of weight loss (between 5-10% of initial body weight) may be beneficial. In older as well as in younger adults, moderate voluntary weight loss may help to prevent the adverse health consequences of obesity.

Zamboni et al. [107] underscored the following conclusions:

- Prevalence of overweight/obesity increases up to 60–69 years in men and women, and then declines. The prevalence of overweight/obesity is, however, increasing in older ages, comparing the period 1999–2000 with the period 1988–94.
- Central adipose tissue and relative loss of fat-free mass may become relatively more important than BMI in determining the health risk associated with overweight/obesity in older ages.
- Indices of fat distribution, such as waist circumference appear to be relatively more important than BMI.
- Weight gain or fat redistribution in older age may still confer adverse health risks (for earlier mortality, comorbidities conferring independent adverse health risks, or for functional decline); evaluation of comorbidity and weight history should be performed in order to generate a comprehensive assessment of potential adverse health effects of overweight or overweight/obesity in the elderly patient.
- Health risks of overweight/obesity in the elderly may be underestimated because elderly people represent 'survivors' in epidemiological studies; in addition to competing mortalities and relatively shortened life expectancy in older persons make it that older obese people may die of non-obese-related disease before the adverse

health effects of overweight/obesity or weight gain in older age become apparent; longitudinal effects of confounding conditions (smoking, weight change, etc.) are difficult to separate from the independent effects of overweight/obesity per se; last but not the least, fat distribution may confer greater health risk than BMI.

- Both in older and in younger adults, voluntary weight loss may have beneficial health effects. Studies on the effect of weight loss in the elderly are scarce, but they suggest that even small amounts of weight loss (more or less 5% of initial body weight) may be beneficial. Treatment should be judicious in order to avoid bone and fat-free mass loss.
- Weight loss not voluntary is always abnormal and deserves careful clinical evaluation for the underlying cause.
- Identification of elderly subjects with sarcopenic obesity is probably clinically relevant. However, clinical identification and definition of sarcopenic obesity and its relation to clinical consequences deserve further studies.

There are actually relatively few data that directly address many of these points, all of which are important areas for future research [108]. Recent findings suggest that survey-based estimates of age patterns in the obesity-mortality relationship are significantly confounded by disparate cohort mortality and age-related survey selection bias. When these factors are accounted for in Cox survival models, the obesity-mortality relationship is estimated to grow stronger with age [108, 109].

Recent observations provide evidence that aging exacerbates obesity-induced oxidative stress and inflammation in the perivascular adipose tissue. The findings support a role for localized perivascular tissue inflammation in exacerbation of vascular oxidative stress and inflammation in aging [108], an effect that likely enhances the risk for development of cardiovascular diseases from overweight/obesity in the elderly individuals.

CONCLUSION

People tend to accumulate fat during all the life span; the age of highest risk is now the childhood. May be the most delicate moment is that of the pregnancy when the effects of maternal epigenetic environment and its lifestyle may be crucial.

Of course, individuals can become overweight at any age, but it is more common at certain times. In recent years, the age at highest risk is now the childhood. The prevalence of childhood overweight/obesity has increased rapidly over recent decades, particularly in some communities and states at the high economic level but also in developing countries. Given such a high prevalence, is now crucial to identify the risk factors best predicting incident overweight/obesity in childhood and what are the contributory characteristics resulting in obesity. The environment is the main accused. Furthermore, the children at highest risk must be accurately targeted for early intervention.

In the adulthood age some predictors of weight gain fare proposed [66], giving from to be overweight at the childhood to menopause, or from low metabolic rate to low level of physical activity. In addition, recent marriage is considered, as are multiple pregnancies; frequently dieting seems important as smoking cessation. Also McAllister EJ [67] proposed some putative contributors to the overweight/obesity epidemic: among these are to be taken into account particularly epigenetics, endocrine disruptors, pharmaceutical iatrogenesis and intrauterine and intergenerational effects.

Overweight/obesity prevalence is growing progressively even among older age groups. Debate persists about the relation between overweight/ obesity in old age and total or disease-specific mortality, the definition of obesity in the elderly, its clinical relevance and about the need for its treatment. Identification of elderly subjects with sarcopenic obesity is probably clinically relevant. However, clinical identification and definition of sarcopenic obesity and its relation to clinical consequences deserve further studies.

References

[1] Poirier, P; Giles, TD; Bray, GA; et al. Obesity and cardiovascular disease: pathophysiology, evaluation, and effect of weight loss: an update of the 1997 American Heart Association Scientific Statement on Obesity and Heart Disease from the Obesity Committee of the Council on Nutrition, Physical Activity, and Metabolism. *Circulation* 2006, 113, 898 –918.

[2] Hedley, AA; Ogden, CL; Johnson, CL; et al. Prevalence of overweight and obesity among U.S. children, adolescents, and adults, 1999–2002. *JAMA* 2004, 291, 2847–50.

[3] Swinburn, BA; Sacks, G; Hall, KD; et al. The global obesity pandemic: shaped by global drivers and local environments. *Lancet* 2011, 378, 804–814.

[4] Mokdad, AH; Bowman, BA; Ford, ES; et al. The continuing epidemics of obesity and diabetes in the United States. *JAMA* 2001, 286, 1195–1200.

[5] Stevens, GA; Singh, GM; Lu, Y; et al. National, regional, and global trends in adult overweight and obesity prevalences. *Popul Health Metr* 2012, 10, 22.

[6] Flegal, KM; Carroll, MD; Ogden, CL; et al. Prevalence and trends in obesity among US adults, 1999–2008. *JAMA* 2010, 303, 235-41.

[7] Flegal, KM; Carroll, MD; Kit, BK; et al. Prevalence of Obesity and Trends in the Distribution of Body Mass Index Among US Adults, 1999-2010. *JAMA* 2012, 307(5), 491-497.

[8] Whitlock, G; Lewington, S; Sherliker, P; et al. Body-mass index and cause-specific mortality in 900 000 adults: collaborative analyses of 57 prospective studies. *Lancet* 2009, 373, 1083–1096.

[9] Murray, CJL; Richards, MA; Newton, JN; et al. UK health performance: findings of the Global Burden of Disease Study 2010. *Lancet* 2013, 381, 997–1020.

[10] Wannamethee, SG; Shaper, AG; Walker, M. Overweight and obesity and weight change in middle aged men: impact on cardiovascular disease and diabetes. *J Epidemiol Commun Health* 2005, 59,134–139.

[11] Manson, JE; Willett, WC; Stampfer, MJ; et al. Body weight and mortality among women. *N Engl J Med* 1995, 333, 677–685.

[12] Booth, HP; Prevost, AT; Gulliford, MC. Impact of body mass index on prevalence of multimorbidity in primary care: cohort study. *Fam Pract* 2014, 31(1), 38–43.

[13] Calle, EE; Thun, MJ; Petrelli, JM; et al. Body-mass index and mortality in a prospective cohort of U.S. adults. *N Engl J Med* 1999, 341 1097-1105.

[14] Murphy, NF; MacIntyre, K; Stewart, S; et al. Long-term cardiovascular consequences of obesity: 20-year follow-up of more than 15,000 middle-aged men and women (the Renfrew–Paisley study). *Eur Heart J* 2006, 27, 96–106.

[15] Hubert, HB; Feinleib, M; McNamara, PM; et al. Obesity as an independent risk factor for cardiovascular disease: a 26-year follow-up of participants in the Framingham Heart Study. *Circulation* 1983, 67, 968-977.

[16] Tsa, AG; Wadden, TA. Obesity. *Ann Intern Med.* 2013, 159(5), ITC3-1. doi:10.7326/0003-4819-159-5-201309030-01003

[17] McAuley, PA; Smith, NS; Emerson, BT; et al. The Obesity Paradox and Cardiorespiratory Fitness. *J Obes* 2012, 9, 515-82.

[18] Casazza, K; Fontaine, KR; Astrup, A; et al. Myths, Presumptions, and Facts about Obesity. *N Engl J Med* 2013, 36,: 446-54.

[19] Jia, H; Lubetkin, EI. Obesity-Related Quality-Adjusted Life Years Lost in the U.S. from 1993 to 2008. *Am J Prev Med* 2010, 39, 220–227.

[20] Stewart, ST; Cutler, DM; Allison, B; et al. Forecasting the Effects of Obesity and Smoking on U.S. Life Expectancy. *N Engl J Med* 2009, 361, 2252-2260.

[21] Lissner, L; Sjöström, L; Bengtsson, C; et al. The natural history of obesity in an obese population and associations with metabolic aberrations. *Int J Obes Relat Metab Disord* 1994, 18(6), 441-447.

[22] Nan, Li; Enqing, Liu; Jia, Guo; et al. Maternal Prepregnancy Body Mass Index and Gestational Weight Gain on Offspring Overweight in Early Infancy. *PLOS ONE* 2013, 8, e77809.

[23] Li1, N<, Liu,LE; Guo1, J; et al. Maternal Prepregnancy Body Mass Index and Gestational Weight Gain on Pregnancy Outcomes. *PLOS ONE* 2013, 8, e778010.

[24] La Merrill, MA; Stein, CR; Landrigan, P; et al. Prepregnancy body mass index, smoking during pregnancy, and infant birth weight. *Ann Epidemiol* 2011, 21, 413–420.

[25] Brion, MJ; Zeegers, M; Jaddoe, V; et al. Intrauterine effects of maternal prepregnancy overweight on child cognition and behavior in 2 cohorts. *Pediatrics* 2011, 127, e202–e211.

[26] Neggers, YH; Goldenberg, RL; Ramey, SL; et al. Maternal prepregnancy body mass index and psychomotor development in children. *Acta Obstet Gynecol Scand* 2003, 82, 235–240.

[27] Tanda, R; Salsberry, PJ; Reagan, PB; et al. The impact of pre-pregnancy obesity on children's cognitive test scores. *Matern Child Health J.* 2011, 17, 222–229.

[28] Nohr, EA; Vaeth, M; Baker, JL; et al. Combined associations of pre-pregnancy body mass index and gestational weight gain with the outcome of pregnancy. *Am J Clin Nutr* 2008, 87, 1750 –1759.

[29] Rasmussen, KM; Yaktine, AL. Weight Gain During Pregnancy: Reexamining the Guidelines. Institute of Medicine and National Research Concil. The National Academic Press, Washington, DC, USA, 2009.

[30] Daniels, SR; Kelly, AS. Pediatric Severe Obesity: Time To Establish Serious Treatments for a Serious Disease. *Child Obes* 2014, 10, 283-284.

[31] Saunders, RP; Evans, MH; Joshi, P. Developing a process-evaluation plan for assessing health promotion program implementation: a how-to guide. *Health Promot Pract* 2005, 6,134-147.

[32] Dubois, L; Girard, M. Early determinants of overweight at 4.5 years in a population-based longitudinal study. *Int J Obes Relat Metab Disord* 2006, 30, 610-617.

[33] Shrewsbury, V; Wardle, J. Socioeconomic status and adiposity in childhood: a systematic review of cross-sectional studies 1990-2005. *Obesity* (Silver Spring) 2008, 16, 275-284.

[34] Semmler, C; Ashcroft, J; van Jaarsveld, CH; et al. Development of overweight in children in relation to parental weight and socioeconomic status. *Obesity* (Silver Spring) 2009, 17, 814-820.

[35] Rey-López, JP; Vicente-Rodriguez, G; Biosca, M; et al. Sedentary behaviour and obesity development in children and adolescents. *Nutr Metab Cardiovasc* 2008, 18, 242-251.

[36] Hills, AP; King, NA; Armstrong, TP. The contribution of physical activity and sedentary behaviours to the growth and development of children and adolescents: implications for overweight and obesity. *Sports Med* 2007, 37, 533-545.

[37] Mo-suwan, L; Pongprapai, S; Junjana, C; et al. Effects of a controlled trial of a school-based exercise program on the obesity indexes of preschool children. *Am J Clin Nutr* 1998, 68,1006-1011.

[38] Trost, SG; Sirard, JR; Dowda, M; et al. Physical activity in overweight and nonoverweight preschool children. *Int J Obes Relat Metab Disord* 2003, 27, 834-839.

[39] Monasta, L; Batty, GD; Cattaneo, A; et al. Early-life determinants of overweight and obesity: a review of systematic reviews. *Obes Rev* 2010, 11, 695-708

[40] Dennison, BA, Erb, TA, Jenkins, PL. Television viewing and television in bedroom associated with overweight risk among low-income preschool children. *Pediatrics* 2002, 109, 1028-1035.

[41] Reilly, JJ, Armstrong, J, Dorosty, AR; et al. Early life risk factors for obesity in childhood: cohort study. *BMJ* 2005, 330, 1357.

[42] Robinson, TN: Television viewing and childhood obesity. *Pediatr Clin North Am* 2001, 48, 1017-1025.

[43] Crawford, D; Jeffery, RW. Obesity Prevention and Public Health. Oxford University Press; New York, 2005.

[44] Report nazionale OKkio alla salute 2012. http://www.epicentro.iss.it/ okkioallasalute/ IndagineNazionale 2012.asp.

[45] Cunningham, SA; Kramer, MR; Narayan, KMV. Incidence of Childhood Overweight/obesity in the United States. *N Engl J Med* 2014, 370, 1660-1661.

[46] Hancock, KJ; Lawrence, D; Zubrick, SR. Higher Maternal Protectiveness Is Associated with Higher Odds of Child Overweight and Obesity: A Longitudinal Australian Study. *PLOS ONE* 2014, 9: e100686.

[47] Verbestel, V; De Henauw, S; Maes, L; et al. Using the intervention mapping protocol to develop a community-based intervention for the prevention of childhood obesity in a multi-centreEuropean project: the IDEFICS intervention. *Int J Behav Nutr Phys Act* 2011, 8, 82-90.

[48] Bronfenbrenner, U. The ecology of human development: Experiments by nature and design. Harvard University Press. Cambridge, MA, 1979.

[49] WHO - Obesity and overweight. Fact sheet N°311 Updated March 2013.

[50] OECD–Obesity and the Economics of Prevention. Fit not fat. 2010, http:// www.oecd.org/els/health-systems/46044572.pdf.

[51] Larson, N; Story, M. A review of environmental influences on food choices. *Ann Behav Med* 2009, 38 (Suppl 1), S56-73.
[52] Story, M; Neumark-Sztainer, D; French, S. Individual and environmental influences on adolescent eating behaviors. *J Am Diet Assoc* 2002, 102 (3 Suppl), S40-51.
[53] Choudhuri, S. From Waddington's epigenetic landscape to small noncoding RNA: some important milestones in the history of epigenetics research. *Toxicol Mech Methods* 2011, 21, 252–274.
[54] Petronis, A. Epigenetics as a unifying principle in the aetiology of complex traits and diseases *Nature* 2010, 465, 721–727.
[55] Nessea. RM; Bergstromb, CT; Ellisonc, PT; et al. Making evolutionary biology a basic science for medicine. *PNAS* 2010, 107 (suppl. 1), 1800-1807.
[56] Jirtle, RL; Skinner, MK. Environmental epigenomics and disease susceptibility. *Nat Rev Genet* 2007, 8, 253-62.
[57] Weaver, IC; Cervoni, N; Champagne, FA; et al. Epigenetic programming by maternal behavior. *Nature Neurosci* 2004, 7, 847–854.
[58] Collins, J; Koplan, JP. Health Impact Assessment. A Step Toward Health in All Policies. *JAMA* 2009, 302, 315-317.
[59] Burdge, GC; Hanson, MA; Slater-Jefferies, JL; et al. Epigenetic regulation of transcription: A mechanism for inducing variations in phenotype (fetal programming) by differences in nutrition during early life? *Br J Nutr.* 2007, 97(6), 1036–1046.
[60] Barker, DJ; Osmond, C. Infant mortality, childhood nutrition, and ischemic heart disease in England and Wales. *Lancet* 1986, 1, 1077–1081.
[61] Dabelea, D; Mayer-Davis, EJ; Lamichhane, AP; et al. Association of intrauterine exposure to maternal diabetes and obesity with type 2 diabetes in youth: the SEARCH Case-Control Study. *Diabetes Care* 2008, 31,1422-6.
[62] Waterland, RA; Jirtle, RL. Early nutrition, epigenetic changes at transposons and imprinted genes, and enhanced susceptibility to adult chronic diseases. *Nutrition* 2004, 20(1), 63-8.
[63] Stein, AD; Zybert, PA; van de, BM; et al. Intrauterine famine exposure and body proportions at birth: the Dutch Hunger Winter. *Int J Epidemiol* 2004, 33, 831–836.
[64] EU Action Plan on Childhood Obesity 2014-2020. http://ec.europa.eu/health/nutrition_physical_activity/docs/childhoodobesity_actionplan_2014_2020_en.pdf.
[65] Maffeis, C; Moghetti, P; Grezzani, A; et al. Insulin Resistance and the Persistence of Obesity from Childhood into Adulthood. *J Clin Endocrinol Metab* 2002, 87, 71–76
[66] Bray, GA. Contemporary Diagnosis and Management of Overweight/obesity. Handbooks in Health Care. Newtown, Pa. 1998.
[67] McAllister, EJ; Dhurandhar, NV; Keith, SW; et al. Ten Putative Contributors to the Obesity Epidemic. *Crit Rev Food Sci Nutr* 2009, 49, 868–913.
[68] Skilton, MR; Siitonen, N; Wurtz, P. et al. High Birth Weight Is Associated With Obesity and Increased Carotid Wall Thickness in Young Adults. The Cardiovascular Risk in Young Finns Study. *Arterioscler Thromb Vasc Biol* 2014, 34,1064-1068.
[69] Sobal, J; Stunkard, AJ. Socioeconomic status and obesity: A review of the literature. *Psychol Bull* 1989, 105, 260–75.
[70] McLaren, L. Socioeconomic status and obesity. *Epidemiol Rev* 2007, 29, 29–48.

[71] Centers for Disease Control and Prevention. National Center for Health Statistics. National Health and Nutrition Examination Survey. Available from: http://www.cdc.gov/nchs/nhanes/nhanes_questionnaires.htm. Accessed November 18, 2010.

[72] Ogden, CL; Lamb, MM; Caroll, MD; et al., Overweight/obesity and Socioeconomic Status in Adults: United States, 2005–2008. NCHS Data Brief , No. 50, December 2010

[73] Report nazionale PASSI 2012. Life Stages 20.12.14 finale 4.docx http:// www.epicentro.iss.it/passi/rapporto2012/R2012Indice.asp.

[74] Sobal, J. Marriage, Obesity and Dieting. *Marriage Fam Rev* 1984, 7, 115-139.

[75] Sobal, J; Rauschenbach, BS; Frongillo, EA Jr. Marital status, fatness and obesity. *Soc Sci Med* 1992, 35, 915–923.

[76] Jeffery, RW; Rick, AM. Cross-Sectional and Longitudinal Associations between Body Mass Index and Marriage-Related Factors. *Obes Res* 2002, 10, 809-815.

[77] Knuiman, MW; Divitini, ML; Bartholomew, HC; et al. Spouse correlations in cardiovascular risk factors and the effect of marriage duration. *Am J Epidemiol* 1996, 143, 48–53.

[78] Reubinoff, BE; Grubstein, A; Meirow, D; et al. Effects of low-dose estrogen oral contraceptives on weight, body composition, and fat distribution in young women. *Fertil Steril* 1995, 63, 516-521.

[79] Williamson, DF; Madans, J; Pamuk, E; et al. A prospective study of childbearing and 10-year weight gain in US white women 25 to 45 years of age. *Int J Obes Relat Metab Disord* 1994, 18, 561-569.

[80] National Task Force on the Prevention and Treatment of Obesity. Weight cycling. *JAMA* 1994, 272, 1196-1202.

[81] Haarbo, J; Christiansen, C. Treatment-induced cyclic variations in serum lipids, lipoproteins, and apolipoproteins after 2 years of combined hormone replacement therapy: exaggerated cyclic variation in smokers. *Obstet Gynecol* 1992, 80, 639-644.

[82] Smith Barnes, A; Coulter, SA. Overweight/obesity and Sedentary Lifestyles. Risk for Cardiovascular Disease in Women. *Tex Heart Inst J* 2012, 39, 224–227.

[83] Hu, FB. Sedentary lifestyle and risk of overweight/obesity and type 2 diabetes. *Lipids* 2003, 38(2), 103-8.

[84] Shields, M; Tremblay, MS. Sedentary behaviour and obesity. Component of Statistics Canada *Catalogue no. 82-003-X Health Reports*, 2008.

[85] Keys, A; Brozek, J; Mickelsen, O; et al. The biology of human starvation. University of Minnessota Press, Minneapolis, MN, 1950.

[86] Leibel, RL; Hirsch, J. Diminished energy requirements in reduced-obese patients. *Metabolism* 1984, 33, 164–70.

[87] Major, GC; Doucet, E; Trayhurn, P; et al. Clinical significance of adaptive thermogenesis. Int J *Obes Relat Metab Disord* 2007, 31 204–12.

[88] Kiortsis, DN; Durack, I; Turpin G. Effects of a low-calorie diet on resting metabolic rate and serum triiodothryronine levels in obese children. *Eur J Pediatr* 1999, 158, 446–50.

[89] Rosenbaum, M; Hirsch, J; Gallagher, DA; et al. Long-term persistence of adaptive thermogenesis in subjects who have maintained a reduced body weight. *Am J Clin Nutr* 2008, 88, 906–12.

[90] Ravussin, E; Lillioja, S; Knowler, WC; et al. Reduced rate of energy expenditure as a risk factor for body-weight gain. *N Engl J* Med 1988, 3, 467–72.
[91] Bosy-Westphal, A; Kossel, E; Goele, K; et al. Contribution of individual organ mass loss to weight loss–associated decline in resting energy expenditure. *Am J Clin Nutr* 2009, 90, 993–1001.
[92] Boyle, CA; Dobson, AJ; Egger, G; Magnus, P. Can the increasing weight of Australians be explained by the decreasing prevalence of cigarette smoking? *Int J Obes Relat Metab Disord* 1994, 18, 55-60.
[93] Flegal, KM; Troiano, RP; Pamuk, ER; et al., The influence of smoking cessation on the prevalence of overweight in the United States. *N Engl J* Med 1995 333, 1165-70.
[94] Department of Health and Human Services. The health benefits of smoking cessation: a report of the Surgeon General, 1990. Washington, D.C.: Government Printing Office, 1990. (DHHS publication no. (CDC) 90-8416.
[95] Wannamethee, G, Shaper, AG. Body weight and mortality in middle aged British men: impact of smoking. *BMJ* 1989, 299, 1497-502.
[96] Little, RE; Sing, CF. Genetic and environmental influences on human birth weight. *Am J Hum Genet* 1987, 40, 512–526.
[97] Stewart, RJ; Sheppard, H; Preece, R; et al. The effect of rehabilitation at different stages of development of rats marginally malnourished for ten to twelve generations. *Br J Nutr* 1980, 43, 403–412.
[98] Stei, AD; Lumey, LH. The relationship between maternal and offspring birth weights after maternal prenatal famine exposure: the Dutch Famine Birth Cohort Study. *Hum Biol* 2000, 72, 641–654.
[99] De Boo, HA; Harding, JE. The developmental origins of adult disease (Barker) hypothesis. *Aust N Z J Obstet Gynaecol* 2006, 46, 4–14.
[100] Reik, W; Santos, F; Dean, W. Mammalian epigenomics: reprogramming the genome for development and therapy. *Theriogenology* 2003, 59, 21–32.
[101] Klebanoff, MA; Secher NJ; Mednick, BR; et al. Maternal size at birth and the development of hypertension during pregnancy: a test of the Barker hypothesis. *Arch Intern Med* 1999, 159, 1607–1612.
[102] Barker, DJ; Shiell, AW; Barker, ME; et al. Growth in utero and blood pressure levels in the next generation. *J Hypertens* 2000, 18, 843–846.
[103] McAuley, PA; Kokkinos, PF; Oliveira, RB; et al. Obesity paradox and cardiorespiratory fitness in 12,417 male veterans aged 40 to 70 years. *Mayo Clin Proc* 2010, 85, 115-21.
[104] Childers, DK; Allison, DB. The 'Obesity Paradox:' a parsimonious explanation for relations among obesity, mortality rate, and aging? *Int J Obes* (Lond), 2010, 34, 1231–1238.
[105] Andres, R; Elahi, D; Tobin, JD; et al. Impact of age on weight goals. *Ann Intern Med,* 1985, 103 1030-3.
[106] Bender, R; Jockel, KH; Trautner, C; et al. Effect of age on excess mortality in obesity. *JAMA* 1999, 281, 1498-1504.
[107] Zamboni, M; Mazzali, G; Zoico, E; et al. Health consequences of obesity in the elderly: a review of four unresolved questions. *Int J Obes* 2005, 29, 1011–1029.

[108] Alam, I; Ng, TP; Larbi, A. Does Inflammation Determine Whether Obesity Is Metabolically Healthy or Unhealthy? The Aging Perspective. *Mediators Inflamm* 2012 ID 456456, 1-14.

[109] Masters, RK; Powers, DA; Link, BG. Obesity and US Mortality Risk Over the Adult Life Course, *Am J Epidemiol* 2013, 177, 431–442.

In: The Different Faces of Being Overweight
Editor: Emilia Manzato
ISBN: 978-1-63483-099-7

Chapter 5

Overweight in Childhood and Adolescence

Andrea Vania, MD *

Former President, ECOG (European Childhood Obesity Group), Belgium
Department of Paediatrics and Paediatric Neuropsychiatry,
"Sapienza" University of Rome, Italy

Abstract

About 40% of children with weight troubles (as well as 60% of adolescents in the same conditions) will remain obese during their adult life. With this in mind, it is clear enough that many cases of adulthood's obesity found their roots in paediatric age.

Belonging to a lineage where obesity runs in the family appears as an important risk factor in the development of childhood obesity, but the relationship between parental and offspring obesity is not limited to genetic factors. Actually, environment can play a major role in both generations.

The concept of environment has widened enough, in the recent years, and scientists look at it now as the "envirome", the total complement of environmental characteristics, conditions, and processes required for life form viability and successful adaptation. Genome and environment coexist, and genomic expression can be modified by environment, leading to the idea that genome and envirome can interact through epigenetic modifications, which are active during the individual life-span, but are suspected to have an inter-generational influence as well.

Should epigenomics' hypothesis be confirmed as reliable, then the whole weighing condition, development, and future of an individual would be really decided during the very first periods of his/her life. According to the hypothesis, epigenetic changes start during the gestational period, and – quite possibly – even before it.

We are still trying to understand which external environmental factors can shape the genomic expression, and what impact each factor can have.

* E-mail: andrea.vania@uniroma1.it.

Introduction

Starting this chapter by speaking of rates and trends of child and adolescent obesity can appear as off-topic in a book targeted to the analysis of risk factors. However, this is not the case: figures can vary according to the studies considered [1, 2]. It is generally accepted that about four out of ten children with weight excess and as many as six out of ten adolescents with the same problem will remain obese during their adult life; being overweight or obese between 14 to 19 years of age is possibly linked with an increased adult mortality rate (from an age as early as 30) from a variety of systemic and/or metabolic diseases [3] to be regarded as complications of the underlying obesity. A huge number of countries are experiencing a very high prevalence of paediatric obesity. The phenomenon affects mostly the developed countries, but the underdeveloped ones are not exempt. This represents a major risk factor for adult obesity, and all efforts made to level it off have to be considered as a very effective way to tackle the epidemics of obesity.

Prevalence of Paediatric Obesity at Different Ages

Prevalence of obesity among children and adolescents has shown a strong positive trend worldwide [4, 5] across the last 30 years. For this reason, it is considered as one of the major issues in public health, in developed countries [6].

Analysing the epidemiology of childhood obesity is not a simple mathematical exercise, it is a basic task that can help to develop and monitor public health interventions effective in dealing with childhood obesity. In turn, this may reduce the risk of developing both obesity later on in life and obese-related co-morbidities.

In spite of the importance of getting strong epidemiological data, and of the numerous articles on the diffusion of childhood obesity [7], comparable prevalence and statistics on trends are lacking worldwide and are quite scarce even in Europe [8]. The main reason for this insufficiency is a lack of harmonization of age group, methods, reference tables and cut-off points used in the different surveys. Last, but not least, the different definitions used to assess nutritional status make a global evaluation more difficult.

On behalf of the European Childhood Obesity Group, Rolland-Cachera recently published a paper trying to clarify what can be a generally accepted definition of overweight and obesity in children and adolescents [9]. The BMI calculation, associated with body composition and risk factors, is generally accepted as a valid indirect measure of adiposity also in children. The terms used to define different levels of weight excess, though, vary considerably, so that the expressions “at risk of overweight”, “overweight” and “obesity”, all found in the literature, may not define the same level of adiposity. As an example, the IOTF terminology to define childhood obesity [10] corresponds to the WHO nomenclature used for adults [11]. A consensus for a single definition is clearly desirable but, for the time being, researchers believe that further studies on the association between childhood BMI levels and adult pathologies are required in order to identify the most suitable definitions in both epidemiological and clinical contexts. Additional consensus for internationally accepted terminology, age ranges, demographic groupings or cut-offs for various anthropometric measurements are also needed. Rolland-Cachera [9] therefore suggests: to use IOTF and

WHO definitions to assess the prevalence of childhood overweight and obesity; to use additional definitions (like CDC and national references) in order to provide more opportunities of comparisons of prevalence between studies; to use the WHO standards in clinical studies involving growth assessment so that comparability between results can be improved; and – which seems quite obvious, yet highly important – always to perform any anthropometric measurement according to standardized procedures.

Keeping in mind all these problems, is there any way a picture of childhood obesity prevalence, with a special focus on Europe, can still be outlined?

Prevalence data from 0 to 6 years of age is insufficient. Available data, collected from the years 1997 (Sweden) to 2007 (France) tends to distort the picture, not allowing a correct evaluation of trends and associated risk factors. A comparative study performed in 2008 in three very different countries (Denmark, Poland, and Italy) on samples that were not nationally representative [12], showed a statistically different prevalence of obesity in all countries, in children 3-6 years of age, with Italy showing the highest rate (21.2%) of overall overweight/obesity as well as the highest rate of obesity alone (9.3% of children, vs. about 2.5 in Denmark and Poland).

Overweight and obesity prevalence in the first 6 years of age is already at alarming level, especially considering the most likely underestimation of the importance of overweight at this age by parents, health workers and paediatricians, even though a growing literature's body is stressing that a rapid weight gain during the first years of age is a risk factor for obesity persistence and its increased severity [13, 14]. Obesity can actually track to older ages: when present in early childhood, it is associated with obesity persistence in adolescence [15] and in adulthood [16], even though with different percentages. In the future this may result in an even higher prevalence and in more severe complications, as well as in a further burden on life expectancy reduction. Prevalence from 7 to 10 years of age may seem easier to define, since this age range is the most surveyed, but again, data is hardly comparable. The first European overview on overweight and obesity prevalence appeared in 2003 [17], collecting data over 9 years (1992-2001) and showing among 20 countries a trend of higher rate of childhood obesity from North to South and from East to West. Afterwards (2008), the European Regional Office of WHO started the project "Childhood Obesity Surveillance Initiative" (COSI) [18], still running and expected to continue for several years with a coverage of at least 12 countries, aimed to get a reliable and comparable picture of overweight and obesity prevalence among children in Europe as well as a picture of the trends along the years. Preliminary results of the first round indicate that on average 24% of the children 6-9 years old in Europe are overweight/obese [19]. The standardized survey detected again a double geographical trend, North to South and East to West. At 7 years of age, the lowest prevalence was found in Czech Republic (20.8%) and the highest in Portugal (38%), while at the age of 8 Belgium showed the lowest value (22.4%) and Italy the highest (45.8%). Considering obesity alone ($\geq$ +2 SD) Sweden was the country with the lowest rate at 7 years of age (6%) and Italy was once again the country with the highest value (22.1%) at 8 years of age. As for ages 11 to 18, the main source of data for adolescents living in as many as 44 European countries comes from the homogeneous and standardized survey "Health Behaviour School Children" (HBSC), led again by WHO. Every 4 years the project assesses health behaviours in 11, 13 and 15 years old subjects. The most recent survey has been conducted in 2009-2010 [20]. The updated prevalence of overweight/obesity among 11 year old teens ranges from 6% in Switzerland and 9% in The Netherlands to 22% in Greece, Ireland,

Portugal and Poland. In 13 and 15 year old subjects it ranges from no less than 9% in The Netherlands, Switzerland and Denmark to 20% in Greece. Data from the survey is however difficult to interpret: no clear geographical trend is present, while gender differences are not always in the same direction even within the same country. More difficulties can be detected. Overweight perception and attitude change dramatically during adolescence: girls are usually more sensitive to this issue and in consequence more prone to lie about their real height and weight, while for boys being a little overweight is sometime considered as "becoming older and stronger" and therefore perceived as a positive factor; this is clearly seen in the self-reports about weight perception in all countries, irrespective of the real BMI situation, and with a clear increase in negative perception from 11 to 13 to 15 years of age. Psychological factors represent a real burden as well and make difficult to affirm with certainty that there is a real decrease of overweight and obesity rates from 11 to 15 years of age. This is even more plausible since self-reported data, like the HBSC ones, tends to underestimate the real prevalence of the facts under study.

Recent Trends in Childhood and Adolescence Overweight/Obesity

After decades of continuous increase in the prevalence of childhood obesity, especially in Europe and in North America, a kind of levelling off has been recently reported in some countries all around the world, either in national or in regional representative samples, but information is still limited and contradictory [20-26]. In the USA, the overall prevalence of childhood and adolescence overweight has not changed significantly in the years 2003 to 2012, and remains at about 17%; on the contrary, the prevalence of obesity among children aged 2 to 5 years has decreased significantly from 13.9% to 8.4% during the same period [26]. Across Europe, a decrease has been observed in some areas of Sweden, with different trends in the 2 genders [24]. Same results come from the largest systematic analysis available until now, which has reviewed studies between 1980 and 2008 [27]. The comparison between 2006 [28] and 2010 [20] results of the HBSC study also shows similar trends among the different countries, as well as similar limits and differences.

When data are analyzed in details, in developed countries the prevalence is lowering in families of upper social class but is still increasing in low SES (social and economical status) classes. This has been assessed in France, for instance, where an increase in overweight prevalence has been observed in children from manual workers parents, while a decrease has been seen in children from more affluent families [29]. This seems to be true also for Sweden, where the gap between high and low SES boys appears to increase over time [30], and for USA, according to the most recent data. Here the school level attained apparently can make the difference, at least among girls [26], with obese girls having a lower education level. Just two years before, another study [31] was partly in contrast with these findings: data from the Pediatric Nutrition Surveillance System (PedNSS, period from 2003 to 2010), which includes 50% of USA preschool children, shows a slight decrease in either obesity or extreme obesity among preschool children coming from families with low income. Possibly due to the contrasting data collected until now, it is not clear whether this apparent levelling off is due to a kind of "saturation" of all sensible children, or to the results of preventive actions taken in the different countries and/or regions. The latter is what WHO suspects: the hypothesis is moulding that more robust measures to tackle childhood obesity has been already taken in those European countries where the problem was more evident and important. A third hypothesis, however, cannot be ruled out: the stop or slowdown might be just temporary, and we might face again a prevalence increase a few years ahead. Most likely, we still miss sufficient data to predict which model the prevalence of obesity will follow in the future. Thus, the initial relief about "the epidemic being over" has to be rethought in terms of more cautious statements and must become a stimulus to implement more intensive intervention, especially in specific population's sub-groups.

What Makes Prevalence Rise

For more than twenty years there has been strong evidence that childhood obesity leads to adult obesity and the developing or worsening of related co-morbidities [32]. Although the presence of obesity during childhood and adolescence represents itself a key risk factor for adult obesity, and its high prevalence simply exacerbate the problem, the following question is: which factors do lead to such an epidemic? Since they represent the roots of many (most?) cases of adult obesity/super-obesity, it is essential to try to identify them. It is widely known and accepted that at every age the core problem of obesity can be summarized as an imbalance between energy intake and energy expenditure over a prolonged period of time [1], with the consequent storage of excess energy in the form of triacyl-glycerol within tissues, primarily but not exclusively the adipose one. But the more we learn about obesity, the more we understand that the factors behind it are complex and that identifying some risk factors as most frequently associated with obesity development (such as parental obesity, wrong birth-weight, low rate of breastfeeding, frequent TV viewing, and low SES [33]) does not exhaust the topic. Genetics has been blamed for impacting obesity development and explains 40 to 60% of the probability to become obese, but, according to the Harvard's School of Public Health [34] "Genes Are Not Destiny", and some findings [35] risk misleading the focus on the whole problem by underscoring the importance of controlling the environment, since almost everything looks like it is already decided. Excluding the forms of obesity caused by mutations in a single gene (the so-called monogenic obesities[1]) and the genetic syndromes caused either by mutations in non-obesity-related genes or by chromosomal abnormalities (also known as secondary obesities)[2] – all of them explaining 5 to 10% of all cases – the so-

[1] At least 8 susceptibility genes identified until now are responsible for rare monogenic forms of non-syndromic obesity, i.e. weight gain with no other clinical symptoms: brain-derived neurotrophic factor (BDNF), leptin (LEP), leptin receptor (LEPR), melanocortin-4 receptor (MC4R), neurotrophic tyrosine kinase receptor type 2 (NTRK2), prohormone convertase 1 (PCSK1), proopiomelanocortin (POMC), and single-minded homolog 1 (SIM1) [36]. All the proteins they code have an integration role of peripheral and neuronal signals through the hypothalamic leptin/melanocortin pathway, thus being responsible for maintaining the homeostasis of energy balance.

[2] About 30 susceptibility genes are probably responsible for rare monogenic forms of syndromic obesity. The best-known examples are: Prader-Willi, Bardet-Biedl, Alstrom, Carpenter, Rubinstein–Taybi, and Cohen syndromes. General features of syndromic obesity are: extreme adiposity, short stature and other physical dysmorphologies, mental retardation, reproductive anomalies, and undefined neuroendocrine abnormalities. These may be responsible for dysfunction of the hypothalamus, the brain appetite centre regulating energy balance, making children with syndromic obesity usually characterized with severe hyperphagia and diminished satiety, which both promotes weight gain.

called "common" obesity represents the vast majority of cases, and is influenced by possibly hundreds of genes.

All the evidences from animal models, twin studies, human linkage studies, and association studies of large populations suggest that our susceptibility to obesity has a genetic component acting in a polygenic way. The twin studies were among the first tools used to find out this genetic component, the oldest of them dating back to 1956 (the Hereditary Abilities Study, started in 1952 on monozygous and dizygous twins [37]); its results were consistent with other studies reported over 20 years later, and indicated a high heritability of body weight among monozygous and dizygous twins. Maes et al. [38] reports the study based on more than 25,000 twin pairs and 50,000 biological and adoptive family members, where a strong correlation (0.74) was found between the values of BMI in monozygotic twins, while the correlation attenuated along the supposedly reduced number of shared genes (with a minimum of 0.06 for adoptive relatives). Although suggesting a strong genetic influence on BMI, all these studies gave no clues about which genes were involved.

Based on the widely accepted hypothesis of "common disease, common variant", stating that genetic risk for common diseases is due to alleles of high frequency, many years later researchers started to use a different tool (the genome-wide association study, GWAS) aimed to identify those minuscule DNA variations, called "gene variants" or "single-nucleotide polymorphisms" by scanning thousands of individuals' complete DNA strands. However, after discovering the first two obesity-related gene variants, one in the so-called "fat mass and obesity-associated" (FTO) gene, on chromosome 16 [39, 40], and the second one close to the gene for melanocortin-4 receptor, on chromosome 18, [41], more than 35 "candidate genes", distributed through 16 chromosomes, and associated with BMI, have been identified until now [42-44]. Unlike genes contributing to monogenic forms of childhood obesity, genes possibly contributing to common obesity have small to modest phenotypic effect. After identifying hundreds of different variants associated with common diseases, those variants in combination accounted for only a small proportion of the estimated percentage of body fat (0.14-0.33% of body fat per risk allele). The FTO is the most promising, probably most widespread, and first identified as a candidate susceptibility gene. Not even it can explain more than a small part of the gene-related propensity to obesity [45]. Most likely, common obesity susceptibility genes function in an additive way to promote positive energy balance resulting in weight gain. It has therefore been hypothesized that children possessing this kind of susceptibility genes associated with early-onset obesity and body fat percentage either possess more than the average number of such genetic factors and/or they may enhance the phenotypic expression of other common obesity susceptibility genes [46].

Anyway, the case-control GWAS allowed to identify 5 obesity susceptibility genes (FTO, MC4R, MAF, NPC1, PTER) for early-onset (less than 6 years of age) and morbid-adult obesity [46]; more recent meta-analysis of several case-control GWAS, collecting about 40,000 individuals, has determined that three of these genes (FTO, MC4R, NPC1) are also associated with body fat percentage in children and adults [47, 48].

A conclusion of all the studies reported is that it cannot be denied that the genetic pool our parents provided us may have strong consequences not only on our physical aspect but on our physical shape as well.

This seems to confirm that "destiny" is ruling whether one person will become and stay lean or fat, and that choosing the right couple of parents would be – if possible – a nice way to start life.

On the other hand, and in spite of the unexpressed hopes and faith by geneticists, it is easy to understand that we cannot elucidate the rapid spread of obesity all around the world in terms of (classical) genetic changes. Genes tend to remain quite stable, and a new mutation or polymorphism needs a long time to spread around. Instead, what has dramatically changed in a few generations is our environment [49]: whilst it takes one million year to have a DNA mutation rate of just 0.5% (which means that in about 10,000 years of known history only 0.05% of our genome has changed), in just one century and especially over the last 40-50 years we have faced striking changes of our lifestyle, including our eating behaviours and styles. It is quite obvious that changes in the physical, social, political, and economic environment will affect what and how much, and even where, we eat as well as how active we are.

What we are starting to understand is that environment can be as powerful as genetics, and sometimes even more powerful, or at least quicker than genetics. We have already learned that the unique genetic pool of any individual (the so-called genome) can be regarded as a whole, and the study of the global properties of genomes is what an entirely new branch of biology, the so-called genomics, does. We are learning that the total set of environmental present and past factors that affect the state, and in particular the disease state, of an organism can also be seen as a whole, the envirome. The study of the environmental components and of their effects is termed enviromics. One of the first things this new discipline taught us about overweight is that an obesity-susceptible genome will not express its potentiality when exposed to a restrictive envirome (such as during famine or a war), but will do so when subject to a more favourable and less restrictive one; in other terms, enviromics tells us that exists something like an "obesogenic environment" [50, 51, 52], in which both the external and the internal milieus can be included, and that such an environment is able to forge our body, sometimes in overt and easy-to-detect ways, most often though in more subtle ones, still not completely understood. It is easy to realize that the comprehension of the ways and pathways involved will throw an entirely new light on the prevention of overweight and obesity.

The work on obesity-related interactions genome-envirome is still at the very beginning, although evidence achieved so far suggests that genetic predisposition is not destiny, and many people carrying "obesity genes" do not become overweight [34]. On one side, it seems that eating a healthy diet and getting enough exercise may counteract some of the gene-related obesity risk; on the other side, the researches on the relationship among at least one of the obesity-related genes (FTO), physical activity, and the outcome "obesity" yielded contradictory results [53, 54, 55]. To reach a more definitive answer, investigators recently meta-analyzed data from 45 studies in adults and 9 studies in children [55], finding that people who carried the FTO gene variant had a 23% higher risk of obesity than those who did not, but also that being physically active lowered such a risk.

The current external obesogenic environment has made it easier for people to overeat and for children to be overfed, and harder for everybody to get enough physical activity and to become less sedentary. All of this plays a key role in triggering the relatively recent raise of paediatric obesity and helping to transform it into the most dangerous non-transmittable epidemics, also known under the name of "globesity" [56].

What is the so-called external obesogenic envirome exactly made of? A non-exhaustive list that includes aspects important for children and adolescents might comprise lifestyles, school habits, eating behaviours, sedentariness and organized physical activities, peer group influence, marketing adverts, mass-medias, family, rhythms and timing of everyday life. Geographical and orographical characteristics are not often included in the list: they are considered as unmodifiable features, even though this is not completely true. Orography can be changed, and actually has been; and geographical position can be changed, or, even if unchanged, somehow modified or counterbalanced by human beings' activities (think, e.g., of temperature control).

A first consideration to be made is that envirome is very similar to genome. It is unique for any person, even though it is made of the same essential components, but the weight of each element composing the puzzle can vary from person to person. The same can be said about the number of nodes that mark the distance between one person and one single element of the environment, thus giving sometimes the impression that one or more elements are missing, or that they are ineffective or unimportant to a single person. A second general consideration is that the "spin" of certain envirome's components may be different according to the general context. There is some evidence that this might be reasonably true for SES, for instance: depending on the macroeconomic environment of a country and on its general cultural background, SES seems to play a different role, with a high one being protective in more developed and richer countries, but obesogenic in less developed and poorer ones [20, 26, 28, 29, 30, 57]. Nonetheless, some single factors are more or less strictly interrelated, even though their effect seems to depend on their positive or negative value, and on the influence of other factors: in families with lower SES the presence of obesity among parents is a negative prognostic marker, while its absence seems to be a protective factor, independently from SES [58].

A logical consequence from these examples – but many more can be easily found in the literature – is that we should always bear in mind that there is an ample number of environmental factors involved, with an even ampler number of interrelations; thinking singularly of each or a few of them may be useful for academic or research's purposes, but does not reflect reality. This is what comes out already from Sørensen in 1992, many years before the idea itself of envirome was proposed [59].

Another essential concept proposed by enviromics is that social (i.e. environmental) policies and processes build a causative network of obesity in which different levels can be recognized: one closer to the individual, such as home and work or school (for children, this includes family, school activities, school hours, school foods), another one at community level (such as public transport facilities, manufactured foods, health care system), a third one at regional or national level (all the policy activities, like those involving education, health, transport, or food), and finally an international one (which includes globalization of the market and development) [60]. The all-inclusive network has probably more strength than we can imagine. This seems to be the most likely explanation for the conflicting results systematic reviews of the literature provide as to effectiveness of preventive lifestyle interventions for childhood obesity. Recent and less recent meta-analyses of prevention programs aimed to pre-school children, school children, and adolescents [61, 62, 63] show sometimes the effectiveness of such programmes, other times a short-term usefulness, or limited to certain ages, other times again a lack of positive results. The uncertainty of these results makes the enticement from JR Speakman [64] even more seductive: "addressing the genetic side of the (gene-environment) interaction is potentially a far more tractable problem than addressing the environmental component by reengineering society, because the level at which interventions might ultimately be made is the individual rather than the society as a whole".

As stated before, referring to an external obesogenic environment means that an internal one must exist as well. Until some years ago, we would have set aside the genetic pool as it is referred to by classical genetics, since this is something that cannot be changed by human intervention, which is somehow in contrast with the principles of enviromics. But the general picture has changed quite a lot recently, and we have started to understand that, although the genes' pool can only be changed by hazard at conception, heritability of body weight and its interaction with environmental factors may occur through "epigenetic" mechanisms. The branches of genetics studying such mechanisms are referred to as "epigenetics" and "epigenomics", and are generally defined as the study of meiotically and/or mitotically heritable/non-heritable changes which affect gene expression or function without modifying the DNA sequence [65]. Epigenetic mechanisms can be considered as mediators between environment and genome.

First, studies on this field have suggested that epigenetic adaptation through increased or decreased methylation of nucleotide bases (primarily cytosine?), together with more generalized histone modifications, could alter the transcription of genes involved in the regulation of energy balance [66, 67]. Other researches then hinted that the methylation status of several genes involved in metabolic or endocrine function results from dietary changes during prenatal or early postnatal life [68, 69], and may be associated with childhood or adulthood adiposity. In mice it has been shown that most of these interactions are short-term ones: methylation patterns are mostly erased and re-established during pre-implantation development and a reprogramming of the genome also happens during the germ-cell maturation, with old epigenetic patterns cleared and replaced by gametespecific ones [70]. But the efficiency of the epigenetic reprogramming events may be quite low for autosomal loci, i.e. most of our genome. Apparently, epigenetic marks may not always be completely erased from the genome in every cell during both gametogenesis and embryogenesis.

This will give as a result that cells of a tissue in a single person can be epigenetically (i.e. functionally) a mosaic, even though their DNA sequence is identical.

The fact that genes involved in metabolic or endocrine function can be epigenetically modified through nutritional changes in the prenatal or early postnatal life seems to be a particularly important risk factor for children: it actually implies that mother's wrong nutritional habits already during pregnancy (and possibly even before, going a few generations back) are likely to affect the future health and outcomes of people. Punning on the already quoted statement made by the School of Public Health in Harvard [34], "Genes Are Not Destiny", we might say: "Genes Are Not Destiny …but Epi-genes Probably Are".

All the same, the definitive role of epigenome-envirome interactions in relation to obesity remains controversial. This partly happens because of the classical chicken and egg situation: does epigenetic modification cause obesity, or does obesity cause epigenetic modification? But it has also to be considered central importance of certain DNA sequences at particular loci. This may lead to a meaningful clinical application of epigenetics to obesity prevention and/or treatment, which is still far beyond our current possibility and knowledge [65].

There is at least one more component of our internal envirome linking it to both genes and elements of the external environment (such as family and food), the role of which we are starting to become aware of: gut microbiota, i.e. the population of bacteria populating our gastrointestinal apparatus. We are in equilibrium, or disequilibrium with such a component depending on the situation. This is not a small part of us, actually, considering that it accounts for 90% of the total number of cells of our body. Bacteroidetes (e.g. Bacteroides), Firmicutes (Clostridium and Lactobacillus, i.a.), Actinobacteria (like Bifidobacterium), Proteobacteria (the well known Escherichia coli), and Verrucomicrobia are the predominant, yet non exclusive, species of the human colonic microbiota [71].

In the last years, many researches in different fields have started to disclose nature, origins, and effects of the symbiosis between gut microbiota and human body. Due to the novelty and freshness of the findings brought by these studies, it is still quite difficult to give specific details about the reciprocal effects of microbiota, quality of food, body weight, and several pathologic conditions, but clues are accumulating that the linkage is even stricter than we thought.

For a start, bacterial catabolites may act as a triggering factor, linking high-fat diet-induced obesity to inflammation in diverse tissues, such as liver, fat tissue, muscle, etc., possibly via increased expression of Toll-like receptor 4 (TLR4) and other receptors, as well as increased TNFα, inducible nitric oxide synthases (iNOS), IL-6, and other metabolites' expression [72, 73, 74]. Evidence suggests that a high-fat diet promotes inflammation in the gastrointestinal tract through the metabolites produced by microbiota [75], so this can be considered as another potential source of inflammation associated with high-fat diet-induced obesity [76].

The conviction that normal non-pathogenic gut microbiota is the pivot of diet-induced inflammation with a key role in the development of adiposity [77] comes from experimental medicine. Germ-free mice have less body fat, and do not become obese when fed a high-fat diet [78], but once conventionalized with a normal microbiota increase in body fat, following a raise in the ileal TNFα levels. These results enhance the possibility that dysbiosis, i.e. a deviation from the normal development of microbiota, and increased inflammation by high-fat diet can play an important role in the onset of obesity and obesity-related metabolic diseases. Beside the role of microbiota in inflammation, its composition can also either shape a healthy immune response or predispose to disease: specific polymorphisms, acting together with diet and physical activity, with the possible modulation by diverse medical practices like vaccines, antibiotics and hygiene are likely to cause dysbiosis; this, in turn, may alter the outcome of immune development [79]. This is in line with the findings that the composition of gut microflora in obese subjects differs from that in lean people, with Bacteroidetes being prevalent here vs. Firmicutes being more widely represented among obese subjects; it has also been shown that gut microbiota composition among overweight adolescents can be changed when energy intake is restricted and physical activity improved [80], thus reinforcing the idea that gut microbiota composition is probably more important to achieve weight loss than expected.

More aspects remain to be disclosed in this field, and some of them are of specific interest as risk factors for childhood obesity. It could be important to know, for instance, to what extent the family microbiota composition influences the one of the children living in the same family; how early such influence starts; if trying to change the composition of gut flora in the obese child would be enough, or rather it should be accompanied by a similar attempt in the whole family.

Another controversial hypothesis that links the internal with the external environments is the old "thrifty gene hypothesis" [81]. In brief, it says that certain groups of people with hunter-gatherer evolutionary lifestyles may have experienced repeated periods of feast and famine, which, through adaptation, would have resulted in the natural selection of thrifty genes, thereby eventually predisposing these population's groups to chronic diseases of civilization such as obesity and diabetes. The thrifty genes would encode proteins involved in maintaining energy balance, e.g. the conversion of food calories into fat in the feasting periods, to be used as an energy source during fasting periods. A key feature of the hypothesis is that the selective advantage of these gene variants becomes a disadvantage when a restrictive environment transforms into an obesogenic one [82].

The hypothesis is consistent with higher frequency gene variants interacting with environmental factors to promote weight gain among certain populations, such as the well known Pima Natives of Arizona, or among the half part of monozygotic and dizygotic twins carrying obesity susceptibility genes when they are living in an obesogenic environment (adopted family) [83], but also with the differences found among populations which are similarly susceptible to gain weight, according to their genomic traits [84].

There have been several criticisms moved across the years to the thrifty gene hypothesis [65], especially the impossibility to find convincing examples of thrifty allelic variants. Nonetheless, the hypothesis is still intriguing, especially if looked at from an epigenetic standpoint [85]. Stöger's hypothesis is that most human genotypes are equally maladjusted for westernized lifestyles. The complex trait metabolic thrift encoded by a highly connected gene network is optimized to meet fluctuating conditions of famine and abundance. According to the author, this trait would have become refractory to allelic variations through genetic canalization, even though the precise molecular mechanisms underlying such canalization are not known, yet. The most important point of his hypothesis, though, is that phenotypic differences among individuals in their tendency to develop type 2 diabetes and obesity are likely to arise from variations in programming events during critical stages of child development, according to the thrifty phenotype hypothesis, but with epigenetic mechanisms having the qualities needed for this kind of programming.

What is clear at the present time is that genes, either unaltered or epigenetically modified, interact with nutrients and the energy they carry, while the intakes of both nutrients and energy is modulated by several factors of the obesogenic envirome. Several studies suggest that sedentary behaviours (like watching TV, playing video games, doing cognitive work such as studying, listening to music, and so on), reduced physical activity, and shorter sleep duration can encourage the overconsumption of macronutrients [86-90]. Fats, above all saturated fatty acids, show not only a strong association with overweight and obesity among children, but also a correlation between their consumption at 6 months of age and body weight one year later [91, 92]. Also refined carbohydrates and their major source, sugar-sweetened beverages, are spotlighted: their increased consumption during the past decades matches quite accurately the increased prevalence of obesity among children and adults [93].

As already said, society intervention programs to fight childhood obesity traditionally focus mainly on guidelines targeted to the general population, but another new branch of genetics, the so-called "nutritional genomics", is studying what kind of gene-diet interactions may help in either prevention or treatment of childhood obesity [94-96]. Understanding these interactions can lead to both correct the paediatric population-based interventions on this aspect and adapt them to single individuals. There are accumulating proves that many susceptibility genes (e.g. FTO and MC4R) interact with, or react to, dietary fats, especially the saturated ones. The same can be said for at least three other candidate obesity susceptibility genes (ADRB2, PLIN1 and PPARG) with respect to dietary carbohydrates [65].

Again, similar connections between at least one candidate susceptibility gene (BDNF rs4923461) and proteins have been made [97]. Several authors are actually convinced that proteins, more than fats and carbohydrates, may play a pivotal role especially in determining early-onset childhood obesity, since several clues suggest that in the very early periods of life unfit protein intakes – mainly from meat and dairy foods [98] – are strictly related to BMI levels not much later in life [99,100], as well as to an earlier than usual adiposity rebound [101].

CONCLUSION

We still lack a unifying theory about risk factors and causes of childhood obesity, even though we are starting to understand that all kinds of environments (internal and external, micro- and macro-, genetic or epigenetic or acquired) are strictly linked, or at least strictly related. This is likely to be the main reason why our efforts to reduce the prevalence of childhood obesity are sometimes discouraging. Trying to modify one single risk factor without taking into consideration the whole complex network around it appears to be like the torture of Tantalus: every time we think we are closer to the core of the problem it seems to recede or becomes even more complex. This largely depends on the fact that the whole reseau of connections will change scatteringly as a consequence of a single alteration. Besides, we have just started to understand the complexity of the topic "childhood and adolescence obesity". All these elements may induce a feeling of frustration: there is always uncertainty about the efficacy of the measures adopted to tackle the epidemics.

Promising aspects rise from the study of the interactions between genome and envirome, especially between genome and food. Understanding the genetic basis of food intake and energy expenditure, i.e. energy balance variations [64] has already been a central task in the last years, but is going to stay that way for the years to come as well.

On the other side of the coin there are the different and sometimes diverging points of view of the specialties involved. Epidemiologists and geneticists have a broader, and apparently privileged, standpoint on causes and networks. This unquestionably helps to define the dimensions of the problem and the importance of the multiple risk factors involved. At the same time, clinicians and paediatricians know that the more the interventions (preventative or therapeutic) are patient-tailored, the better the individual outcome can be, and this is definitively of much greater importance in children than in adults, considering the longer life-span the formers have to cope with.

Maximal effort shall therefore be devoted, from now on, to put together the varied pieces of the puzzle composing the picture of "childhood obesity", not forgetting the thinnest of them: in the light of what we know today, they might be as important as any other piece.

ACKNOWLEDGMENT

I would like to thank my friend and colleague Margherita Caroli for her critical, yet very helpful comments on this chapter. I would also like to apologize to a great number of unquoted authors: even though relevant, their work was not cited here, or was simply addressed to through other more general papers, due to text size limitations.

REFERENCES

[1] Lakshman R., Elks C. E., Ong K. K. Childhood Obesity. Circulation. 2012; 126(14):1770-1779. Available from: http://circ.ahajournals.org/content/126/14/1770.full.pdf

[2] The N. S., Suchindran C., North K. E., Popkin B. M., Gordon-Larsen P. Association of adolescent obesity with risk of severe obesity in adulthood. *JAMA,* 2010; 304(18):2042–2047. Available from: http:// jama.jamanetwork.com/article.aspx?articleid=186874

[3] Bjorge T., Engeland A., Tverdal A., Smith G. D. Body mass index in adolescence in relation to cause-specific mortality: a follow-up of 230,000 Norwegian adolescents. *Am. J. Epidemiol.*, 2008(1); 168:30-7. Available from: http://aje.oxfordjournals.org/content/168/1/30.full.pdf

[4] Magkos F., Manios Y., Christakis G., Kafatos A. G. Age-dependent changes in body size of Greek boys from 1982 to 2002. Obesity (Silver Spring). 2006;14(2):289-294. Available from: http:// onlinelibrary.wiley.com/doi/10.1038/oby.2006.37/pdf

[5] Matusik P., Malecka-Tendera E., Klimek L. Nutritional status of Polish prebubertal children assessed by population-specific and international standards. *Acta Paediatrica*, 2007; 96(2):276-280.

[6] Ebbeling C. B., Pawlak D. B., Ludwig D. S. Childhood obesity: public-health crisis, common sense cure. *Lancet,* 2002; 360(9331):473-82. Availble from: http://www.thelancet.com/pdfs/journals/lancet/PIIS0140-6736%2802%2909678-2.pdf

[7] Ahrens W., Pigeot I., Pohlabeln H., et al. Prevalence of overweight and obesity in European children below the age of 10. *Int. J. Obesity,* 2014;38:S99-S107. Available from: http://www.nature.com/ijo/journal/ v38/n2s/pdf/ijo2014140a.pdf

[8] Wijnhoven T. M. A., van Raaij J. M. A., Spinelli A., et al. WHO European Childhood Obesity Surveillance Initiative: body mass index and level of overweight among 6–9-year-old children from school year 2007/2008 to school year 2009/2010. *BMC Public Health*, 2014; 14:806-22. Available from: http://www.biomedcentral.com/1471-2458/14/806

[9] Rolland-Cachera M. F. Childhood obesity: current definitions and recommendations for their use. *IJPO*, 2011; 6(5-6):325-31. Available from: http://informahealthcare.com/doi/pdf/10.3109/ 17477166.2011.607458

[10] Cole T. J., Bellizzi M. C., Flegal K. M., Dietz W. H. Establishing a standard definition for child overweight and obesity worldwide: international survey. *BMJ,* 2000;320:1240-3. Available from: http://www.bmj.com/content/320/7244/1240.full.pdf+html

[11] World Health Organization. Physical status: the use and interpretation of anthropometry: report of a WHO Expert Committee. Geneva: WHO Technical Report Series, No. 854; 1995. Available from: http://whqlibdoc.who.int/trs/WHO_TRS_854.pdf?ua=1

[12] Caroli M., Malecka-Tendera E., Epifani S., et al. Physical activity and play in kindergarten age children. *IJPO*, 2011; 6(S2):47-53.

[13] Botton J., Heude B., Maccario J., Ducimetière P., Charles M. A. Postnatal weight and height growth velocities at different ages between birth and 5 y and body composition in adolescent boys and girls. *Am. J. Clin. Nutr.,* 2008; 87(6):1760-8. Available from: http:// ajcn.nutrition

[14] Baird J., Fisher D., Lucas P., Kleijnen J., Roberts H., Law C. Being big or growing fast: systematic review of size and growth in infancy and later obesity. *BMJ,* 2005; 331:929-35. Available from: http:// www.bmj.com/content/bmj/331/7522/929.full.pdf

[15] Vogels N., Posthumus D. L., Mariman E. C., et al. Determinants of overweight in a cohort of Dutch children. *Am. J. Clin. Nutr.,* 2006; 84:717-724. Available from: http://ajcn.nutrition

[16] Freedman D. S., Khan L. K., Serdula M. K., Dietz W. H., Srinivasan S. R., Berenson G. S. Racial differences in the tracking of childhood BMI to adulthood. *Obes. Res*., 2005; 13(5):928-35.

[17] Lobstein T., Frelut M. L. Prevalence of overweight among children in Europe. *Obes. Rev*., 2003; 4(4):195-200. Available from: http:// www.easo.org/docs/report70.pdf

[18] Wijnhoven T. M. A., van Raaij J. M. A., Spinelli A., et al. WHO European Childhood Obesity Surveillance Initiative 2008: weight, height and body mass index in 6-9-year-old children. *Pediatr. Obes.,* 2013; 8 (2):79-97.

[19] de Onis M., Onyango A. W., Borghi E., Siyam A., Nishida C., Siekmann J. Development of a WHO growth reference for school-aged children and adolescents. *Bull. World Health Organ*., 2007; 85(9):660-7.

[20] WHO Regional Office for Europe. Health Policy for Children and Adolescents, no. 6. Social determinants of health and well-being among young people. Health behaviour in school-aged children (hbsc) study: international report from the 2009/2010 survey. WHO Regional Office for Europe, Copenhagen (DK), 2012. Available from: http://www.euro.who.int/__data/assets

[21] Ervin R. B., Ogden C. L. Trends in intake of energy and macronutrients in children and adolescents from 1999-2000 through 2009-2010. *NCHS Data Brief.,* 2013; 113:1-8. Available from: http://www.cdc.gov/nchs/ data/databriefs/db113.pdf

[22] Salanave B. Peneau S., Rolland-Cachera M. F., Hercberg S., Castetbon K. Stabilization of overweight prevalence in French children between 2000 and 2007. *Int. J. Pediatr. Obes*., 2009; 4(2):66-72.

[23] Péneau S., Salanave B., Maillard-Teyssier L., et al. Prevalence of overweight in 6- to 15-year old children in central/western France from 1996 to 2006: trends toward stabilization. *Int. J. Obesity*, 2009; 33:401-7. Available from: http:// www.nature.com/ijo/journal/v33/n4/pdf/ ijo200931a.pdf

[24] Lissner L., Sohlström A., Sundblom E., Sjöberg A. Trends in overweight and obesity in Swedish schoolchildren 1999-2005: has the epidemic reached a plateau? *Obes. Rev*., 2010; 11(8):553-9.

[25] ISS. [An aye to health: National data 2012]. [homepage on the Internet]. c2013 https://www.okkioallasalute.it/?q=node/74. Italian. Available from: http:// www.epicentro.iss.it/okkioallasalute/pdf/OKkio%20alla%20SALUTE%20sintesi%202012_finale_14marzo2013aggiornata.pdf

[26] Ogden C. L., Carroll M. D., Kit B. K., Flegal K. M. Prevalence of Childhood and Adult Obesity in the United States, 2011-2012. *JAMA,* 2014; 311(8):806-14. Available from: http://jama.jamanetwork.com/ article.aspx?articleid=1832542

[27] Finucane M. M., Stevens G. A., Cowan M. J., et al. National, regional, and global trends in body-mass index since 1980: systematic analysis of health examination surveys and epidemiological studies with 960 country-years and 9·1 million participants. *Lancet,* 2011; 377(9765): 557-67.

[28] WHO Regional Office for Europe. Health Policy for Children and Adolescents, no. 5.Inequalities in young people's health. Health behaviour in school-aged children: international report from the 2005/2006 survey. WHO Regional Office for Europe, Copenhagen (DK), 2008. Available from: http://www.euro.who.int/__data/assets

[29] Direction de la Recherche, des Etudes, de l'Evaluation et des Statistiques (DREES), Ministère de la Santé. [Young people, their relationship with health, and their health status. Eating, or feeding themselves? Overweight, obesity and body image.] In: [Health status of French population. Publication of the objects added to the Act on public health: report 2009-2010.] [document on the Internet] Paris (F), 2010; p. 33-35. French. Available from: http://www.ladocumentationfrancaise.fr/var/ storage

[30] Sundblom E., Petzold M., Rasmussen F., Callmer E., Lissner L. Childhood overweight and obesity prevalence levelling off in Stockholm but socioeconomic differences persist. *Int. J. Obes.*, 2008; 32(10):1525-30. Available from: http://www. nature.com/ijo/journal/v32/n10/pdf/ ijo2008104a.pdf

[31] Pan L., Blanck H. M., Sherry B., Dalenius K., Grummer-Strawn L. M. Trends in the Prevalence of Extreme Obesity Among US Preschool-Aged Children Living in Low-Income Families, 1998-2010. *JAMA,* 2012;.308(24):2563-5. Available from: http://jama.jamanetwork.com/ article.aspx?articleid=1487493

[32] Serdula M. K., Ivery D., Coates R. J., Freedman D. S., Williamson D. F., Byers T. Do obese children become obese adults? A review of the literature. *Prev. Med.*, 1993; 22(2):167–177.

[33] Roditis M. L., Parpalani E. S., Tzotzas T., Hassapidou M., Krassas G. E. Epidemiology and predisposing factors of obesity in Greece: from the second world war until today. *J. Ped. Endocrin. Met.*, 2009; 22(5):389-405.

[34] Harvard's School of Public Health. Genes Are Not Destiny [homepage on the Internet] 2014. Available from: http://www.hsph.harvard.edu/ obesity

[35] Qi Q., Chu A. Y., Kang J. H., et al. Fried food consumption, genetic risk, and body mass index: gene-diet interaction analysis in three US cohort studies. *BMJ,* 2014; 348:g1610. Available from: http:// www.bmj.com/content/348/bmj.g1610.full.pdf+html

[36] Hu F. Genetic predictors of obesity. In: Hu F, editor. Obesity Epidemiology. New York City: Oxford University Press, 2008; p. 437-60.

[37] Clarck P. J. The heritability of certain anthropometric characters as ascertained from measurements of twins. *Am. J. Hum. Genet.,* 1956; 8(1):49-54. Available from: http://www.ncbi.nlm.nih.gov/pmc/articles/ PMC1716621/pdf/ajhg00404-0054.pdf

[38] Maes H. H., Neale M. C., Eaves L. J. Genetic and environmental factors in relative body weight and human adiposity. *Behav. Genet.,* 1997; 27 (4):325-51.

[39] Frayling T. M., Timpson N. J., Weedon M. N., et al. A common variant in the FTO gene is associated with body mass index and predisposes to childhood and adult

obesity. *Science*, 2007; 316(5826):889-94. Available from: http:// www.ncbi.nlm.nih.gov/pmc/articles/ PMC2646098/pdf/nihms45574.pdf

[40] Dina C., Meyre D., Gallina S., et al. Variation in FTO contributes to childhood obesity and severe adult obesity. *Nat. Genet.,* 2007; 39(6): 724-6.

[41] Loos R. J., Lindgren C. M., Li S., et al. Common variants near MC4R are associated with fat mass, weight and risk of obesity. *Nat. Genet.,* 2008; 40(6):768-75. Available from: http://www.ncbi.nlm.nih.gov/pmc/ articles/PMC2669167/pdf/ukmss-4362.pdf

[42] Speliotes E. K., Willer C. J., Berndt S. I., et al. Association analyses of 249,796 individuals reveal eighteen new loci associated with body mass index. *Nat. Genet.,* 2010; 42(11):937-48. Available from: http:// www.ncbi.nlm.nih.gov/pmc/articles/ PMC3014648/

[43] Heid I. M., Jackson A. U., Randall J. C. Meta-analysis identifies 13 novel loci associated with waist–hip ratio and reveals sexual dimorphism in the genetic basis of fat distribution. *Nat. Genet.*, 2010;42(11):949-60. Available from: http:// www.ncbi.nlm.nih.gov/pmc/articles/ PMC3000924/

[44] Garver W. S., Newman S. B., Gonzales-Pacheco D. M., et al. The genetics of childhood obesity and interaction with dietary macronutrients. *Genes Nutr.,* 2013; 8(3):271-87. Available from: http:// www.ncbi.nlm.nih.gov/pmc/articles/PMC3639324/pdf/ 12263_2013_Article_339.pdf

[45] Walley A. J., Asher J. E., Froguel P. The genetic contribution to non-syndromic human obesity. *Nat. Rev. Genet.*, 2009; 10(7):431-42.

[46] Meyre D., Delplanque J., Chevre J. C., et al. Genome-wide association study for early-onset and morbid adult obesity identifies three new risk loci in European populations. *Nat. Genet.,* 2009;41(2):157-9. doi: 10.1038/ ng.301. Epub 2009 Jan 18. Also available in http://www.nature.com/ng/journal/v41/n2/pdf/ng.301.pdf

[47] Kilpeläinen T. O., Qi L., Brage S., et al. Physical activity attenuates the influence of FTO variants on obesity risk: a meta-analysis of 218,166 adults and 19,268 children. *PLoS Med.,* 2011; 8(11):e1001116. doi:10.1371/journal.pmed.1001116. Epub 2011 Nov 1. Available from: http://www.plosmedicine.org/article/ fetchObject.action?uri=info%3Adoi%2F10.1371%2Fjournal.pmed.1001116&representation=PDF

[48] den Hoed M., Luan J., Langenberg C., et al. Evaluation of common genetic variants identified by GWAS for early onset and morbid obesity in population-based samples. *Int. J. Obes.,* 2013;37(2):191-6. doi: 10.1038/ijo.2012.34. Epub 2012 Mar 20. Available from: http:// www.ncbi.nlm.nih.gov/pmc/articles/PMC3680864/pdf/emss-53282.pdf

[49] Perrone L., Miraglia Del Giudice E. [Genetic Aspects]. In: Iughetti L., Bernasconi S., editors. [Obesity in paediatric age]. Milano: McGraw Hill Education Italy, 2005; p. 46-57. Italian.

[50] Egger G., Swinburn B. An "ecological" approach to the obesity pandemic. *BMJ,* 197;315(7106): 477-80. Available from: http:// www.ncbi.nlm.nih.gov/pmc/articles/ PMC2127317/

[51] Ravussin E., Bouchard C. Human genomics and obesity: finding appropriate drug targets. *Eur. J. Pharmacol.,* 2000; 410(2-3):131-45. Available from: http:// www.sciencedirect.com/science

[52] Qi L., Cho Y. A. Gene-environment interaction and obesity. *Nutr. Rev.,* 2008; 66:684-94. Available from: http://www.ncbi.nlm.nih.gov/pmc/ articles/PMC3683966/

[53] Rampersaud E., Mitchell B. D., Pollin T. I., et al. Physical activity and the association of common FTO gene variants with body mass index and obesity. *Arch. Intern. Med.*, 2008; 168(16):1791-7. Available from: http://www.ncbi.nlm.nih.gov/pmc/articles/PMC3635949/

[54] Ruiz J. R., Labayen I., Ortega F. B., et al. Attenuation of the effect of the FTO rs9939609 polymorphism on total and central body fat by physical activity in adolescents: the HELENA study. *Arch. Pediatr. Adolesc. Med.*, 2010; 164(4):328-33. Available from: http:// archpedi.jamanetwork.com/article.aspx?articleid=383015

[55] Jonsson A., Renstrom F., Lyssenko V., et al. Assessing the effect of interaction between an FTO variant (rs9939609) and physical activity on obesity in 15,925 Swedish and 2,511 Finnish adults. *Diabetologia,* 2009; 52(7):1334-8. Available from: http://download.springer.com/static/pdf/ 315/art%253A10.1007%252Fs00125-009-1355-2.pdf?auth66=1418808994_9c20529934b72ac2ed1e9303d49e5fd0&ext=.pdf

[56] World Health Organization. Obesity: Preventing and Managing the Global Epidemic. Report of a WHO consultation on obesity. Geneva, 1997, June 3-5. *World Health Organ Tech. Rep. Ser.,* 2000; 894:i-xii,1-253. Available from: http://apps.who.int/iris

[57] Due P., Damsgaard M. T., Rasmussen M., et al. Socioeconomic position, macroeconomic environment and overweight among adolescents in 35 countries. *Int. J. Obes.*, 2009; 33(10):1084-93. Available from: http:// www.nature.com/ijo/journal/v33/n10/pdf/ijo2009128a.pdf

[58] Semmler C., Ashcroft J., van Jaarsveld C. H. M., Carnell S., Wardle J. Development of Overweight in Children in Relation to Parental Weight and Socioeconomic Status. *Obesity*, 2009; 17(4):814-20. Available from: http://onlinelibrary.wiley.com/doi/10.1038/oby.2008.621/pdf

[59] Lissau-Lund-Sørensen I., Sørensen T. I. Prospective study of the influence of social factors in childhood on risk of overweight in young adulthood. *Int. J. Obes. Relat. Metab. Disord.*, 1992; 16(3):169-75.

[60] Kumanyika S., Jeffery R. W., Morabia A., Ritenbaugh C., Antipatis V. J. Obesity prevention: the case for action. *Int. J. Obes.*, 2002; 26(3):425-36. Available from: http://www.bvsde.paho.org/texcom/cd050644/ kumanyik.pdf

[61] Ho M., Garnett S. P., Baur L., et al. Effectiveness of lifestyle interventions in child obesity: systematic review with meta-analysis. *Pediatrics,* 2012; 130(6):e1647. doi: 10.1542/peds.2012-1176. Available from: http://pediatrics.aappublications.org/content/130/6/e1647.full.pdf

[62] Waters E., de Silva-Sanigorski A., Hall B. J., et al. Interventions for preventing obesity in children. *Cochrane Database Syst. Rev.,* 2011; (12):CD001871. doi: 10.1002/14651858.CD001871.pub3. Available from: http://www.scielo.br/pdf/spmj/v132n2/1516-3180-spmj-132-02-00128.pdf

[63] Miller W. C., Koceja D. M., Hamilton E. J. A meta-analysis of the past 25 years of weight loss research using diet, exercise or diet plus exercise intervention. *Int. J. Obes.,* 1997; 21(10):941-7. Available from: http://www.iub.edu/~k562/articles/obesity

[64] Speakman J. R. Obesity: the integrated roles of environment and genetics. *J. Nutr.*, 2004; 134(8 Suppl.):2090S–2105S. Available from: http://jn.nutrition

[65] Garver W. S., Newman S. B., Gonzales-Pacheco D. M., et al. The genetics of childhood obesity and interaction with dietary macronutrients. *Genes Nutr.,* 2013; 8:271-87.

Available from: http:// www.ncbi.nlm.nih.gov/pmc/articles/PMC3639324/pdf/ 12263_2013_Article_339.pdf

[66] Russo P., Lauria F., Siani A. Heritability of body weight: moving beyond genetics. *Nutr. Metabol. Cardio. Dis.*, 2010; 20(10):691-7.

[67] Herrera B. M., Keildson S., Lindgren C. M. Genetics and epigenetics of obesity. *Maturitas,* 2011; 69(1):41-9. Available from: http:// www.ncbi.nlm.nih.gov/pmc/ articles/PMC3213306/

[68] Tobi E. W., Lumey L. H., Talens R. P., et al. DNA methylation differences after exposure to prenatal famine are common and timingand sex-specific. *Hum. Mol. Genet.*, 2009; 18(21):4046-53. Available from: http://www.ncbi.nlm.nih.gov/pmc/ articles/PMC2758137/pdf/ddp353.pdf

[69] Godfrey K. M., Sheppard A., Gluckman P. D., et al. Epigenetic gene promoter methylation at birth is associated with child's later adiposity. *Diabetes,* 2011; 60(5):1534. Available from: http:// www.ncbi.nlm.nih.gov/pmc/articles/PMC3115550/ pdf/1528.pdf

[70] Wells J. C. The thrifty phenotype as an adaptive maternal effect. *Biol. Rev. Camb. Philos. Soc.,* 2007; 82(1):143-72. Available from: http://onlinelibrary.wiley.com/doi/ 10.1111/j.1469-185X.2006.00007.x/ pdf

[71] Chassard C., Lacroix C. Carbohydrates and the human gut microbiota. *Curr. Opin. Clin. Nutr. Metab. Care,* 2013; 16(4):453-60. doi: 10.1097/ MCO.0b013e3283619e63

[72] Ghanim H., Abuaysheh S., Sia C. L., et al. Increase in plasma endotoxin concentrations and the expression of Toll-like receptors and suppressor of cytokine signaling-3 in mononuclear cells after a high-fat, high-carbohydrate meal: implications for insulin resistance. *Diabetes Care,* 2009; 32(12):2281-87. doi: 10.2337/dc09-0979. Available from: http:// www.ncbi.nlm.nih.gov/pmc/articles/PMC2782991/pdf/zdc2281.pdf

[73] Weisberg S. P., McCann D., Desai M., et al. Obesity is associated with macrophage accumulation in adipose tissue. *J. Clin. Invest.,* 2003; 112(12):1796-1808. doi: 10.1172/jci19246. Available from: http://www.ncbi.nlm.nih.gov/pmc/ articles/ PMC296995/pdf/JCI0319246.pdf

[74] Cancello R., Tordjman J., Poitou C., et al. Increased infiltration of macrophages in omental adipose tissue is associated with marked hepatic lesions in morbid human obesity. *Diabetes,* 2006; 55(6):1554-61. doi: 10.2337/db06-0133. Available from: http:// diabetes

[75] Ding S., Chi M. M., Scull B. P., et al. High-fat diet: bacteria interactions promote intestinal inflammation which precedes and correlates with obesity and insulin resistance in mouse. *PLoS One*, 2010; 5(8):e12191. doi: 10.1371/journal.pone.0012191. Available from: http:// www.ncbi.nlm.nih.gov/pmc/articles/PMC2922379/pdf/ pone.0012191.pdf

[76] de La Serre C. B., Ellis C. L., Lee J., et al. Propensity to high-fat diet-induced obesity in rats is associated with changes in the gut microbiota and gut inflammation. *Am. J. Physiol. Gastrointest. Liver Physiol.,* 2010; 299(2):G440-8. doi: 10.1152/ ajpgi.00098.2010. Available from: http:// www.ncbi.nlm.nih.gov/pmc/articles/ PMC2928532/

[77] Backhed F., Ding H., Wang T., et al. The gut microbiota as an environmental factor that regulates fat storage. *Proc. Natl. Acad. Sci. U S A,* 2004; 101(44):15718-23. doi:

10.1073/pnas.0407076101. Available from: http://www.ncbi.nlm.nih.gov/pmc/articles/PMC524219/pdf/pnas-0407076101.pdf

[78] Backhed F., Manchester J. K., Semenkovich C. F., Gordon J. I. Mechanisms underlying the resistance to diet-induced obesity in germ-free mice. *Proc. Natl. Acad. Sci. U S A*, 2007; 104(3):979-84. doi: 10.1073/pnas.0605374104. Available from: http://www.ncbi.nlm.nih.gov/pmc/articles/PMC1764762/pdf/zpq979.pdf

[79] Marcos A. [Food science and technology for our small tenants]. Round-table presentation at: [4th Workshop on Probiotics, Prebiotics and Health: Scientific evidence]; 2013 Jan. 31-Feb. 1; Spain. Spanish.

[80] Santacruz A., Marcos A., Wärnberg J., et al. Interplay between weight loss and gut microbiota composition in overweight adolescents. *Obesity,* (Silver Spring). 2009; 17(10):1906-15. doi: 10.1038/oby.2009.112. Epub 2009 Apr 23. Available from: http://onlinelibrary.wiley.com/doi/ 10.1038/oby.2009.112/pdf

[81] Neel J. V. Diabetes mellitus: a "thrifty" genotype rendered detrimental by "progress"? *Am. J. Hum. Genet.,* 1962; 14(4):353-62. Available from: http:// www.ncbi.nlm.nih.gov/pmc/articles/PMC1932342/pdf/ajhg00558-0047.pdf

[82] Neel J. V. The "thrifty genotype" in 1998. *Nutr. Rev.*, 1999; 57(5 Pt. 2):S2–S9. Available from: http://deepblue.lib.umich.edu/bitstream/ handle/2027.42/74010/j.1753-4887.1999.tb01782.x.pdf?sequence=1

[83] Silventoinen K., Rokholm B., Kaprio J., Sorensen T. I. A. The genetic and environmental influences on childhood obesity: a systematic review of twin and adoption studies. *Int. J. Obes.*, 2010; 34(1):29-40. doi: 10.1038/ijo.2009.177. Epub 2009 Sep 15. Available from: http:// www.nature.com/ijo/journal/v34/n1/full/ijo2009177a.html

[84] Casazza K., Hanks L. J., Beasley M., Fernandez J. R. Beyond thriftiness: independent and interactive effects of genetic and dietary factors on variations in fat disposition and distribution across populations. *Am. J. Phys. Anthro.,* 2011; 145(2):181-91. doi: 10.1002/ajpa.21483. Epub 2011 Mar 1. Available from: http:// www.ncbi.nlm.nih.gov/pmc/ articles/PMC3099307/pdf/nihms288256.pdf

[85] Stöger R. The thrifty epigenotype: an acquired and heritable predisposition for obesity and diabetes? *Bioessays*, 2008; 30(2):156-66. doi: 10.1002/bies.20700. Available from: http://onlinelibrary.wiley.com/ doi/10.1002/bies.20700/pdf

[86] Graves L., Stratton G., Ridgers N. D., Cable N. T. Energy expenditure in adolescents playing new generation computer games. *Br. J. Sports Med.,* 2008; 42(7):592-4. Available from: http://bjsm.bmj.com/content/42/7/ 592.full.pdf+html

[87] Chaput J. P., Drapeau V., Poirier P., Teasdale N., Tremblay A. Glycemic instability and spontaneous energy intake: association with knowledge-based work. *Psychosom. Med.,* 2008; 70(7):797-804. doi: 10.1097/ PSY.0b013e31818426fa. Epub 2008 Aug. 25.

[88] Stroebele N., de Castro J. M. Listening to music while eating is related to increases in people's food intake and meal duration. *Appetite,* 2006; 47(3):285–289. Epub 2006 May 24. Available from: http:// www.sciencedirect.com/science

[89] Temple J. L., Giacomelli A. M., Kent K. M., Roemmich J. N., Epstein L. H. Television watching increases motivated responding for food and energy intake in children. *Am. J. Clin. Nutr.*, 2007; 85(2):355-61. Available from: http://ajcn.nutrition

[90] Westerlund L., Ray C., Roos E. Associations between sleeping habits and food consumption patterns among 10–11-year-old children in Finland. *Br. J. Nutr.,* 2009;

102(10):1531-7. doi: 10.1017/ S0007114509990730. Epub 2009 Aug. 7. Available from:https://www.researchgate.net/publication/26726185_Associations_between_sleeping_habits_and_food_consumption_patterns_among_10-11-year-old_children_in_Finland

[91] Aeberli I., Beljean N., Lehmann D., l'Allemand D., Spinas G. A., Zimmerman M. B. The increase of fatty acid-binding protein aP2 in overweight and obese children: interactions with dietary fat and impact on measures of subclinical inflammation. *Int. J. Obes.,* 2008; 32(10):1513-20. doi: 10.1038/ijo.2008.128. Epub 2008 Aug 5. Available from: http://www.nature.com/ijo/journal/v32/n10/pdf/ijo2008128a.pdf

[92] Lin P. H., Wang Y., Grambow S. C., Goggins W., Almirall D. Dietary saturated fat intake is negatively associated with weight maintenance among the PREMIER participants. *Obesity,* 2012; 20(3):571-5. doi: 10.1038/oby.2011.17. Epub 2011 Feb 17. Available from: http:// onlinelibrary.wiley.com/doi/10.1038/oby.2011.17/pdf

[93] Malik V. S., Popkin B. M., Bray G. A., Despres J. P., Willet W. C., Hu F. B. Sugar-sweetened beverages, and risk of metabolic syndrome and type 2 diabetes: a meta-analysis. *Diabetes Care,* 2010; 33(11):2477-83. doi: 10.2337/dc10-1079. Epub 2010 Aug. 6. Available from: http:// www.ncbi.nlm.nih.gov/pmc/articles/PMC2963518/pdf/zdc2477.pdf

[94] Hetherington M. M., Cecil J. E. Gene-environment interactions in obesity. *Forum Nutr.,* 2010;63:195-203. doi: 10.1159/000264407. Epub 2009 Nov. 27

[95] Kaput J. Diet–Disease Gene Interactions. Nutrition. 2004;20:26-31 doi: 10.1016/j.nut.2003.09.005. Available from: http://web

[96] Abumrad N. A. The gene-nutrient-gene loop. *Curr. Opin. Clin. Nutr. Metab. Care,* 2001; 4(5):407-10.

[97] Rukh G. 1., Sonestedt E., Melander O., et al. Genetic susceptibility to obesity and diet intakes: association and interaction analyses in the Malmö Diet and Cancer Study. *Genes Nutr.,* 2013;8(6):535-47. doi: 10.1007/s12263-013-0352-8. Available from: http://www.ncbi.nlm.nih.gov/pmc/articles/PMC3824829/pdf/12263_2013_ Article_352.pdf

[98] Günther A. L. B., Remer T., Kroke A., Buyken A. E. Early protein intake and later obesity risk: which protein sources at which time points throughout infancy and childhood are important for body mass index and body fat percentage at 7 y of age? *Am. J. Clin. Nutr.,* 2007; 86(6):1765-72. Available from: http://ajcn.nutrition

[99] Koletzko B., von Kries R., Monasterolo R. C., et al. Can infant feeding choices modulate later obesity risk? *Am. J. Clin. Nutr.,* 2009; 89(5): 1502S-1508S. doi: 10.3945/ajcn.2009.27113D. Available from: http:// ajcn.nutrition

[100] Rolland-Cachera M. F., Péneau S. Stabilization in the prevalence of childhood obesity: a role for early nutrition? *Int. J. Obes. (Lond.),* 2010; 34(10):1524-5. doi: 10.1038/ijo.2010.64. Epub 2010 Mar 30. Availabl from: http://www.nature.com/ijo/journal/v34/n10/full/ijo201064a.html

[101] Péneau S., Thibault H., Rolland-Cachera M. F. Massively obese adolescents were of normal weight at the age of adiposity rebound. *Obesity*, 2009; 17(7):1309-10. doi: 10.1038/oby.2009.93.

In: The Different Faces of Being Overweight
Editor: Emilia Manzato
ISBN: 978-1-63483-099-7

Chapter 6

EATING DISORDERS AND BIASED EATING BEHAVIORS AS RISK FACTORS FOR OVERWEIGHT

Emilia Manzato *

Psychiatrist, University of Ferrara, Italy
National Council Member,
Italian Society for the Study of Eating Disorder (SISDCA), Italy

ABSTRACT

Eating disorders and biased eating behavior could be risk factors leading to overweight and obesity or encouraging such as status.

In this chapter we deal particularly with binge eating disorder, the most frequent eating disorder in the overweight and obese population, because the presence of binge episodes without compensatory behaviors. Furthermore, the presence lifetime of any eating disorder (anorexia, bulimia or binge eating disorder) represents a risk factor for weight gain. We describe also night eating syndrome, a particular disorder included, for the first time, between the Eating Disorders in DSM5th in the "Other specified feeding or eating disorder" section. These eating disorders, if present, could play an important role in the development of overweight and obesity.

We describe also some other biased eating behavior such as grazing- not included in eating disorders but important because its contribution to the weight gain- and emotional eating.

They are still object of researches programs.

In the last part of the chapter we'll also deal with a particular eating behavior such as "Hyperphagia" as risk factor for overweight and obesity.

Keywords: eating disorders, binge eating disorder, bulimia, night eating syndrome, grazing, emotional eating, hyperphagia

* emilia.manzato@gmail.com.

INTRODUCTION

Disturbed eating behaviors could be an important risk factor for weight gain in normal or overweight individuals and it could also worsen obesity.

Moreover it is important to recognize eating disturbances and their psychological antecedents because in many cases weight management programs are not developed for treating symptoms of eating disturbances and consequently, dieting could have the opposite effect that is weight gain.

Obese individuals may display different eating behaviors in the absence of hunger, it is important to detect these eating behavior disturbances also in overweight and in any patient seeking treatment.

Eating disturbances range from eating disorders, such as binge eating disorders, bulimia nervosa, night eating syndrome, to altered eating behaviors such as grazing.

Currently different models can explain the different eating disturbances: the dietary restraint theory, the theory of affection regulation or the theory of food addiction.

While dieting is targeted to a concrete reduction in calories intakes by means of a real weight control procedures (i.e. the consumption of less than 1200 kcal over a minimum period of 3 days), the dietary restraint is a cognitive process raised by concerns about weight, shape, body image etc. without an effective reduction in calories intake and consequent weight loss.

Because dietary restraint could be an effect of repeated attempts of dieting, it is a common disturbed eating behavior not only in obese patients but also in overweight individuals.

In fact many overweight people tend to do specific efforts to control their weight, especially because of social pressure to thinness.

In dieting prescriptions many dietitians recommend "keeping one's diet under control" facilitating the shift from reliance on physiological cues of hunger and satiety to cognitive control over eating behavior. Studies demonstrate that the cognitive control often fails resulting in an increased risk of overeating and consequently weight gain.

Also a too rigid dieting cause distress which promotes loss of control behavior such as binge eating disorder.

Within this scope an interesting theory on dieting failures is the "Thought suppression" theory.

"Thought suppression" theory is seen as a mental control process that leads the dieting patient to a special cognitive process and describes how human brain is unable "not to think" about a forbidden food e.g. if dieting prescriptions ban chocolate the patient's brain actives trigger images of chocolate, and paradoxically promotes an unwanted behavior such as eating more snacks with chocolate. In fact in clinical setting dieting patients often refer obsessive thoughts about forbidden foods that pull them to " loss of control behavior" [1, 2].

So what should induce weight loss may end up producing weight gain!

The shift from dieting to loss of control behavior is widely treated in the chapter 3.

Another interesting theory for explaining the eating behavior in obese people is the "Food addiction" theory that consider the loss of control on food as a result of a food addiction behavior.

The theory of food addiction is widely treated in a specific chapter (see chapter 2).

In this chapter we'll describe Eating Disorders related to overweight and obesity, such as Binge Eating Disorder, Bulimia Nervosa, Night Eating Syndrome.

EATING DISORDERS

In "Diagnostic and Statistical Manual of mental Disorders" in its 5th edition (DSM 5) "Feeding and eating disorders" are defined as “disorders characterized by a persistent disturbance of eating or eating related behaviour that results in the altered consumption or absorption of food and that significantly impairs physical health or psychosocial functioning” [3]

Obesity is not included in DSM5 as a mental disorder even if it is specified that there are robust associations between obesity and a number of mental disorders especially in the mood disorders area. On the other hand, obesity may be a risk factor for the development of some mental diseases.

ED classified in DSM5 are: Anorexia Nervosa, Bulimia Nervosa, Binge Eating Disorder, Other Specified ED and Other Unspecified ED.

Literature shows strong evidence that the lifetime presence of an episode of any ED - also an episode of Anorexia Nervosa -is an important risk factor for weight gain [4, 5].

In fact, an episode of Anorexia Nervosa can commonly evolve into Bulimia Nervosa thus causing a loss of control behavior and consequently weight gain. Bulimia Nervosa is generally associated with normal weight or overweight.

Furthermore, Anorexia Nervosa and Bulimia Nervosa in the majority of the cases are preceded by dietary restrictions. In literature repeated failure of dietary restrictions are associated with weight gain and with a high risk of developing an ED even if it is claimed that weight loss dieting might be necessary but not a sufficient condition for developing an eating disorder.

The initial suggestion that dieting and weight loss cause negative psychological consequences including eating disorders and depressive symptoms came from the pioneering study by Keys et al. in 1950's [6]. Findings from this study of adverse effects of caloric restriction in normal weight individuals are often applied to those who are overweight.

In a review about dieting and the development of eating disorders in overweight and obese adults [7] the authors found that moderate caloric restriction with behavioral weight loss treatment does not seem to cause clinically significant binge eating in most overweight adults without preexisting binge eating problems.

On the other hand, weight loss treatment with concomitant dietary restriction, might trigger the development of an ED or exacerbate an ED in already affected patients.

It has been widely shown that social pressures to thinness could lead to body discomfort or body dissatisfaction also in normal weight or in mild overweight people, especially if associated with low self-esteem. Further, all these could encourage them to be engaged on dieting treatment (See chapter7).

Unfortunately, in many cases these treatments result in a temporary weight loss with a subsequent weight gain together with an increased body dissatisfaction feeling.

Furthermore, exposure to unrealistic media images and messages has been identified as a risk factor for Eating Disorders.

Given the relation between failure to meet desired society ideals and higher body dissatisfaction it is not surprise that overweight and obesity people can show depressive symptoms. So overweight people with history of dieting, restraint dietary, weight concerns and body image concerns may risk to experience- more than normal weight people- Eating Disorders and Depression disorders [8, 9]. Also overweight children show these aspects. In fact, data suggest that binge eating and its correlates- such as concerns about eating, body shape and weight- are more prevalent among overweight children than among normal weight children [10].

Many researches have focused on identifying the factors associated with the onset and maintenance of a state of obesity particularly on the presence of Binge Eating Disorder (BED) [11, 12, 13].

The presence of BED in overweight patients can be a serious risk factor for the progression to obesity. In particular, binge behaviour seems to have a direct role in weight gain in "binge first" patients, that is patients showing an unregulated food consumption prior their dieting [14].

The "binge first" group has a significantly earlier age of onset than the "diet first" group [15]. Additionally, in these individuals the use of restrictive diets is just a compensatory behaviour to prevent weight gain caused by binge eating. The subgroup of "binge first" would amount to 35-54% of patients with BED [16, 17, 18, 19]. Literature shows that obese patients with BED typically have greater psychiatric comorbidity than obese patients without BED, particularly in the area of mood and personality disorders [20, 21, 22, 23].

Psychiatric symptoms often are a barrier for compliance to weight treatment. Literature data also report that body checking behaviour, avoidance of body exposure (expression of an intense body dissatisfaction), episodes of hyperphagia or the loss of eating control, can be found in overweight patients and that may be a risk factor for the onset of ED and for obesity [24]. Attitudes about loss of eating control were studied in groups of not-treatment-seeking overweight patients, in particular in the developmental age [25]. It is important to recognize eating disturbances and their psychological antecedents in children as in many cases weight management programmes are not developed for treating symptoms of eating disturbances [26].

Research studies on adolescents show a higher frequency of abnormal attitudes and behaviours toward food in individuals who are already overweight compared to normal weight subjects. Unregulated food consumption, over eating and unhealthy eating habits to control weight are a significant threat to the physical and psychosocial wellbeing of overweight teenagers and are risk factors for further weight gain or for the development of ED [27]. Even a study on a sample of children treated for severe overweight shows that 15% had episodes of loss of control over food, even if they had not had a diagnosis of BED [28]. The overweight and obesity in children and adolescents are widely treated in the chapter 5.

BINGE EATING DISORDER

IN DSM 5TH Binge eating Disorder (BED) is characterized by :

A. Recurrent episodes of binge eating. An episode of binge eating is characterized by both of the following:

- eating, in a discrete period of time (e.g., within any 2-hour period), an amount of food that is
- definitely larger than most people would eat during a similar period of time and under similar circumstances
- a sense of lack of control over eating during the episode (e.g., a feeling that one cannot stop eating or control what or how much one is eating)

B. Binge eating episodes are associated at least with three typical features like:

1. eating much more rapidly than normal,
2. eating until feeling uncomfortably full,
3. eating large amounts of food when not feeling physically hungry,
4. eating alone because of feeling embarrassed by how much one is eating,
5. feeling disgusted with oneself, depressed or very guilty afterward

C. Marked distressed regarding binge eating is present
D. The binge eating occurs, on overage, at least during once a week for 3 months
E. The binge eating is not associated with inappropriate compensatory behaviors (e.g. purging) as in BN and does not occur exclusively during the course of bulimia nervosa or anorexia nervosa.

The BED could be in.

- "Partial Remission" if- after full criteria for BED were previously met- BE occurs at an average frequency of less than one episode per week for a sustained period of time
- "Full remission" if- after full criteria for BED were previously met- none of the criteria have been met for a sustained period of time.

In DSM 5TH the severity has been specified and the level of severity is based on the frequency of episodes of binge eating:

Mild: 1-3 binge eating episodes per week
Moderate: 4-7 binge eating episodes per week
Severe: 8-13 binge eating episodes per week
Extreme: 14 or more binge eating episodes per week.

Most Eating Disorders in overweight and obese adults involve Binge Eating Disorder, in fact the BED is the most common eating disorder seen in obesity treatment setting [29].

Results of studies from the United States indicate that the prevalence of BED in adult community samples is less than 3% [30]. The prevalence in overweight individuals is higher; the higher the BMI is the more frequent BED's are in patients.

Nevertheless it is hard to know the real percentage of BED in overweight or obese people due to the insufficient awareness about their ED's [31].

Furthermore, patients with binge eating episodes could not recognize them as real "binge eating" episodes [32].

Some authors linked this insufficient awareness about binge episodes with the lack of purging behavior as in Bulimia Nervosa. In fact, the binge/ purging episodes are more easily recalled by patients because vomiting is a strong symptom which can be identified more clearly by patients.

BED's are present also in children, in fact Binge eating episodes are reported in 9% of normal weight children and up to 36% of children who are overweight and obese [33].

In European epidemiologic studies in obese/overweight teenagers prevalence rates are around 10-24% for BED's and 9% for BN [34, 35, 36].

Binge Eating episodes are characterized by overeating, but the amount of calories intake is still unclear.

Fairburn and Cooper in 1993 [37] distinguished between objective bulimic episodes- loss of control with a large amount of food intake - and subjective bulimic episodes, loss of control with consumption of an amount of food that is not unambiguously large but is subjectively perceived as large.

Hilbert e Wilfley et al. in 2011, studied the binge size in the BED's to assess the clinical significance, the prognostic validity and the associated comorbility. The results showed that the presence of both types of episodes accounted for higher psychopathology whereas the presence of objective bulimic episodes accounted for greater body mass index [38].

In a study on a large sample, Field et al. [39] tried to investigate whether loss of control during an overeating episode could be predictive of becoming overweight or obese or predictive of binge drinking or substance abuse etc.

The "growing up today study" (GUTS) used seven follow up assessments over 9 years and recruited more than 7,200 female, at the baseline the main age of the participants was 12 years. Weight status, weight control behaviors, binge eating, binge drinking, drug use, depressive symptoms have been assessed every 12-18 months.

During 9 years of follow-up approximately 20% became overweight or obese. Binge eating increased over time as the girls aged, but the prevalence of overeating remained constant. Although binge eating was more common than overeating without loss of control, both were predictive of becoming overweight or obese over the subsequent 1-2 years.

The association was more evident with girls who engaged in binge eating at least once a week. Also girls who showed sub-threshold BED (according DSMIV) had 2, 3 times the odds of becoming overweight or obese in the next 1-2 years compared whit their peers who did not binge eat. Excessive concerns about physical shape and weight are not included in the diagnostic criteria of BED; most studies reported such concerns in overweight patients with BED, differently from non-BED overweight individuals.

A study compared features of eating disorders, psychological distress and BMI among overweight BED patients who over-value their shape /weight, overweight bed patients with subclinical levels of overvaluation and overweight non-BED comparison group [40].

The overweight BED patients over-valuing their shape/weight reported greater eating concerns and depressive symptomatology than the subclinical counterparts. Both BED groups also reported a major overall eating pathology and negative feelings in comparison with the overweight individuals without ED.

Bulimia Nervosa

Even if the most frequent ED in overweight and obesity is Binge Eating Disorder, also Bulimia Nervosa (BN) could be present in overweight patients, but it is uncommon in obese patients.

BN can be an evolution of an episode of AN, or BN can begin during or after an episode of dieting to lose weight.

Childhood overweight and obesity may be risk factors for BN [41].

BN is characterized by recurrent episodes of binge eating, recurrent inappropriate compensatory behavior to prevent weight gain and unduly influence of body shape and weight on self-evaluation. The features of binge eating episodes are the same as those described in binge eating disorder.

In DSM5 for diagnosis of BN the frequency of binge eating episodes and inappropriate behaviour is at least once per week for 3 months.

Weight status is not a diagnostic criterion for BN and DSM IV states that moderate and morbid obesity are uncommon comorbid conditions within this diagnostic group, whereas the association of BN with overweight status could be present.

Many studies have focused on the onset of BN or on the clinical features of BN, previous presence of AN or psychiatric comorbility etc. but only few studies have focused on differential weight status. Furthermore, since the publication of the DSM IV classification there has been a rapid escalation of overweight and obesity in the general population.

Mitchell and colleagues [42] found that only a small percent (4%) of patients with BN were also overweight and this subgroup differed considerably from patients with normal weight BN.

They found that the overweight BN group was older, and had less frequent binge eating and vomiting episodes.

A recent study compared BN in overweight [43] and normal weight women.

The overweight BN group reported less frequent binge eating and less restraints than normal weight BN group.

Furthermore BMI was significantly related to depression (as measured by the Beck's Depression Inventory) in the overweight BN group but not in the normal weight BN group.

Interestingly the study reported higher rate of ethnic minorities in the overweight BN group (about 29%) than the normal weight BN group (about 13%).

Night Eating Syndrome

Night Eating Syndrome (NES) was first characterized by Stunkard as one of several behavioral patterns thought to contribute to weight gain and obesity. After a long period of neglect, only recently researchers have begun to focus on night eating in efforts to understand the contribution of this disturbed eating pattern to the risk for developing overweight and obesity.

Until DSM5 Edition NES was not included in Eating Disorders section.

In the DSM5 it has been included in the "Other specified feeding or eating disorders" section and it has been defined as an eating disorder characterized by:

- Recurrent episodes of night eating, as manifested by eating after awakening from sleep or by excessive food consumption after evening meal.
- There is awareness and recall of the eating.
- The night eating is not better explained by external influences such as changes in the individual's sleep-wake cycle or by local social norms.
- The night eating causes significant distress and/or impairment in functioning.
- The disordered pattern of eating is not better explained by binge eating disorder or another mental disorder, including substance use, and is not attributable to another medical disorder or to an effect of medication".

In DSM 5, the diagnostic criteria of NES are still vague and the matter about differential diagnosis with others Eating Disorders still remains pending.

Stunkard for the first time described night eating disorder in 1955 [44] and distinguished two distinct eating patterns, night eating and binge eating, which could contribute to understanding the etiology of obesity. Although binge eating, the core feature of Bulimia Nervosa and Binge Eating Disorder, has been extensively studied, few research has been focused on NES.

Stunkard defined NES as involving morning anorexia, evening hyperphagia, and insomnia. Morning anorexia was defined as negligible (i.e. coffee or juice) or no food intake at the traditional breakfast time. Evening hyperphagia was defined as consuming at least 25% of the total daily calories intake after the evening meal. Insomnia was required to occur three or more times a week.

Since then, many various definitions of NES have been suggested, but only in 1999 a study of Birketved et al. [45] about neuro-endocrinological features of NES renewed the interest in this eating behavior.

In 2006 Strieghel-Moore [46] contended that the lack of empirical data prevent a valid diagnosis of NES, because the core features, the threshold of frequency of episodes and the duration of symptoms had not been clear defined.

But in 2008 Stunkard et al. [47] proposed again the need of a deep analysis about NES because its negative effect on treatment and outcome of obesity and overweight as well as its association with depression and anxiety.

In the First International Night Eating Symposium held in 2008 April in Minneapolis [48] the recommendations suggested to clarify some clinical features of NES, such as the calories intakes, the differential diagnosis with sleep related disorders and the identification of subtypes.

Because all these unresolved problems, NES has been included in the DSM5th edition only in the "Other Specified Eating Disorders" section.

In some studies BMI was significantly higher in patients with NES because NES was associated with increased food intake which may cause unwanted weight gain [49].

In the general population the prevalence of NES is estimated to be 1,5% and among obese patient the prevalence ranges between 6% to 16% [50].

NES amounts to 8-42% in obese patients non-responding to weight loss treatments.

NES accounts for 9.7% in diabetics patients and in such individuals it is usually associated with their poor metabolic control or severe medical complications. NES –as grazing- has been studied overall in obese patients required bariatric surgery: in these samples its presence has been estimated to be 8-42%, moreover NES appears to be more frequent among male individuals [51].

In general female population NES amount to 1.6%, 91% is represented by black women [52]. Furthermore, NES seems to have family aggregation: mothers with NES are more likely to have children with NES [53].

In a study on overweight patients with serious mental illness, NES was present in 25% of the sample [54].

Depression, male gender, and BMI are risk factors for NES [55].

Aronoff and colleagues [56] also showed a strong relationship between overweight status and NES; furthermore obese patients with NES reported an earlier onset of obesity than obese individuals without NES. Moreover, 52% of obese with NES reported the onset of NES before the development of obesity, that means that the presence of NES in normal weight or overweight people could be a severe risk factor for weight gain.

The serotonin system may be active in the pathophysiology of NES.

Elevations in serotonin transporter levels lead to decreased postsynaptic serotonin transmission and should impair circadian rhythms and satiety. These deficits suggest that improvement in serotonin function should alleviate night eating syndrome, and explain the therapeutic response of NES to selective serotonin reuptake inhibitors (SSRI) [57].

The prevalence of NES is high also among psychiatric outpatients within this group 12.3% of subjects met the criteria for NES [58].

The link between NES and mood disorders has been highlighted by many studies. Gluck et al. found higher rate of depression in patients with NES than in general population [59].

Furthermore, NES patients reported lower self-esteem than non-NES [60].

NES need also a differential diagnosis with "Sleeping Related Eating Disorder" (SRED). SRED patients are included in "Parasomnias "disorders characterized by abnormal behavioral events occurring in association with sleep. In DSM5 SRED's are defined as "unwanted recurrent episodes of eating with varying degrees of amnesia, ranging from no awareness to full awareness without the ability to not eat. During these episodes, inappropriate foods may be ingested. SRED individuals may find evidence of their eating only in the next morning".

The prevalence of SRED in general population is 5% and this disorder does not improve with SSRI. Also SRED is associated with high levels of obesity.

OTHER BIASED EATING BEHAVIORS

Grazing

Grazing called also nibbling or picking is a biased eating behavior not included in ED.

It is a new studied eating behaviour increasingly cited in the literature particularly in the area of bariatric surgery, it is characterized by eating in an unplanned and repetitious manner between meals and snacks.

Unfortunately it remains unclear if grazing is accompanied by a sense of loss of control, what amount or type of food is consumed or how frequently this behavior occurs.

Despite the inconsistent definitions of this concept, the existing literature seems to point to a high prevalence of such a behavior and supports its association with loss of control eating.

Busetto and colleagues [61] identified nibbling as "eating small quantities of foods repetitively between meals, typically triggered by inactivity and/or loneliness".

Grazing also is defined as "the repeated consumption of smaller amounts of food over an extended period of time with a loss of control" [62], but researchers have differed whether grazing includes feelings of loss of control.

Instead Saunders defined grazing as "smaller, subjective episodes of overeating" point out the feelings of poor control over eating behavior [63].

As a potential contributor to weight gain grazing has received minimal attention.

Grazing has been studied in bariatric surgery because preoperative patients with BED may convert their ED in grazing, this eating behavior could be a risk factor for bariatric surgery failures.

The question remains as whether grazing is a disordered eating behaviour, a maladaptive, or perhaps even normative eating behaviour outside the spectrum of eating disorder behaviour. Furthermore it remains unclear whether grazing is a problematic eating behaviour and if its assessment provides useful clinical information.

It is also difficult to develop a better understanding of grazing because postsurgical patients may perceive grazing as a healthy eating pattern, following physicians recommendations. This eating pattern may be viewed as unhealthy only when the frequency and the amount and type of food consumed is similar to previous bad habits [64].

It could be important to investigate the minimum frequency of grazing and the impact on psychological distress. In DSM 5 the frequency of bulimia nervosa and binge eating disorder has been specified (it is once a week in the last three months) but in literature there are no clear data regarding the frequency of grazing.

In a recent study, grazing is considered present when reported from 1 to 5 days in the previous 28 days investigated in a sample with eating disorders [65]. Furthermore grazing is associated with less weight loss in weight loss treatments [66].

Patients with eating disorders reported more frequent grazing episodes [67]. In fact grazing has a prevalence of 56.8% in patients with BN, 50.4% in BED and only 31.8% in a control group [68].

The data in literature show a lack of association with ED psychopathology, compensatory behaviors or BMI and support the concept that grazing is outside the spectrum of eating disorder behavior.

In a study explored eating behaviors among post bariatric surgery patients [69] grazing was present in 26.4 % of pre-surgical patients.

After surgery, grazing was present in 38% of patients with an increased prevalence by 31%. Furthermore, over 60% of baseline BED patients reported recurrent post-surgical grazing. In addition, pre-surgical grazers were highly likely to continue grazing (91%). Both preoperative and post-operative grazing independently predicted poorer post-surgical weight loss.

Grazers reported less dietary restraints, great hunger, a higher number of daily eating episodes and more symptoms of depression.

So grazing could be a risk factor for weight gain if present in overweight individuals, but up to now there aren't clear data about its prevalence in general population and particularly in overweight patients.

It could be important to organize research with well-designed protocols and reliable methods for measuring this biased eating behavior in overweight population to better understand the impact of grazing in weight gain.

EMOTIONAL EATING

Emotional eating refers to the tendency to overeat in response to negative emotions.

External eating refers to the overeating tendency resulting from susceptibility to tempting food cues, a notion derived from Schachter's externality theory of obesity [70].

Emotional and/or external eating can therefore complicate the association between dietary restraint, food intake, and change in body weight.

Many studies reported an association of dietary restraint (a form of inhibition) with overeating tendencies (disinhibition), as in emotional eating or external eating [71].

Emotional eating is a biased eating behavior characterized by consuming "comfort food" such as high calories foods with high fat and sugar percentage as a kind of avoidant stress coping.

It refers to the tendency to overeat in response to negative emotions as a result from poor "interoceptive" awareness, a notion derived from Bruch's psychosomatic theory [72].

Distress arises when the demand of a situation exceeds an individual's ability to cope with the problem so that the individual feels emotional, behavioral and cognitive malaises.

Distress can affect also eating behavior.

Emotional eating has been seen as an effort to regulate aversive mood using food to reduce anxiety, to provide a more balanced psychological level and to shade negative effects of distress.

In 2007 an U.S. survey found that 50% of people reported feeling greater stress than five years before and 43% reported using food to cope with stress [73]. The higher prevalence of stress-related eating could have an important role in the increasing prevalence of overweight and obesity.

Emotional eating could be linked also with low self-esteem, negative mood, body dissatisfaction or social isolation.

Many studies show that individuals under distress eat more and tend to choose unhealthy foods in absence of hunger in 30 % of cases [74, 75, 76, 77].

For adolescents with a genetic risk for overweight, the emotional eating is considered as an important risk factor for weight gain [78, 79, 80].

Moreover, when the stress is accompanied by feeling of loss of control it can lead to binge eating episodes even in the absence of dietary restraints.

So emotional eating can play an important role in weight gain in normal weight people as well as in overweight people who show particular psychological functioning and can complicate the association with dietary restraints, food intake and change in body weight [81].

A South Korean [82] study showed that emotional eating along with high restrained eating was an indicator for long term (4 year follow-up) weight gain in a large sample of healthy twins and their families.

Following studies showed that emotional eating was associated with weight gain only in connection with negative life events.

As for external eating in overweight individuals the data are controversial.

Some studies found that overweight people did not differ from normal weight people in their degree of external eating and this call into question the possible role of environmental food cues in the development of overweight, as that is described in the "obesogenic environment" theory.

In many studies, external eating is not associated with weight gain but the role of physical activity has not been assessed.

A Dutch study [83] using a perspective 2 year follow-up design, examined risk factors for developing overweight and its association with behavioral lifestyle. It found out that BMI change was also associated with emotional and external eating.

The study also highlighted how physical activity considerably influenced weight change, in fact increased physical activity was associated with weight loss.

HYPERPHAGIA

It is also interesting to recall an eating behavior, without psychopathological comorbility, that could have an important role on weight gain.

Hyperphagia (overeating) derives from a Greek word and it refers to excessive hunger or increased appetite that leads to an abnormally large intake of food.

Hyperphagia can be refer to sporadic episodes, for example many people overeat during festivities or in holiday, but when overeating became an usual eating pattern there is an excess food consumption in relation to the expended energy leading to weigh gain.

This eating behavior has been studied overall in obese patients.

Apfendolfer [84] a French psychiatrist, for the first time described the "hyperphagia" as eating a great amount of food during the mean meals not accompanied by loss of control.

Eating is typically experienced as pleasurable and rewarding (see the chapt. 2, Food addiction).

Hyperphagia behavior is not limited to the act of eating but also consists of preparatory, consumption and post-consumption phases.

During eating, the immediate, direct pleasure is derived from mainly gustatory and olfactory sensations. The length of the consumption phase is highly variable between glutter and great-eaters. Rather than the pleasure of tasty and eating food, there is a general feeling of satisfaction that lingers on long after termination and most likely contributes to the reinforcing power of meals.

The individuals with hyperphagia like eating with other people, like choosing elaborate foods and they do not feel psychological malaises linked with the eating behavior.

Apfendolfer distinguished between "gluttons" and "great-eaters" (over-consumers).

The gluttons are gourmet, expert in cooking, they focus on the "quality" of food so that they like cooking and eating elaborated foods. They can eat great amount of food but they eat slowly with pleasure, tasting the different type of food. The great eaters tend to prefer the "amount" instead the quality (property), they eat in a voracious manner but they don't feel loss of control over eating behavior.

Hyperphagia is often the result of family habits, and if it becomes a habitual eating pattern could facilitate the development of overweight and obesity because the high calories intake.

It could be difficult to evaluate the amount of food intake because often the individuals with hyperphagia are not aware about their eating behavior.

In a study on the presence of overeating in obese BED patients, using Nutritional Data System for Research (NDS-R) to gather nutritional intake, overeating has been defined as consuming 1.000 calories or more in one meal [85]. The study reported the presence of overeating both in obese BED and obese non BED, but greater rates of hyperphagia have been found in obese BED patients.

Furthermore, high over-consumers differed from low over-consumers in that they were more often overweight, had higher degrees of dietary restraint, emotional eating and external eating, and were better educated.

Given the wide variations in cultural values, practice and norms concerning food it is difficult to assess hyperphagia as biased eating patterns and clarify its role for weigh gain also in normal weight individuals.

REFERENCES

[1] Soetens, B; Braet, C. 'The weight of a thought': food-related thought suppression in obese and normal-weight youngsters. *Appetite*, 2006 46 (3), 309-17.

[2] Bryant, EJ; King, NA. Blundell Disinhibition: its effects on appetite and weight regulation *JE Obes. Rev.,* 2008 9(5), 409-19.

[3] Diagnostic and statistical manual of Mental disorders 5th edition. Arlington, VA American Psychiatric Association 2013.

[4] Bed 30- Mond, J; Hay, P; Rodgers, B et al. Use of extreme weight control behavior with and without binge eating in a community sample: implications for the classification of bulimic type eating disorders. *Int. J. Eat. Disord.* 2006 39, 294-302.

[5] Hebebrand, J; Fichter, M; Gerber, G; Görg, T; Hermann, H; Gelle, F; Schäfer, H; Remschmidt, H; Hinney, A. Genetic predisposition to obesity in bulimia nervosa: a mutation screen of the melanocortin-4 receptor gene. *Mol. Psychiatry*. 2002 7(6), 647-51.

[6] Keys, A; Brozek, J; Henschel, A et al. The biology of human starvation. University of Minnesota Minneapolis 1950.

[7] National Task Force on the Prevention and Treatment of Obesity. Dieting and the development of Eating Disorders in Overweight and Obese Adults. *Arch. Intern. Med.* 2000 160, 2581-2589.

[8] Ting, WH; Huang, CY; Tu,YK; Chien, KL. Association between weight status and depressive symptoms in adolescents: role of weight perception, weight concern and dietary restrain. *Eur. J. Pediatr,* 2012 171, 1247-1255.

[9] Jeffers, AJ; Cotter, EW; Snipes, DJ; Benotsch, EG. BMI and depressive symptoms: the role of media pressures. *Eat Behav.*, 2013 14, 468-47.

[10] Tanofsky-Kraff, M; Yanovsky, SZ; Wilfley, DE; et al. Eating disordered behaviours, body fat, and psychopathology in overweight and normal weight children. *J. Consult. Clin. Psychol.,* 2004, 72, 53-68.

[11] Barnes, RD; Blomquist, KK; Grilo, CM. Exploring Pretreatment Weight Trajectories in Obese Patients with Binge Eating Disorder. *Compr. Psychiatry,* 2011 52(3), 312-318.

[12] Stunkard, AJ. Eating disorders and obesity. *Psychiatr. Clin. North Am.* 2011 34(4), 765-71.

[13] Schag, K; Schönleber, J; Teufel, M; Zipfel, S; Gie, KE. Food-related impulsivity in obesity and Binge Eating Disorder – a systematic review. *Obes. Rev.* 2013 14(6), 477-495.

[14] Dingemans, AE; Bruna, MJ; van Furth, EF. Binge eating disorder: a review. *Int. J. Obes Relat. Metab. Disorder,* 2002 26(3), 299-307.

[15] Manwaring, JL; Hilbert, A; Wilfley, DE; Pike, KM; Fairburn, CG; Dohm, FA; Striegel-Moore, RH. Risk Factors and Patterns of Onset in Binge Eating Disorder. *Int. J. Eat. Disord.,* 2006 39(2), 101-107.

[16] Grilo, CM; Masheb, RM. Onset of dieting vs binge eating in outpatients with binge eating disorder. *Int. J. Obes. Realt. Matab. Disord.,* 2000 24(4), 404-9.

[17] Abbott, DW; de Zann, M; Mussell, MP; Raymond, NC; Seim, HC; Crow, SJ; Crosby, RD; Mitchell, JE. Onset of binge eating and dieting in overweight women: implication for ethiology, associated features and treatment. *J. Psychosom. Res.,* 1998 44(3-4), 367-374.

[18] Spurrell, EB; Wilfley, DE; Tanofsky, MB; Brownwll, KD. Age of onset for binge eating: are there different pathways to binge eating? *Int. J. Eat. Disord.,* 1997 21(1), 55-65.

[19] Mussell, MP; Mitchell, JE; Weller, CL; Raymond, NC; Crow, SJ; Crosby, RD. Onset of binge eating, dieting, obesity, and mood disorder among subjects seeking treatment for binge eating disorder. *Int. J. Eat. Disord* 1995 17(4), 395-401.

[20] Grilo, CM; White, MA; Masheb, RM. DSM-IV psychiatric disorder comorbidity and its correlates in binge eating disorder. *Int. J. Eat. Disord.,* 2009 42(3), 228–234.

[21] Grilo, MA; White, RD; Barnes, RM. Masheb Psychiatric disorder co-morbidity and correlates in an ethnically diverse sample of obese patients with binge eating disorder in primary care settings. *Compr. Psychiatry,* 2013 54(3), 209-216.

[22] Yanovski, SZ; Nelson, JE; Dubbert, BK; Spitzer, RL. Association of binge eating disorder and psychiatric comorbility in obese subjects. *Am. J. Psychiatr,* 1993 150, 1472-1479.

[23] Manzato, E; Zanetti, T; Simoni, M. Atteggiamenti alimentari e caratteristiche temperamentali di madri e rispettive pazienti con bulimia nervosa e "Binge Eating Disorder". *Quaderni Italiani di Psichiatria,* 2006 XXV, 17-25.

[24] Reas, DL; Grilo, CM; Masheb, RM; Wilson, T. Body Checking and Avoidance in Overweight Patients with Binge Eating Disorder. *Int. J. Eat. Disord,* 2005 37(4), 342-346.

[25] Neumark-Sztainer, D; Story, M; Hannan, PJ; Perry, CL; Irving, LM. Weight-related concerns and behaviours among overweight and non-overweight adolescents:

implications for preventing weight-related disorders. *Arch. Pediatr. Adolesc. Med.*, 2002 156 (2), 171-8.
[26] Epstein, LH; Paluch, RA; Saelens, BE; Ernst, MM; Wifley, DE. Changes in eating disorder symptoms with pediatric obesity treatment. *J. Pediatr.*, 2001 139, 58-65.
[27] Goldschmidt, A; Aspen, PV; Sinton, MM; Tanofsky-Kraff, M; Wilfley, DE. Disordered Eating Attitudes and Behaviors in Overweight Youth. *Obesity,* 2008 16(2), 257-64.
[28] Levine, MD; Ringham, RM; Kalarchian, MA; Wisniewski, L; Marcus, MD. Overeating among seriously Overweight Children seeking treatment: results of the Children's Eating Disorders Examination. *Int. J. Eat. Disord.,* 2006 39(2), 135-140.
[29] Udo, T; McKe, SA; White, M A; Masheb, RM; Barnes, R D; Grilo, C M. Sex Differences in Biopsychosocial Correlates of Binge Eating Disorder: A Study of Treatment-Seeking Obese Adults in Primary Care Setting. *Gen. Hosp Psychiatry* 2013 35(69), 1-9.
[30] Hudson, JI; Hiripi, E; Pope, HG Jr; Kessler RC. The prevalence and correlates of eating disorders in the National Comorbidity Survey Replication. *Biol. Psychiatry*, 2007 61, 348–58.
[31] De Zwaan, M; Mitchell, JE; Specker, SM; Pyle LR; Mussell; MP; Seim, HC.
[32] Binge eating disorder: Level of agreement between self-report and expert-rating. *Int. J. Eat. Disord.,* 1993 14, (3), 289–295.
[33] Engels, SG; Kalher, KA; Lystad, CM; et al. Eating behavior in obese binge eating disorder, obese non-binge eating disorder, and non-obese control participants. *Behav. Res. Ther.,* 2009 47, 897-900.
[34] Levine, MD; Ringham, RM; Kalarchian, MA; Wisniewski, L; Marcus, MD. Overeating among seriously overweight children seeking treatment: results of the children's eating disorder examination. *Int. J. Eat. Disord.*, 2005 39, 135-140.
[35] Nicholls, D; Bryant- Waugh, R. Eating disorders of infancy and childhood: definition, symptomatology, epidemiology and comorbidity. *Child. Adolesc. Psychiatr. Clin. N. Am.*, 2009 18 (1), 17-30.
[36] Hilbert, A; Czaja, J. Binge eating and obesity in children. *Psychoter Psychosom Med. Psychol.*, 2007 57 (11), 413-419.
[37] Braet, C; O'Malley, G; Weghuber, D; Vania, A; Erhardt, E; Nowincka, P; Mazur, A; Frelut, ML; Ardelt-Gattinger, E. The assessment of eating behaviour in children who are obese: a psychological approach. A position paper from the European childhood obesity group. *Obesity Facts*, 2014 7, 153-164.
[38] Fairburn, CG; Cooper, Z. The Eating Disorder Examination (12th edition). In edited Fairburn, CG; Wilson, GT." Binge Eating: Nature, Assessment and Treatment"Ed. Guilford New York 1993.
[39] Hilbert, A; Wilfley, DE; et al. Characterization, significance and predictive validity of binge size in binge eating disorder. In Strieghel-Moore, RH; Wonderlich, SA; Walsh, BT; Mitchell, JE. "Developing an evidence-based classification of eating disorders" APA, Arlington, Virginia 2011.
[40] Field, AE; Corliss, HL; Skinner, HH; Horton, NJ. Loss of control eating as a predictor of weight gain and the development of overweight, depressive symptoms, binge drinking and substance abuse. In "Developing an evidence-based classification of eating disorders" Strieghel-Moore, RH; Wonderlich, SA; Walsh, BT; Mitchell, JE.

"Developing an evidence-based classification of eating disorders" APA, Arlington, Virginia 2011.

[41] Grilo, MC; Hrabosky, JI; Withe, MA; Allison, KC; Stunkard, AJ; Masheb, RM. Overvaluation of shape and weight in binge eating disorder and overweight controls: refinement of a diagnostic construct. *J. Abnorm. Psychol.* 2008 117(2), 414- 419.

[42] Croll, J; Neumark-Sztainer, D; Story, M; Ireland, M.. Prevalence and risk and protective factors related to disordered eating behaviors among adolescents: relationship to gender and ethnicity. *J. Adolesc. Health,* 2002 31*(2),* 166–175.

[43] Mitchell, JE; Pyle, RL; Eckert, ED; Hatsukami, D; Soll, E. Bulimia nervosa in overweight individuals. *J. Nerv. Ment. Dis.,* 1990 178 (5), 324-327.

[44] Masheb, RM; White, MA. Bulimia nervosa in overweight and normal weight women. *Compr Psychiatry,* 2012 53 (2), 181-186.

[45] Stunkard, A; Grace, WJ; Wolff, HG. The night-eating syndrome; a pattern of food intake among certain obese patients. *Am. J. Med.,* 1955 19, 78–86.

[46] Birketvedt, G; Florholme, J; Sundsfjord, J; Osterud, B; Dinges, D; Bilker, W; et al. Behavioral and neuroendocrine characteristics of the night eating syndrome. *J. Am. Med. Assoc.,* 1999 282, 657-663.

[47] Striegel-Moore, RH; Franko, DL; May, A; Ach, E; Thompson, D; Hook, JM. Should night eating syndrome be introduced in the DSM? *Int. J. Eat. Disord.*, 2006 39, 544-549.

[48] Stunkard, AJ; Allison, KC; Lundgren, JD. Night eating syndrome in DSM-V. *Am. J. Psychiatry,* 2008 165-4.

[49] Allison, KC; Lundgren, JD; O'Reardon, JP; Geliebter, A; Gluck, ME; et al. Proposed diagnostic criteria for night eating syndrome. *Int. J. Eat. Disord.* 2010 43, 241-247.

[50] Kucukgoncu, S; Tek, C; Bestepe, E; Musket, C; Guloksuz, S. Clinical features of Night Eating Syndrome among depressed patients. *Eur. Eat. Disorders Rev.*, 2014 22,102-108.

[51] Ceru-Bjork, C; Andersson, I; Rossner, S. Night eating and nocturnal eating- two different or similar syndromes among obese patients? *Int. J. Obes. Relat. Metab. Disord.*, 2001 25, 3,365-372.

[52] Rand, CSW; Macgregor, MD; Stunkard, AJ. The night eating syndrome in the general population and among post-operative obesity surgery patients. *Int. J. Eat. Disord.,* 1997 22, 65-69.

[53] Striegel-Moore, RH;Dohm, FA; Hook, JH; Schreiber, GB; Crawford, PB; Daniels, SR. Night Eating Syndrome in Young Adult Women: Prevalence and Correlates. *Int. J. Eat. Disord.,* 2005 37, 200–206.

[54] Lundgren, JD; Allison, KC; Stunkard, AJ. Familial aggregation in the night eating syndrome. *Int. J. Eat. Disord.,* 2006 39 (6), 516-518.

[55] Lundgren, JD; Rempfer, MV; Brown, CE; Goetz, J; Hamera, E. The prevalence of night eating syndrome and binge eating disorder among overweight and obese individuals with serious mental illness. *Psychiatry Res,* 2010 175(3), 233-236.

[56] Özlem Orhan, F; Özer, UG; Özer, A; Altunören, O; Çelik, M; Karaaslan, MF. Night Eating Syndrome Among Patients With Depression. *Isr. J. Psychiatry Relat. Sci.*, 2011 48, 3, 212-7.

[57] Aronoff, NJ; Geliebter,A; Zammit, G. Gender and body mass index as related to the night-eating syndrome in obese outpatients. *J. Am. Diet. Assoc.,* 2001 101, 102-104.

[58] Miyaoka, T; Yasukawa, R; Tsubouchi, K; Miura, S; Shimizu, Y; Sukegawa, T; et al. Successful treatment of nocturnal eating/drinking syndrome with selective serotonin reuptake inhibitors. *Int. Clin. Psychopharmacol.,* 2003 18, 175-177.

[59] Lundgren, JD; Allison, KC; Crow, S; O'Reardon, JP; Berg, KC; Galbraith, J; et al. Prevalence of the night eating syndrome in a psychiatric population. *Am. J. Psychiatry,* 2006 163,156-158.

[60] Gluck, ME; Geliebter, A; Satov, T. Night eating syndrome is associated with depression, low self-esteem, reduced daytime hunger, and less weight loss in obese outpatients. *Obes. Res,* 2001 9, 264-267.

[61] de Zwann, M; Burgard, MA; Schenck,CH; Mitchell, JE. Night time eating: a review of the literature. *Eur. Eat. Disord. Rev.*, 2003 11, 7-24.

[62] Busetto L, Segato G, De Marchi F, et al. Outcome predictors in morbid obese recipients of an adjustable gastric band. *Obes. Surg.* 2002 12, 89, 83-92.

[63] Carter, FA; Jansen, A. Improving psychological treatment for obesity. Which eating behaviours should we target? *Appetite* 2012 58, 1063-1069.

[64] Saunders, R. Grazing: a high-risk behaviour. *Obes. Surg.* 2004 14, 98-102.

[65] Zunker, C; Karr, T; Saunders, R. Eating Behaviors Post-Bariatric Surgery: a qualitative study of Grazing. *Obes. Surg.* 2012 22, 1225-1231.

[66] Conceicao, EM; Crosby, R; Mitchtell, JE et al. Picking or nibbling: Frequency and associated clinical features in bulimia nervosa, anorexia nervosa, and binge eating disorder. *Int. J. Eat. Disord.* 2013 46, 8, 815-818.

[67] Saunders, R.A. Grazing a high-risk behavior. *Obes. Surg.* 2004 14, 1, 98-102.

[68] Masheb, RM; Grilo, CM; White, MA. An examination of eating patterns in community women with bulimia nervosa and binge eating disorder. *Int. J. Eat. Disord.* 2011, 44, 618-624.

[69] Masheb, RM ,; Roberto CR; White, MA. Nibbling and picking in obese patients with Binge Eating Disorder. *Eat. Behav.* 2013 14, 424-427.

[70] Colles, SL; Dixon, JB; O' Brien, PE. Grazing and loss of control related to eating: two high-risk factors following bariatric surgery. *Obesity* 2008 16, 3, 615-622.

[71] Schachter, S. Obesity and Eating. *Science* 1968, 161, 751-756.

[72] Herman, CP; Povy J. External cues in the control of food intake in humans. The sensory - normative distinction. *Physiol. Behav.*, 2008 94, 722-728.

[73] Bruch, H. Psychological aspects in overeating and obesity. *Psychosomatics* 1964 5, 269-274.

[74] American Psychiatric Association Press Releas. Stress a major health problem in the U.S. warns. APA 2007 Oct 24 (http://www.apa.org/news/press/release/2007/10/ stress.aspx

[75] Epel, ES; Lapidus, R; McEwen, B; Brownell, K. Stress may add bite to appetite in women: a laboratory study of stress-induced cortisol and eating behavior. *Psychoneuroendocrinology,* 2011 26, 37-49.

[76] Newman, E; O'Connor, DB; Conner, M. Daily hassles and eating behavior: the role of cortisol reactivity status. *Psychoneuroendocrinology,* 2007 32, 125-132.

[77] Rutters, F; Nieuwenhuizen, AG; Lemmens, SG; Born, JM; Westerterp-Plantega, MS. Acute stress-related changes in eating in the absence of hunger. *Obesity,* 2009 17, 72-77.

[78] Groesz, L; McCoy, S; Carl,J; Saslow, L; Stewart, J; Adler, N; Laraia, B; Epel, E. What is eating you? Stress and the drive to eat. *Appetite*, 2012 58 (2), 717-721.

[79] Neumark-Sztainer, D; Wall, M; Story, M; Sherwood, NE. Five-year Longitudinal predictive factors for disordered eating in a population-based sample of overweight adolescents: implications for prevention and treatment. *Int. J. Eat. Disord.*, 2009 42, 664-672.

[80] Puder, JJ; Munsch, S. Psychological correlates of childhood obesity. *Int. J. Obes.*, 2010 34, S37-S41.

[81] 80. Braet, C; O'Malley, G; Weghuber, D; Vania A; Erhardt, E; Nowicka, P; Mazur, A; Frelut, ML, Ardelt-Gattinger, E. The assessment of eating behavior in children who are obese: a psychological approach. A position paper from the European childhood obesity group. *Obes. Facts*, 2014 7, 153-164.

[82] Koenders, PG; van Strien, T. Emotional eating rather than lifestyle behavior drives weight gain in a prospective study in 1562 employees. *Int. J. Occup. Environ. Med.*, 2011 53, 1287-1293.

[83] Sung,J; Lee, K; Song, Y. Relationship of eating behavior to long term weight change and body mass index. The healthy twin study. *Eat and weight disorder*, 2009 14, 98-105.

[84] van Strien, T; Herman, CP; Verheijden, M W. Eating style, overeating and weight gain. A prospective 2- year follow-up study in a representative Dutch sample. *Appetite* 2012 59, 782-789.

[85] Apfeldorfer, G. Je mange donc je suis. ED Payot France 1993.

[86] Engel, AG; Kahle, KA; et al. Eating behavior in obese binge eating disorder, obese non-binge eating disorder and non-obese control participants. *Behavior Research and Therapy*, 2009 47, 897-900.

In: The Different Faces of Being Overweight
Editor: Emilia Manzato
ISBN: 978-1-63483-099-7

Chapter 7

NEGATIVE BODY-IMAGE AND BODY DISSATISFACTION IN OVERWEIGHT

Antonia Bolognesi*

Psychologist, Psychotherapist,
Member of the Italian Society for the Study of Eating Disorder (SISDCA), Italy

ABSTRACT

Body image disorder can be included among the multiple factors, which develop and maintain the overweight condition.

With the term "body image" we refer to the mind representation that an individual has of their body. Although it is structured upon specific individual physical characteristics, it is influenced by psychological, relational and cultural factors. Body image is multifactorial and dynamic construct and it includes- and at the same time overcomes- the physical characteristics.

In such a complex construct, the breaking points may be various: a disturbed body image can be expressed as 'misperception' (body shape is wrongly evaluated), as dissatisfaction (consequence of the gap between perception and a thin ideal) or as excessive evaluation of body shape and weight.

Some authors suggest to give a nosographic validity to body image disorder, placing it in the Diagnostic and Statistics Manual of Mental Disorders5th edition (DSM5). At the moment, body image disorder is not universally recognized as *a* diagnosis, we refer therefore to negative body image to indicate a condition which is more uncomfortable and inhibiting than ordinary body anxiety. Subjects with negative body image can be dissatisfied with their weight and complain that they are too fat, seeing weight loss as a solution strategy.

Sex is an important modulator as far as it concerns the thin ideal, the type of worries and the tendency to express or hide anxiety. In cultures where western influence is more consistent, the ideal of woman beauty is oriented to thinness, while man to muscularity. Since this kind of ideal is almost unreachable for most people, the levels of dissatisfaction in both men and women increase.

---

* Email: antoniabolognesi@libero.it.

Body image is a moderator in the relationship the individual has with eating, physical activity and the consequent evolution of weight and health conditions in life. Literature also stresses how body image mediates the relationship between Body Mass Index (BMI) and psycho-social variables such as self-esteem and life quality.

The sociocultural, individual and relational factors, which play a role in the construction and evolution of body image in overweight people in their lifetime, are numerous.

In a society where the stress on thinness is constant, especially for young women, being overweight or obese is a risk factor FOR the creation and development OF negative body image.

Other factors which cause negative body image are linked to the individual dimension (i.e. low self-esteem and binge eating) as well as relational dimension (family and extra family relationships).

The chapter explores the contributions in literature about body image in overweight people with and without eating disorders, paying particular attention to the factors which play a role in the creation of negative body image and body dissatisfaction among these people.

Introduction

The prevalence of overweight and obesity conditions in lifetime makes topical the study on risk factors for development and maintainance of ponderal excess.

Among these, body image is an important moderator in the way an individual relates to eating [1,2,3,4], to physical activity [5,6] and to the subsequent evolution of weight and health conditions in their lifetime. Literature shows how body image constitutes a mediator in the relationship between Body Mass Index (BMI) and psycho-social variables such as self-esteem and life quality [6].

Body image disorder has been included among the factors causing weight increase both in treated overweight patients and in not treated [7,8].

Body image disorder is one of the diagnostic criteria for Anorexia Nervosa (AN) and Bulimia Nervosa (BN), in particular AN diagnosis requires an 'alteration of the way the person lives his or her own weight and the shape of their body, excessive influence of weight or body shape on the levels of self-esteem, or the person persistently refuses to admit the gravity of present at the moment underweight condition".

Excessive influence of weight and body shape on the levels of self-esteem is also a criteria for diagnosis of BN. Body image disorder, indeed, is not among the criteria for Binge Eating Disorder (BED), which is often associated to overweight and obesity [9].

However, Stunkard in the Sixties, underlined the importance of considering body image in the evaluation of profiles of psychopathologic obese individuals with and without Eating Disorders (ED) [10]. More recent studies have underlined the role of negative body image, in particular the role of the focus on the body and shapes in the evaluation of one-self in the BED, so that an integration of diagnostic criteria was suggested [11,12,13].

The only specific diagnostic category of DSM5 that refers to body image disorder is Muscle Dysmorphia, although it is not placed among ED but among Obsessive-Compulsive Disorders and related disorders [9]. If in ED the disease is focused on weight and body shape, in particular about specific body areas such as tummy, thighs and bottom, in the Body

Dysmorphic Disoder, dissatisfaction is related to physical imperfection real or assumed (often the face) which shows imperfect or disgusting aspect.

Under this category we suggest to point out whether Muscle Dysmorphia is present: a recently defined disorder [14] (studied especially among men) in which the symptoms core is the fear of being too thin even with muscular body and for this reason named "reverse anorexia" [15].

In the chapter the contributions of literature are explored, on the topic of body image in overweight individuals with and without ED, paying specific attention to the factors which play a role in the creation of negative body image and body dissatisfaction.

What Is Body Image? Body Image As a Multidimensional Construct

The concept of body image is to be distinguished from other constructs about the topic of body; Paillard [16] underlines how this concept is still confused with body scheme and the two terms are often interchanged.

Body scheme and body image refer to different study areas; body scheme to the neurological area and it refers to the topographic representation that the individual perceives and creates, the conscious self-representation of one's own body. It is the result of cortical projections from the sensory-motor system which merge to form a unitary, topographic and constantly updated representation of the body, of its position in space and the relative position of its different parts.

Body image refers to the psychological area and therefore to the inner world and meaningful relations with the outer world. It does not recall an objective photograph of the real body, but its subjective, affective and symbolic representation, which is largely unconscious, built upon the basis of affective relational experiences [17, 18].

Dolto, distinguishing between body scheme and body image, defines body scheme as a mind construct identical for all human beings while body image refers to an individual's own identity [19].

We should also separate the concept of body image from physical appearance. The latter recalls the outside appearance as perceived by others, while body image refers to the mind representation an individual has of his/her own body.

Body image, although it is structured upon specific individual physical characteristics, depends also on other factors. These may be of psychological, relational and cultural nature. It is therefore a multifactorial and dynamic construct, which comprehends and at the same time overcomes the physical characteristics [20].

Schilder, in the Thirties of the XX century, for the first time introduced the concept of body image as a mind image in constant evolution in which perceptions, emotions and socio-cultural influences merge. [21].

Since this moment, contributions have been several, by authors belonging to psychoanalytical, phenomenological and cognitive-behavioural approaches. From the symbolic function of body representation from psychoanalysis, to the body conceptualized as "*vehicle*" ("*obstacle*" in the pathology) of "*being in the world*" of fhenomenology.

Most contemporary research on body image derives from cognitive paradigms; they tend to focus on social learning processes and the role of cognitive mediation in behaviours and emotions. Cognitive-emotional schemes related to body representation are the basis of personality management and the process of identity construction. The concepts of scheme and body image are distinct, the former referring to direct perception of physical self, the latter conceptualized as "cognitive filter" through which reality is interpreted. Body image cannot be led only to the sensory dimension, rather to the cognitive and emotional interpretation operated by the individual [20].

Multidimensionality in the body image construct is underlined in Cash's model [22]; the author points out two main dimensions: perceptive experiences (evaluation of one's own body dimensions and proportions) and attitudes and opinions (cognitive, affective and behavioural dimension). The latter component, besides cognitive evaluations and emotions about physical appearance, includes the importance given to physical appearance by the individual. Cash underlines how the factors which contribute to body image development can be defined as historical/evolution influences and proximal events; the former working as organizational central constructs interacting with emotional and behavioural processes which come true in environmental contexts. Such historical influences play an important role in the creation of schemes and attitudes about the body and they include:

cultural messages: they have a crucial role in the definition of aesthetic standards distinguished according to gender, suggesting at the same time methods in order to modify one's own appearance according to social expectations (e.g. dieting, physical exercise, fashion);

interpersonal experiences: interactions, expectations and family or extra-family opinions about the topic of physical appearance.

physical characteristics: physical appearance influences the way a person is considered and treated. Thinking for example of the stereotypes connected to weight in our society, they tend to relate thinness to positive connotations (strength, self-control, determination, intelligence, success) while obesity to negative characteristics, such as scarce self-control abilities.

personality characteristics: good self-esteem is a protection factor against body dissatisfaction; while perfectionism - exasperating the body control dimension -and the need for social approval - making the individual more sensitive to socially recognized aesthetic standards - are risk factors.

In such a complex construct, the breaking points can be multiple; disorder body image may express as misperception (sense deficit which can lead to misevaluate one's own body shape to the extent of low awareness of one's own sensations and inner states), as dissatisfaction (consequence of the gap between personal perception and the aesthetic ideal) or as excessive evaluation of shape and weight of one's own body [20].

Thompson [23] suggests to include body image disorder in DSM; he defines it as characterised by "persistent dissatisfaction, anxiety and uneasiness towards physical appearance; there has to be, moreover, some damage in interpersonal relationships, social activities and work activities".

At the moment, body image disorder is not universally recognized as diagnosis, we refer therefore to negative body image as it was suggested by Rosen [24] who defines it as a condition which is more uncomfortable and inhibiting than ordinary body anxiety. Subjects with negative body image can be dissatisfied with their weight and complain that they are too fat, other complaints may be about appearance not related to body weight (such as the face shape or shape and size of breast), or they are not physically fit, or they look old. Weight loss is seen by these people as a way to change these aspects [24].

We should underline that sex is an important modulator as far as it concerns the aesthetic ideals, the type of worries and the tendency to express or hide worries. In cultures where western influence is more consistent, the ideal of woman beauty is oriented to thinness, while man to muscularity (muscular V-shaped body). Since this kind of ideal is almost unreachable for most people, the level of dissatisfaction in both men and women increases [25]

Which Factors Influence Body Image in Overweight?

1. Sociocultural Factors: Evolution of Aesthetic Models and Stereotypes Related to Overweight and Obesity Conditions

The concept of beauty or the aesthetic model related to a "canon", that is a set of rules shared by a social group that is more or less homogeneous, has evolved remarkably in the course of history.

From mediterranean Venere images dating 120.000 years ago, changes of the socially desirable aesthetic ideal have been many in time. Such evolution has been influenced by historical and cultural factors. In particular the nutrition trends of population have influenced the definition of body shapes considered as socially desirable. Along with reduced availability of food, massive aesthetic ideals tended to develop, recalling generative potentials and well-being. On the contrary, when food availability did not represent threat to survival, a slender and long limbed body came along, which recalled a life of privileges, in which hand work was not needed and physical strength was not required [27].

The arts and media (in more recent times) represent the main source of testimony about the aesthetic models of every period in history. Very different ways of portraying man and woman evince that the concept of beauty has profoundly changed over the course of history.

Since the Seventies, the ideology of thinness has setteled, with subsequent tendency to iponutrition.

In industrialized countries there is pressure towards thinness in particular for women. The weight stigma is widely spread among adults and children and it is well documented in literature; being thin is related to intelligence and success, while overweight and obese people are considered lazy, unmotivated and with scarce self-control abilities [28,29,30, 31,32,33,34].

In nearly all areas of living, including interpersonal relationships, education, employment, and health care, obese persons are often mischaracterized and mistreated [30,31]. Despite the ubiquity of weight stigma, there is little consensus on why heavier individuals are universally maligned [30]. Research suggests that it is often greater among individuals who embrace certain etiological views of obesity or ideological views of the world [33,35,36]. For instance, Allison et Al. [33] found that people who consider being overweight and obese as totally depending in individual control tend to have more negative attitudes toward overweight or obese people compared to those who do not consider body weight under the person's complete control. Crandall [35,36] found a link between negative attitudes towards obese people and ideological beliefs such as “people get what they deserve in life and that hard work and determination lead to good things”. People who embrace ideologies of this kind believe that obese persons "deserve" their condition or haven't engaged enough in order to avoid it. Strikingly, differently from other stigmatized groups - i.e. minorities - [37], internalized weight stigma was found even among overweight and obese people themselves [38,39].

Money and psychological engagement about internalized weight stigma and discrimination connected to obesity are remarkable[40,41,42,43]. Obese people have less chances of employment, work promotion and more likely receive poorer salaries [40,43,44]; stigmatizing experiences put obese people at risk of binge eating, psychological stress, body image disorder and low self-esteem. [41,42,45]. Moreover, it was underlined how in overweight and obese women, stigmatizing experiences are factors predicting physical exercise avoidance [46].

Most studies about obesity stigma have explored beliefs and discrimination towards obese people compared to non-obese [47]. The impact of stigmatizing experiences on the psychological well-being of overweight and obese individuals has also been explored [41,42]. Less examined are the factors connected to internalized weight stigma in overweight and obese people who requested treatment for ponderal loss [39,41,42,48]. Carels et Al. [48] studied the relation between the level of internalized weight stigma, perception of weight on one side and world beliefs on the other. It was shown how, even among overweight people, internalized stigma related to weight was present; it varied according to the individuals' world belief and in particular it increased if they believed weight was under a person's complete control.

Recent studies pointed out that negative weight-based implicit attitudes may be strengthened by stereotypical portrayals of obesity [48].

Therefore, given that implicit anti-fat attitudes are resistant to change [50] associated with prejudiced behaviors [51] they may have a negative impact on successful weight loss among treatment-seeking adults [52].

This study provides preliminary support for the recommendation that changes in media practices toward more positive portrayals of obesity and overweight could have an impact on public attitudes and health.

Given the strength and ubiquity of these stereotypes, it is likely that obese individuals, similar to other stereotyped groups, may experience disrupted performance on relevant tasks when their actions could be seen as confirming negative stereotypes associated with being overweight. This experience is commonly referred to as stereotype threat [53,54]. Previous research has consistently shown that individuals often perform poorly on stereotype-relevant tasks when they are reminded of the stereotype beforehand [54,55,56]. Preliminary research suggests that stereotype threat can impact the behavioral intentions of overweight/obese adults [57]. Shapiro [58] proposed that a number of factors are associated with the emergence of stereotype threat. One such factor is group identification, which is apparent when individuals perceive themselves as similar to other in-group members [59]. Generally speaking, the stronger an individual identifies with his or her group (i.e., other overweight individuals), the more likely the individual is to fear confirming and supporting the negative stereotype about overweight persons.

Similarly, the Multi-Threat Framework suggests that stereotype endorsement is a critical factor in the emergence of stereotype threat [58]. The more an individual believes (or trusts that others believe) that a stereotype is true (stereotype endorsement), the more likely he or she will be to experience stereotype threat. Shapiro demonstrated that individuals in high stereotype-endorsing as well as low identifying groups (i.e., overweight state, mental illness) were more likely to view themselves, rather than their group, as the target of the threat. Preliminary findings show that individuals who are overweight or obese have lower group identification and greater stereotype endorsement than other stigmatized groups, such as racial or religious minorities. As a result, they are more likely to perceive their self as a target of threat compared to the group. Thus, individuals who are overweight or obese would endorse perceiving threat from situations in which they themselves are the target of the stereotype more so than when their group (overweight people in general) was the target of the threat [58,59].

Research by Carels et al. [60], examined how these different forms of perceived stereotype threat were related to concepts, such as group identity, stereotype endorsement, stigma consciousness, etc., among 216 overweight and obese adults. Findings revealed that individuals who are overweight or obese reported a significant history of being threatened by stereotypes related to weight. Whether real or imagined, the fear that one's actions could lead to harsh judgment or the confirmation of negative stereotypes is a real concern for overweight and obese individuals. Unlike other stigmatized groups with stronger group identity, such as racial minorities, overweight/obese individuals are more concerned that their behaviors will reflect poorly on him or herself than on obese people in general. The results of the present study support two of the primary tenets of the Multi-Threat Framework: that the emergence of stereotype threat is strongly associated with group identification (a perceived similarity to other in-group members) and stereotype endorsement (a belief that the stereotype is true); furthermore it suggests that, among overweight/obese individuals, those individuals identifying as part of the 'overweight' group and who believe in common stereotypes about overweight individuals were more likely to perceive that stereotype threat had occurred in stigmatizing situations. Particularly female participants and participants with higher BMIs reported a greater likelihood of experiencing stereotype threat. Finally, experiencing low self-esteem was related to higher levels of stereotype threat. As shown in other studies, self-esteem has been found to be negatively related to the greater frequency of stigmatizing situations [61].

Although the presence of stereotype about overweight and obese conditions has been widely documented, besides pshychological consequences which derive from these conditions [28,29] [30,31,29,32,33,34], little is known about the psychological state of those who leave a stigmatized group. In a research on 20649 overweight Americans who later became normoweight, Levy e Pilver [62] found that the likelihood of any anxiety disorder and any depressive disorder for the formerly overweight group was significantly greater than for the consistently normal-weight group, and not significantly different from the consistently overweight group. Further, the formerly overweight group was significantly more likely to attempt suicide than the other groups. Data suggest that losing a self-image shaped by stigma is a more protracted process than losing weight.

Research examining how body weight is depicted in the mass media has shown repeatedly that the media portray what many authors have termed a "thin standard" or a "thin ideal", that is, a tendency to emphasize the importance of one's weight, to show underweight persons or characters in far greater numbers (or in the alternative, highly-muscularized males) than their normal- weight or overweight counterparts, and to portray the former in a much more flattering manner than the latter [63,64,65,66]. Such messages have become more prevalent over time and that today, more than ever before, the media provide highly-unrealistic–some would even say highly-unattainable– portrayals of body weight [63].

Moreover, researchers have also demonstrated that many persons internalize the "thin ideal" or the "thin standard" propagated by the media, and that people who do this are prone to developing eating disorders [67].

In exemplary studies examining two samples of female students in the Fiji Islands in 1995 (before the introduction of satellite television) and in 1998 (afer three years of exposure to satellite television) increase in the frequency of self-induced vomit was found, from 0% to 11% and an increase of rating in the Eating Attitude Test, a test showing altered eating behaviour (from 12,7% to 29,2% the rating was at least 20). Media exposure seems to have promoted the value of social thinness [68].

Analogue research among university students explored the influence of television with specific attention to body representations. After exposure to videos in which the visual message focused on the socially accepted female model, tendency to overevaluation of their own shapes was revealed, with consequent increase of body dissatisfaction and lower self-esteem. Body image, besides being a dynamic construct, seems to be defined upon the interaction of multiple factors: objective physical shape, interiorized ideal body and socially represented ideal body [69].

Some authors have studied the content related to weight which are proposed by the media. Fouts et al. [70], for example, studied how male characters were shown in primetime television situation comedies. They reported that overweight males were underrepresented in these programs compared to their numbers in the general population and that being overweight was a subject for self-deprecating comedic jokes among such characters. They found that underweight females were overrepresented and that negative comments were made about those females whose weight was considered unacceptably- high [71].

Social learning theory [72,73] posits that people acquire their beliefs, attitudes, and propensity to engage in behaviors, directly based on firsthand experiences they have with others who exhibit particular behaviors and/or indirectly, based on what they observe others – including others appearing in the mass media - doing or saying.

The social learning theory would predict that people of all ages (and young people in particular) will learn a great deal about body weight, social expectations for what is a "proper" body weight, the accepted or expected steps that can or should be taken to maintain that "appropriate" weight, and the social consequences of being overweight just from being exposed to weight-related media content.

Beside the learning theory, the cultivation theory [74,75] offers interesting contributions to understand the role of media in orienting people's choices. Cultivation theory would posit that media messages serve as agents of socialization regarding what to think about thinness, being overweight, and weight-related behaviors. This would be particularly true for young viewers who are exposed rather heavily to such media messages through the types of programming that they tend to view.

Klein e Shiffman [76] investigated body weight-related messages in animated cartoons. Exposition to these begins early and protracts in time. The message is clear:" *Thin is in and stout is out*." On virtually all dimensions examined, socially-desired traits were associated with thinness and socially-disapproved characteristics were associated with being overweight. Compounding these findings, we also discovered that underweight characters were more likely to perform prosocial acts–that is, to do things that are designed specifically to benefit others–than other characters are, and conversely, that overweight characters were more likely to engage in antisocial acts when compared to others. Animated cartoons both reflect and shape social values about body weight, and help to form children's initial notions of what it means to be thin or heavy. These messages are reinforced by other media to which they are exposed (since those media, too, typically portray similar messages about thinness and heaviness), by their peers, by their parents, and by other role models around them. The adverse effects of internalizing such messages about body weight have been shown in numerous studies that have linked them to problems like low self-esteem [77,78], poor body image [79,80], eating disorders[67,81,82,83], and depression [79,80].

Early and pervasive exposition to aesthetic models oriented to thinness, contributes to increase body dissatisfaction of overweight people, especially if such condition emerged early.

2. Interpersonal Experiences

2.1. Family Relationships

The study of family influence on children's body image has received particular attention in literature: the role of family context and the quality of relationships, parents attitudes towards body and eating and the role of parents' awareness of children's overweight condition have been explored.

*Psychoanalitical Authorshav*e underlined the influence of early interactions in structuring body image. In particular, the stress was on the quality of primary relation for the construction of accurate and balanced self.

In such early stage, quality is expressed through sensory and kinetic contact of mother to her child, in the capability to establish empathic relation with the newborn body even before word and language time. From the quality of this relation the unity of mind and body arise. Through sense stimulation the baby can distinguish their own body from what surrounds it. The contact with their mother facilitates the perception of the baby's own body surface limits, while the mother's empathy acts as a mirror, organizing and giving meaning to the newborn sensations. The way a mother holds, touches and feeds her baby will deeply affect the attitudes they will develop toward their own body [20].

The roots of this experience can be traced during maternity; the mother represents her baby not as what he/she actually is, an embryo, but as a whole individual. The baby's imagined body is affectively endowed by the mother. The characteristics of such maternal representations and the affective investment which accompanies them, contribute to the individual's construction of body image after birth. [17].

During infancy, the body holds high communicative value, the baby expresses anxieties and conflict especially through it; examples of this are psychosomatic diseases in early years of life [17]. According to the model by the Paris psychosomatics and psychoanalysis school, in the mother-child dyad, the mother represents the mind unit, the child is the somatic one. Alexithymic characteristics in the mother expose the child to higher risks of developing symptoms and psychosomatic disease such as cholics in the first three months, anorexy, psychogenic vomiting, laryngospasm or bronchial asthma [84]. The alexithymic construct relates to difficulties in identifying, describing and communicating emotions, in distinguishing between emotive experiences and physiological activation of emotions, to poor imaginative processes, to a cognitive style oriented to factual and outside reality, to conformist social adjustment [85].

Several studies have focused on the role played by interpersonal modeling in the setting of the individual body image construction. The theory of social learning states that parents are among the first important agents of socialization, which come into the baby's life, they influence body image through processes of modeling, feedback and teaching. Parents who are particularly focused on appearance, or take special care in making the child's appearance perfect, reinforce the belief that good appearance is needed, in order to be socially accepted. Parents expectations about the imagined child influence the construction of body image, they are expressed through attitudes, comments and behaviours [20].

The level of accuracy of the children's weight perception in parents has also been explored in literature; the acknowledgement of overweight conditions in children is a variable which plays an important role in the decisions for changes in the surrounding context and lifestyle. These represent crucial aspects for the prevention and treatment of obesity in infancy and adolescence. [86,87].

Several studies have underlined the parents' tendency to underestimate overweight and obesity conditions in their own children [88,89,90,91].

In a 2009 review of literature, Towns et Al. observed that parents of overweight children tend to underestimate their children's weight with following risks for their health. Several factors related to parents' underestimation of overweight children have been underlined; the main being age, gender, ethnic group they belong to. Underestimation was more frequent when children were little, as with growing up, self-perception and comments by peers became the facilitators for adequate acknowledgement of overweight states also by parents. Even the child's gender proved to be a discriminating variable: both mothers and fathers were at risk of underestimating overweight children when they were males; moreover, it was more acceptable to have an overweight boy than an overweight girl. These differences related to gender may influence, even in early phases, the construction of healthy self-esteem and positive or negative body image and access to programs for weight management. These studies pointed out stronger tendencies in Latin-Hispanic and Americans (African American and Native Americans) to prefer abundant body shapes, as they did not identify overweight children as a problem. Also the BMI of both parents and children proved to be a variable: the probability that mothers acknowledged overweight children raised with their own low BMI and a child's high BMI. [89].

Several studies focused on the mother's perception, especially the body patterns they refer to when defining overweight children and individuate a "risk threshold" which describes the overweight state. Parents' underestimation of overweight conditions in children may be a risk factor in their evolution towards obesity. A study on 531 children (6-8 years old) and their mothers showed that half of them underestimated their children's BMI and identified overweight conditions when obesity had already been reached. Waist measuring and skinfolds were the most frequently used parameters, probably being more visible (despite BMI and fat scores). Although other studies showed the opposite, girls were less likely to be identified as overweight, compared to boys. Contrasting data in literature may relate to the target age, in fact tendency to underestimate overweight children increased as their age decreased. The study also pointed out that the mother's BMI related to her ability to identify overweight states in children: mothers with higher BMI were less likely to identify excessive weight in children but they stated more frequent preoccupation about the evolution of children's weight towards overweight or obesity [90].

The relation between body underestimation in parents and children has also been explored [91] [92].

In a study on 151 children and their parents, Tremblay et al. tried to investigate body perception in children and possible relations to the parents' perception of their children's body. Children were between 3 and 5 years old (48% girls and 52% boys), underweight children were not included in the study. The majority of overweight children underestimated their body shape. This work also underlines how underestimation in overweight children was present in their parents who tended to underestimate their children's body shapes not recognizing their overweight state [91]. These results match what emerged in a work by Cramer and Steinwert. The authors considered body misperception as the individuals' try to guard their own self-esteem instead of internalizing negative attitudes related to being overweight. Along with this hypothesis, the children who perceived themselves as 'thin' showed more negative stereotypes about being obese.

The study by Tremblay et al. points out gender differences related to body dissatisfaction, matching what resulted from studies on adolescents and adults. Body dissatisfaction is stronger in girls than in boys, and especially among the girls who overestimate their body shapes. Therefore, negative body image and the desire for thinness in girls is pointed out, already at pre-school age [92].

Data substantiate the importance for prevention programs aimed at increasing the parents' capability to early acknowledge overweight and obesity states in children, to perceive the risks for health, and at the same time promoting better body satisfaction in healthy weight pre-school children involving the relating adults.

One more variable focus on is the age when overweight conditions appear; it remarkably influences the structuring of negative body image. It influences more deeply if the overweight state appeared early. In individuals who have been overweight since birth, deeper altering was found in body image, compared to individuals who developed overweight or obesity conditions in adult age. In the former, body image structured with an actual overweight condition. Most probably, since infancy they had undergone teasing by peers and pressure by parents on reducing eating and losing weight. These factors may have contributed to the creation of negative body image. In a study by Adami et Al., individuals who had had early obesity, even when thanks to bariatric surgery they could lose weight to normal range, they continued to perceive themselves as 'too fat', maintaining high levels of body dissatisfaction. On the contrary, individuals who had developed obesity in adulthood, when they lowered their weight to normal levels, experienced better attitudes toward their own body and they were remarkably more satisfied about it. These individuals may have probably had access, after the weight loss, to a positive body image they had acquired during development, on the contrary, those who had developed the excessive weight problem early, did not have a positive body image to access and refer to. [93].

Research on pre-adolescents stress the fact that worries about body image are more present in girls, and they correlate positively with the BMI: in a study Hausenblas et al. [94] on 395 middle school students (49,5% girls) it is shown how high BMI was a strong predictor of body dissatisfaction. This, although prevailing among girls, resulted to be a relevant dimension for both genders.

Adolescence represents a crucial moment for the reorganization of body image, following important physical changes of puberty. Adolescents see their pre-puberal image disappear and have to elaborate the physical transformation of it. During these years, the influence of context factors, family and cultural values and especially the role of peers become stronger. The component of ideal body image plays a crucial role; the degree of body satisfaction is conditioned by comparisons to the peers' physical appearance and to the aesthetic model which is socially suggested. This process of restructuring is usually accompanied by experiences of dissatisfaction and inadequacy. The body changes from being a reassuring anchor in the continuing experience of the self, to a signal of catastrophic change. Ambivalence and adolescent conflict often find expression in the "theatres of the body" [95].

When an individual's body image is extremely weak, the idealized image tends to prevail over the basic image with the risk of pathologic consequences. The body image disorder in adolescence is more common among girls rather than boys, in late adolescence, among those who have internalized more deeply the ideal of thinness and among those who have been teased about their physical appearance and their weight.

In this developing context, the overweight state is a factor of risk for psychological and clinical problems, besides being related to more unhealthy behaviours about weight [96].

Several studies have examined the factors influencing attitudes towards body and eating and behaviours for weight check in overweight adolescents. Parenting models, the type of family managing and the quality of parents-children relationships proved important factors influencing attitudes and behaviours in adolescents [97,98].

The model offered by parents in terms of attitudes toward the body and eating (i.e. body dissatisfaction and strict dieting to monitor weight) proved to be predicting analogue behaviours in adolescent girls [97]. Beside the parenting behavioural model, it was shown that even the representation young people had of their parents' attitudes towards eating and weight (i.e. the perception that parents' attitudes were altered) could influence their behaviour [98].

About the influence impressed by the family context, overweight states in adolescents seem to be related to higher levels of family conflicts and lower levels of family cohesion [99].

Good family cohesion and the habit of eating meals in a serene atmosphere are the variables, which inversely relate to body dissatisfaction [100].

A study on 130 overweight/obese teenagers and their parents (90,3% of which were mothers), showed how behaviours of weight check in children were not entirely conditioned by the parenting model. Nevertheless, adolescents who perceived body dissatisfaction in their parents and weight check behaviours (especially when extreme and unhealthy), more likely adopted similar behaviours in order to lose weight. However, other variables such as body satisfaction and self-esteem levels in parents proved to be relevant in influencing adolescents behaviours toward body and eating: parents with lower self-esteem levels were related to teenagers who considered thinness more important. Moreover, parents' body dissatisfaction correlated children's. This data confirms similar results in literature, which point out relations between body dissatisfaction levels in daughters and parents. Moreover, aspects related to family functioning (poor cohesion and adaptation) correlated overeating in children. Even though, in other studies we see that individual variables (such as body image and, partially, self-esteem levels) play a more consistent role compared to context variables (such as family encouragement and the level of instruction) in mediating the relationship between BMI the quality of life [102].

2.2. Peer Relations: The Influence of Comments and Teasing

In western society, where the ideal of beauty, especially for women, identifies with thinness, overweight and obese people can not surprisingly, be objects of comments and teasing.

This aspect gets more relevant in developmental age, especially pre-adolescence and adolescence, when a need for structuring body image appears, integrating the somatic changes occurred during the puberty phase.

This evolution is part of a main developmental duty: this phase in the life cycle is the reach of individual stable and cohesive identity.

Body for adolescents has special value, in fact it represents a way for symbolic expression of their own conflicts and their relational modalities, a way to communicate belonging and separation, and their new identity. Equally important during this phase is the group of peers, which acquires diverse functions: it helps define personality and the new sex roles, support movements of separation from the family and from one's own infant self; moreover it is an important source of emotional safety [103].

Inside this evolution frame where body and the group acquire remarkable importance, we can understand how sensitive adolescents are towards comments and teasing about weight and body shape, when these come from peers.

Weight teasing is rather popular among teenagers; in a study by Neumark-Sztainer, teasing was reported by 26% of girls and 22% of boys. Differences in the weight condition emerged though: teasing targeted 19% of normal weight against 45% of overweight girls, and 13% of normal weight against 50% of overweight boys. [104].

Overweight and obese teenagers are more likely to be judged and teased for their body shapes and their weight, both by family members and by peers. This makes them more vulnerable for altered eating attitudes, low self-esteem and depression

In a research on 4796 adolescents from different ethnic groups, comments and weight teasing were explored, both intra-family and among peers; it showed that weight teasing is a common problem, targeting obese and overweight young people remarkably more frequently than normal weight people. Differences related to ethnicity were not reported [105].

Evidence shows how overweight girls are much more teased compared to boys, causing their relationships much more difficult in peers milieu [106].

In a behavioural intervention aimed at weight monitoring, little weight loss in obese teenagers allowed improvement in the relational dimension, reducing the fear of judgement and weight teasing episodes. It was underlined that when the individual's interpersonal sensitivity decreased, teasing attitude decreases along time [107].

Several studies have explored the relation between weight teasing and the presence of altered eating attitudes.

The Project SAL (Successful Adolescent Weight Losers), examined the risk of weight teasing in overweight adolescents. The sample included more girls (65,5%), was composed of 130 overweight teenagers between 12 and 20 years of age, belonging to different ethnic groups. It showed how being exposed to a source – family or peers - of comments and weight teasing is a factor of risk for altered eating attitudes; being teased by two different sources – family and peers – was related to more strict eating practices. No relation between teasing and healthy tries of weight loss was reported (increase of fruit and vegetables consumption or increase of physical activity). More frequency in teasing corresponded to higher levels of binge eating, eating in secret and depression [108].

NEGATIVE BODY IMAGE IN OVERWEIGHT ADULTS WITH AND WITHOUT EATING DISORDER

The cognitive core of body image disorder is characterised by the tendency to consider one's own appearance as the main referent for self-esteem; as a consequence, being overweight cannot only influence negatively one's own body image, but in individuals affected by body image disorder it can reveal self-inadequacy. [26]

Although negative body image is not among the diagnostic criteria of BED [9], several contributions in literature underlined the role of focus on weight and body shapes in the evaluation of themselves in BED, as to suggest integration of current diagnostic criteria [12,13].

Contrasting data about the relation between BMI and the levels of body dissatisfaction in overweight and obese people are reported in literature [109-113]. Variability in body dissatisfaction in this group lets us believe it is not entirely explainable through the overweight degree, but that the presence of negative body image is an important mediator.

Among overweight people there are subgroups who experience a more negative body image, among which: women, people who encountered obesity in early age or have received critics about their body, people who suffer from BED, people who state a history of weight cycling or have been stigmatized because of their excessive weight [113-118]. Various research have observed relations between body dissatisfaction increase, depression symptoms increase and self-esteem decrease in obese women requesting treatment for weight loss [110, 112, 114] and the relation seems to be independent from the obesity degree. Nevertheless, while there is a difference in body image dissatisfaction between obese and non-obese women, there is no difference in the two samples about depression symptoms, self-esteem and anxiety [116, 119]. The acknowledgement of an individual's own overweight condition plays an important role in the decision to undertake weight loss treatment; the perceived weight seems to have stronger impact on this decision compared to actual weight. [120].

Heinberg et al. [119] suggested that people with moderate body dissatisfaction are usually motivated to lose weight or better their health, changing eating habits and physical activity. On the contrary, people with high levels of dissatisfaction don't seem to be willing to change these behaviours.

Underestimation of their overweight condition is also a factor obstructing motivation to change. Such underestimation refers to a body image disorder, in particular to an alteration of the perceptive component. Such alteration relates to the presence of discrepancy between physical appearance and the mind representation the person has of his/herself, for instance obese people, even when they have lost weight, may continue to see themselves as fat as they were before.

Literature points out some conditions which may lead to alter the perception process and overestimate one's own body shape, among which are bad mood, [121], being exposed to images of thin women [23], pre-menstruation period [122] or weight fluctuation [123].

Several studies have explored the relation between BMI and the perceptive component, reporting discordant results; some report tendency to overestimate body shape, [123,124], others underline good grades of esteem [125].

Recent contributions in literature show the tendency to underestimate their own weight and body shapes in overweight and obese individuals. [126,120,127,128,129].

A Spanish study on a wide sample of 9320 adults waiting for dieting counseling, showed the diffused tendency to underestimate their weight; such tendency was higher in men [129] and increased with age for both genders [120].

Literature underlines the role of factors such as gender and ethnicity in the modulation of body perception: women tend to perceive themselves as overweight more than men, even with the same BMI. Men are less accurate in estimating their body shape and weight. [127,130]. In a recent review of literature, Gardner points out how the introduction of computer methods has helped clarify the role of sensor and non-sensor variables in the perception of body shape. Studies where men were asked to insert their weight into one of several discrete categories ranging from thin to overweight. Most men who are thin or who are in the normal weight range are accurate in categorizing themselves, while overweight and obese men consistently report underestimation of their size. The findings have been consistent across several nationalities. Distinct differences have also been found between cultures where smaller versus larger body size are seen as preferred. Body size underestimations occurring in cultures where a larger body is found to be desirable [131].

A study on overweight and obese Pakistan adults who attended a general practitioner room, analyzed the factors related to disperception; the tendency to underestimate their weight was higher in people in advance age (older or equal to 40 years of age), in men, in those who presented good levels of body satisfaction and did not know their healthy weight. Especially obese people underestimated their condition (73%), half of them believed they were only overweight[127].

Similar results were found in a study on a sample of general population in the surroundings of Nairobi. Even there, more than half of overweight and obese people underestimated their weight, (53%), although in this case women clearly prevailed (34,6% F vs 16,9% M). More than one third of the subjects (belonging to all BMI categories) with no relevant difference between genders, showed preference for overweight and obesity sizes, placing in this area their aesthetic ideal [128].

In the same weight conditions, affection by ED influences the degree of body satisfaction; adults with BED refer more body dissatisfaction compared to those without ED [132-134], higher dissatisfaction for specific areas in their body and higher levels of depression [135]. Moreover, body dissatisfaction seems to be positively related to the seriousness of binge eating [136]. In a follow-up, Striegel-Moore et al., assessed body dissatisfaction and BMI in individuals with and without BED. The former showed a remarkable increase of both variables in time compared to the latter. Individuals with BED show frequent behaviours of avoidance and body checking which represent expressions of negative body image, they express body dissatisfaction and at the same time they contribute to maintaining it. [137].

A recent study compared women with and without BED who had requested treatment for weight loss; not significantly different for BMI, the women with BED showed higher levels of body dissatisfaction which had led them, in time, to undertake dieting. Overweight and obese individuals with BED showed a psychopathologic core similar to people with other ED, characterized by excessive estimation of weight and body shape, and eating monitoring. Such core was not present in obese individuals without BED. This data is in line with what the transdiagnostic theory of ED expresses [140]. Women with BED, compared to women without BED, showed better internalization of the thin ideal experiencing a remarkable gap between actual and ideal body shapes. Such gap, besides encouraging body dissatisfaction, exposed it to higher risks of hypereating compared to women without BED [139].

Most research on overweight and obese patients with ED focused on BED [141]; however, excessive weight was found also in bulimia nervosa (BN) and in eating disorders not otherwise specified (EDNOS) [135]. Research comparing samples of ED patients with diverse weight conditions (healthy weight, overweight and obese) is scarce. [143,144]. The results of some studies suggest that ED patients with higher BMI or with a history of obesity present higher levels of specific psychopathologies (worries about weight, binge eating episodes) and general psychopathology (anxiety and depression) [141,142,143,144]. In recent studies undertaken in Sweden on 3798 adults attending clinics for diagnosis and treatment of ED, the following variable were examined in BN, EDNOS and BED (in the study, underweight people were excluded): self-esteem, specific and general psychopathology. More than 28% of the sample was overweight and obese. Overweight and obese ED patients did not score higher levels of general psychopathology compared to healthy weight patients. However, they reported more negative image of themselves (especially in the self-control and self-neglect dimensions) and more negative eating behaviours [145].

REFERENCES

[1] Sarwer, DB; Thompson, JK; Cash, TF. Body image and obesity in adulthood. *Psychiatr Clin. North Am,* 2005 28, 69-87.

[2] Farhat, T; Iannotti, RJ; Caccavale, LJ. Adolescent overweight, obesity and chronic disease-related health practices: mediation by body image. *Obes. Facts*, 2014 7(1), 1-14.

[3] Wiedemann, AA; Saules, KK. The relationship between emotional eating and weight problem perception is not a function of body mass index or depression. *Eat Beahav,* 2013 14(4), 525-528.

[4] Eichen, DM; Cinner, BT; Daly, BP; Pauber, RL. Weight perception, substance use, and disordered eating behaviors: comparing normal weight and overweight high-school students. *J. Adolesc. Young Adult Oncol,* 2012 41(1), 1-13.

[5] Hausenblas, HA; Fallon, EA. Body image satisfaction of physically active versus nonactive individuals: A meta-analytic review. *Paper presented at the Association for the Advancement of Applied Sport Psychology, Orlando*, FL, October, 2001.

[6] Pesa, JA; Syre, TR; Jones E. Psychosocial differences asssociated with body weight among female adolescents: the importance of body image. *J. Adolesc. Health*, 2000 26, 330-337.
[7] Reas DL; Grilo CM; Masheb RM; Wilson T. Body Checking and Avoidance in Overweight Patients with Binge Eating Disorder. *Int. J. Eat Disord*, 2005 37(4), 342-346.
[8] Ohsiek S; Williams M. Psychological factors influencing weight loss maintenance: An integrative literature review. *J. Am. Acad. Nurse Pract,* 2011 23, 592-601.
[9] American Psychiatric Association. Diagnostic and Statistical Manual of Mental Disorders (5th ed.). *The American Psychiatric Association*: Washington, DC, 2013.
[10] Stunkard, AJ; Allison, KC; Binge Eating Disoder: disoder or marker. *Int. J. Eat Disord*, 2003 34,107-116.
[11] Hrabosky, JI; Masheb, RM; White, MA; Grilo, CM. Overvaluation of shape and weight in binge eating disorder. *J. Consult Clin. Psychol.*, 2007 75, 175–180.
[12] Mond, JM; Hay, PJ; Rodgers, B; Owen, C. Recurrent binge eating with and without the "undue influence of weight or shape on self-evaluation": Implications for the diagnosis of binge eating disorder. *Behav. Res. Ther,* 2007 45, 929–938.
[13] Hrabosky, JI; Masheb, RM; White, MA; Grilo, CM. Overvaluation of shape and weight in binge eating disorder. *J. Consult. Clin. Psychol*, 2008 75, 175-180.
[14] Pope, CG; Pope, HG; Menard, W; Fay, C; Olivardia, R; Philips KA. Clinical features of muscle dysmorphia among males with body dysmorphia. *Body Image*, 2005 2(4), 395-400.
[15] Murray, SB; Rieger, E; Touyz , SWDe la Garza Garcia Y. Muscle Dysmorphia and the DSM-V comundrum: Where does it belong? A review paper. *Int. J. Eat Disord*, 2010 43, 483-491.
[16] Paillard, J. Body Schema and Body Image: a double dissociation in deafferented patients. In S. Gantchev & J. Mori. *Motor control; today and tomorrow.* Sophia: Accademic Publishing House, 1999.
[17] Cuzzolaro, M., Piccolo F., Speranza, A.M. *Anoressia, bulimia, obesità: disturbi dell'alimentazione e del peso corporeo da 0 a 14 anni*. Carrocci Faber, Roma, 2009.
[18] Head, H. Studies in neurology. Vol. II. London: Oxford University Press 1920.
[19] Dolto, F. *L'immagine inconscia del corpo*. Ed. Bompiani Milano, Italia, 1998.
[20] Zappa, L. *Alice in fuga dallo specchio*. Ed. Franco Angeli Milano, Italia, 2009.
[21] Schilder, P. I*mmagine di sé e schema corporeo.* Ed. Franco Angeli Milano, Italia 1973.
[22] Cash, T.F. *The Body Image Woorbook.* New Harbinger Oakland, 1997.
[23] Thompson, JK. Body image: extent of disturbance, associated features, theoretical models, assessment methodologies, intervention strategies and a proposal for a new DSM-IV diagnostic category- Body Image Disorder. *Progress behavior modification.* Vol 28:3-54. Sycamore. IL: Sycamore 1992.
[24] Rosen, J.C. Improving body image in obesity. In Thompson, KT. (Eds.). *Body image, eating disorders and obesity.* 425-440. Washington DC: American Psychological Association 1996.
[25] Thompson, J.K., & Heinber, L.J; Altabe M., & Tantleff-Dunn S. Sociocultural theory: the media and society. In J.K. Thompson, & L.J. Heinberg, & M.N. Altable, &; Tantleff-Dunn, S. (Eds.), *Exacting Beauty: theory, assessment, and treatment of body*

image disturbance (pp 85-124). Washington, DC: American Psychological Association. 1999.

[26] Dalle Grave, R. *Terapia cognitivo-comportamentale dell'obesità*. Positive Press. Verona, Italia, 2013.

[27] Consiglio, C., Scaini, V. (2003). *Evoluzione e alimentazione. Il cammino dell'uomo*. Ed. Bollati Boringhieri Milano, Italia, 2003.

[28] Puhl, RM, Heuer, CA. The stigma of obesity: a review and update. *Obesity,* 2009 17(5),1-24.

[29] Wadden, TA; Stunkard, AJ. Psychcopathology and obesity. *Annals of the New York Accademy of Science*. 1985 499, 55-65.

[30] Puhl, RM; Brownell KD. Psychosocial origins of obesity stigma: toward changing a powerful and pervasive bias. *Obes. Rev.*, 2003 4, 213-227.

[31] Puhl, RM; Latner, JD. Stigma, obesity, and the health of the nation's children. *Psychol. Bull,* 2007 133, 557-580.

[32] Allon, N. The stigma of overweight in every-day life. In B.B Wolman, & S. DeBerry (Eds.), *Psychological Aspects of Obesity: a handbook*. (130-174). New York: Van Nostrand Reinhold 1982.

[33] Allison, DB; Basile, VC; Yuker, HE. The measurement of attitudes toward and beliefs about obese persons. *Int. J. Eat Disord*, 1991 10, 599-607.

[34] Puhl, RM, Moss-Racusin, CA, Schwartz, MB, Brownell, KD. Weight stigmatization and bias reduction: perspectives of overweight and obese adults. *Health Educ. Res.,* 2008 23, 347–358.

[35] Crandall, CS. Prejudice against fat people: ideology and self-interest. *J. Pers Soc. Psychol.*, 1994 66, 882-894.

[36] Crandall, CS; Schiffhauer, KL. Anti-fat prejudice: Beliefs, values, and American culture. *Obes. Res.*, 1998 6, 458-460.

[37] Rudman, LA; Feinburg, J; Fairchild, K. Minority members' implicit attitudes: automatic ingroup bias as a function of group status. *Soc. Cogn*, 2002 20, 294-320.

[38] Blumber, P. et Al. Medical students' attitudes toward the obese and the morbility obese. *Int. J. Eat Disor*. 1985 4, 169-175.

[39] Wang, SS; Brownell, KD; Wadden, TA. The influence of the stigma of obesity on overweight individuals. *Int. J. Obes*, 2004 28, 1333-1337.

[40] Rothblum, ED; Brand, PA; Miller, CT; Oetjen, HA. The relationship between obesity, employment discrimination, and employment-related vicitimization. *J. Vocat Behav.*, 1990 37, 251-266.

[41] Friedman, KE; Reichmann, SK; Costanza, PR; Zelli, A; Ashmore, JA; Musante, GJ. Weight stigmatization and ideological beliefs: relation to psychological functioning in obese adults. *Obesity*, 2005 13, 907-916.

[42] Ashmore, JA; Friedman, KE; Reichmann, SK; Musante, GJ. Weight-based stigmatization, psychological distress, and binge eating behavior among obese treatment-seeking adults. *Eat Behav.*, 2008, 9, 203-209.

[43] Pagan, JA; Davila, A. Obesity, occupational attainment, and earnings. *Soc. Sci.* Q, 1997 78, 756-770.

[44] Register, CA; Williams, DR. Wage effects of obesity among young workers. *Soc. Sci.* Q, 1990 71, 130-141.

[45] Puhl RM, Moss-Racusin CA; Schwartz MB. Internalization of weight bias: Implications for binge eating and emotional well-being. *Obesity*, 2007 15, 19-23.

[46] Vartanian, LB, Shaprow, JG. Effects of weight stigma on exercise motivation and behavior. *J. Health Psychol.*, 2008 13, 131-138.

[47] Greenleaf, C; Starks, M; Gomez, L; Chambliss, H; Martin, S. Weight-related words associated with figure silhouettes. *Body Image*, 2004 1, 373-384.

[48] Carels, RA; Young, KM; Wott, CB; Harper, A; Gumble, M; Wagner Hobbs, M; Clayton, AM. Internalized weight stigma and its ideological correlates among weight loss treatment seeking adults. *Eat Weight Disord*, 2009 14, 92-97.

[49] Carels, RA; Hinman, NG; Burmeister, JM; Hoffmann, DA; Ashrafioun, L; Koball AM. Stereotypical images and implicit weight bias in overweight/obese people. *Eat Weight Disord*, 2013 18, 441-445.

[50] Teachman, BA; Gapinkski, K; Brownell, KD; Rawlins, M; Jeyaram, S. Demonstrations of implicit ant-fat bias: the impact of providing causal information and evoking empathy. *J. Health Psychol.*, 2003 22, 68-78.

[51] Dovidio, JF; Kawakami, K; Gaertner, SL. Implicit and explicit prejudice and interracial interaction. *J. Pers. Soc. Psychol.*, 2002 82, 62-68.

[52] Carels, RA; Young, KM; Wott, CB; Harper, J; Gumble, A; Oehlof, MW; Clayton, AM. Weight bias and weight loss treatment outcomes in treatment seeking adults. *Ann. Behav. Med.*, 2009 37, 350-355.

[53] Shapiro, JR; Neuberg, SL. From stereotype threat to stereotype threats: implications of a multi-threat framework for causes, moderators, mediators, consequences, and interventions. *Pers. Soc. Psychol. Rev.*, 2007 11, 107–130.

[54] Steele, CM; Aronson, J. Stereotype Threat and the intellectual test-performance of African-Americans. *J. Pers. Soc. Psychol.*, 1995 69, 797–811.

[55] Schmader, T; Johns, M; Forbes, C. An integrated process model of stereotype threat effects on performance. *Psychol. Rev.*, 2008 115, 336–356.

[56] Schmader, T; Johns, M. Converging evidence that stereotype threat reduces working memory capacity. *J. Pers. Soc. Psychol.*, 2003 85,440–452.

[57] Seacat, JD; Mickelson, KD. Stereotype threat and the exercise/dietary health intentions of overweight women. *J. Health Psychol.*, 2009 14, 56–567.

[58] Shapiro, JR. Different groups, different threats: a multi-threat approach to the experience of stereotype threat. *Pers. Soc. Psychol. Bull*, 2011 37, 464–480.

[59] Ashmore, RD; Deaux, K; McLaughlin-Volpe, T. An organizing framework for collective identity: articulation and significance of multidimensionality. *Psychol. Bull*, 2004 130, 80–114.

[60] Carels, RA; Domoff, SE; Burmeister, JM; Koball, AM; Hinman, NG; Davis, AK; Wagner Oehlhof, M; Leroy, M; Bannon, E; Hoffmann, DA. Examining Perceived Stereotype Threat among Overweight/Obese Adults Using a Multi-Threat Framework. *Obes. Facts*, 2013 6(3), 1-12.

[61] Myers, A; Rosen, JC. Obesity stigmatization and coping: relation to mental health symptoms, body image, and self-esteem. *Int. J. Obes*, 1999 25, 1525–1531.

[62] Levy, BR; Pilver, CE. Residual stigma: Psychological distress among the formerly overweight. *Soc. Sci. Med.*, 2012 75(2), 297-299.

[63] Malkin, AR; Wornian, K; Chrisler, JC. Women and weight: Gendered messages on magazine covers. *Sex Roles*, 1999 40, 647-655.

[64] Nemeroff, CJ; Stein, RI; Diehl, NS; Smilack, KM. From the Cleavers to the Clintons: Role choices and body orientation as reflected in magazine article content. *Int. J. Eat Disord*, 1994 16, 167-176.

[65] Petrie, TA; Austin, LJ; Cowley, BJ; Helmcamp, A; et al. Sociocultural expectations of attractiveness for males. *Sex Roles*, 1996 35, 581-602.

[66] Spitzer, BL; Henderson, KA; Zivian, MT. Gender differences in population versus media body sizes: A comparison over four decades. *Sex Roles*,1999 40, 545-565.

[67] Stice, E. Risk and maintenance factors for eating pathology: A meta-analytic review. *Psychol. Bull,* 2002 128,825-848.

[68] Becker, AE. Television, disordered eating, and young women in Fiji: negotiating body image and identity during rapid social change. *Cult Med. Psychiatry*, 2004 28(4), 533-59.

[69] Myers, PN; Biocca, FA. The elastic body image: the effect of television advertising and programming on body image distorsion in young women. *J. Commun.*, 1992 42(3), 108-133.

[70] Fouts, G; Vaughan, K. Television situation comedies: Male weight, negative references, and audience reactions. *Sex Roles,* 2002 46, 439-442.

[71] Fouts G, Burggraf K. Television situation comedies: Female weight, male negative comments, and audience reactions. *Sex Roles*, 2000 42, 925-932.

[72] Akers, R.L. *Deviant behavior*. Belmont, CA, Wadsworth. 1973.

[73] Bandura, A. *Social learning theory*. General Learning Press New York, 1971.

[74] Gerbner, G; Gross, L. Living with television: The violence profile. *J. Commun.*, 1976 26, 173-199.

[75] Signorielli, N. & Morgan, M. *Cultivation analysis: New directions in media effects research*. Sage Publications Newbury Park, CA, 1990.

[76] Klein, H; Shiffman, KS. Thin is “in” and stout is “out”: What animated cartoons tell viewers about body weight. *Eat Weight Disord*, 2005 10,107-116.

[77] Henderson-King, D; Henderson-King, E; Hoffman, L. Media images and women’s self-evaluations: Social context and importance of attractiveness as moderators. *Pers. Soc. Psychol. Bull,* 2001 27, 1407-1416.

[78] Wilcox, K; Laird, JD. The impact of media images of super-slender women on women’s self-esteem: Identification, social comparison, and self-perception. *J. Res. Pers.*, 2000 34, 278-286.

[79] Durkin, SJ; Paxton, SJ. Predictors of vulnerability to reduced body image satisfaction and psychological wellbeing in response to exposure to idealized female media images in adolescent girls. *J. Psychosom. Res.,* 2002 53, 995-1005.

[80] Lin, LF; Kulik, JA. Social comparison and women’s body satisfaction. *Basic Appl. Soc. Psych.,* 2002 24, 115-123.

[81] Murray, SH; Touyz, SW; Beumont, PJV. Awareness and perceived influence of body ideals in the media: A comparison of eating disorder patients and the general community. *Eat Disord,* 1996 4, 33-46.

[82] Stice, E. Modeling of eating pathology and social reinforcement of the thin-ideal predict onset of bulimic symptoms. *Behav. Res. Ther.*, 1998 36, 931-944.

[83] Thomsen, SR; McCoy, JK; Williams, M. Internalizing the impossible: Anorexic outpatients’ experiences with women’s beauty and fashion magazines. *Eat Disord*, 2001 9, 49-64.

[84] Kreisler, L., & Fain, M. & Soule M. *L'enfant et son corps*. Presses Universitaires de France, Paris, France, 1999.

[85] Carretti, V., & La Barbera D. *Alessitimia: valutazione e trattamento*. Ed. Astrolabio Roma, Italia, 2005.

[86] Pinhas, L; Toner, BB; Ali, A; Garfinkel, PE; Stuckless, N. The effects of the ideal of female beauty on mood and body satisfaction. *Int. J. Eat Disord,* 1999 25, 223-226.

[87] Rhee, KE; De Lago, CW; Arscott-Mills, T; Mehta, SD; Davis, RK. Factor associated with parental readiness to make chiane for overweight children. *Pediatric*, 2005 116, 94-101.

[88] Doolen, J; Alpert, PT; Miller, SK. Parental disconnect between perceived and actual weight status of children: a metasynthesis of the current research. *J. Am. Acad. Nurse Pract*, 2009 21,160-166.

[89] Towns, N; D'Auria, J. Parental perceptions of their child's overweight: an integrative review of the literature. *J. Pediatr. Nurs*, 2009 24(2),115-30.

[90] Parkinson, KN; Drewett, RF; Jones, AR; Dale, A; Pearce, MS; Wright, CM; Adamson, AJ; and the Gateshead Millennium Study core team. When do mothers think their child is overweight? *Int. J. Obes*, 2011 35(4), 510-516.

[91] Tremblay, L; Lovsin, T; Zecevic, C; Lariviere, M. Perception of self in 3-5 years old children: a preliminary investigation into the early emergence of body dissatisfaction. *Body Image*, 2011 8, 287-292.

[92] Cramer, P; Steinwert, T. Thin is good, fat is bad: How early does is begin? *J. Appl. Dev. Psychol.,* 1998 19, 429-451.

[93] Adami, G; Bauer, B; Gandolfo, P; Scopinaro, N. Body image in early-onset obese patients. *Eat Weight Disord*, 1997 2, 87-93.

[94] Hausenblas, H.A; Symons Downs, DS; Fleming DS; Connaughton DP. Body image in middle school children. *Eat Weight Disord*, 2001 7,244-248.

[95] McDougall J. *Theatres du corps. Le psychosoma en psychanalyse*. Ed. Gallimard Paris, France, 1989.

[96] Maggiolini A., & Pietropolli Charmet G. *Manuale di psicologia dell'adolescenza: compiti e conflitti*. Ed. Franco Angeli Milano, Italia, 2004.

[97] Wertheim, E; Mee, V; Paxton, S. Relationships among adolescent girls' eating behaviors and their parents' weight-related attitudes and behaviors. *Sex Roles*, 1994 41, 169-187.

[98] Boutelle, K; Birkeland, R; Hannan, P; et al. Associations between maternal concern for healthful eating and maternal eating behaviors, home food availability, and adolescent eating behaviors. *J. Nutr. Educ.*, 2007 39, 248-256.

[99] Zeller, M; Reiter-Purtill, J; Modi, A; et al. Controlled study of critical parent and family factors in the obesigenic environment. *Obesity*, 2007 15,126-136.

[100] Fulkerson, JA; Strauss, J; Neumark-Sztainer, D; et al. Correlates of psychosocial well-being among overweight adolescent: the role of the family. *J. Consult Clin. Psychol.*, 2007 75,181-186.

[101] Cromley, TR; Neumark-Sztainer, D; Story, M; Boutelle, K. Parent and family associations with weight-related behaviors and cognitions among overweight adolescent. *J. Adolesc. Health*, 2010 47(3), 263-269.

[102] Kolodziejczyk, JK; Gutzmer, K; Wright, SM; Arredondo, EM; Hill, L; Patrick, K; Huang, JS; Gottschalk, M; Norman, GJ. Influence of specific individual and

environmental variables on the relationship between body mass index and health-related quality life in overweight and obese adolescents. *Qual Life Res* 1, 2014 (epub ahead of print).

[103] Maggiolini, A., & Pietropolli Charmet G. *Manuale di psicologia dell'adolescenza: compiti e conflitti*. Ed. Franco Angeli Milano, Italia, 2004.

[104] Neumark-Sztainer, D; Falkner, N; Story, M; et Al; Weight-teasing among adolescents: correlation whit weight status and disordered eating behaviors. *Int. J. Obes. Relat. Metab. Disord,* 2002 26, 123-131.

[105] Van den Berg, P; Neumark-Sztainer, D; Eisenberg, ME; Haines, J. Racial/ethnic differences in weight-related teasing in adolescents. *Obesity*, 2008 2, 3-10.

[106] Tang-Peronard, JL; Heitmann, BL. Stigmatization of obese children and adolescent, the importance of gender. *Obesity*. 2009 4, 3-11.

[107] Rancourt, D; Barker, DH; Sato, Af; Lloyd-Richardson, EE; Hart, CN; Jelalian, E. Longitudinal association among change in overweight status, fear of negative evaluation, and weight-related teasing among obese adolescents. *J Pediatr Psychol*, 2014 Pii:jsu 033(Epub ahead of print).

[108] Libbey, HP; Story, MT; Neumark-Sztainer, DR; Boutelle, KN.Teasing, disordered eating behaviors, and psychological morbidities among overweight adolescents. *J. Obesity*, 2008 6, 24-29.

[109] Eldrige, KL; Agras, WS. Weight and shape overconcern and emotional eating in binge eating disorder. *Int. J. Eat Disord* 1996 19, 73–82.

[110] Foster, GD; Wadden, TA; Vogt, RA. Body image before, during, and after weight loss treatment. *Health Psychol.*, 1997 16, 226–229.

[111] Matz, PE; Foster, GD; Faith, MS; et al. Correlates of body image dissatisfaction among overweight women seeking weight loss. *J. Consult Clin. Psychol.*, 2000 70, 1040–1044.

[112] Sarwer, DB; Wadden, TA; Foster, GD. Assessment of body image dissatisfaction in obese women: specificity, severity and clinical significance. *J. Consult Clin. Psychol.,* 1998 66(4), 651–654.

[113] Wilfley, DE; Schwartz, MB; Spurrell, EB; et al. Using the eating disorder examination to identify the specific psychopathology of binge eating disorder. *Int. J. Eat Disord*, 2000 27, 259–269.

[114] Grilo, CM; Wilfley, DE; Brownell, KD; et al. Teasing, body image, and self-esteeming a clinical sample of obese women. *Addict Behav.*, 1994 9, 443–450.

[115] Jackson, TD; Grilo, CM; Masheb, RM. Teasing history, onset of obesity, current eating disorder psychopathology, body dissatisfaction, and psychological functioning in binge eating disorder. *Obes. Res.*, 2000 8,451–458.

[116] Annis, NM; Cash, TF; Hrabosky JI. Body image and psychosocial differences among stable average-weight, currently overweight, and formerly overweight women: the role of stigmatizing experiences. *Body Image*, 2004 155-67.

[117] Friedman, MA; Schwartz, MB; Brownell, KD. Differential relation of psychological functioning with the history and experience of weight cycling: psychological correlates of weight cycling. *J. Consult. Clin. Psychol.*, 1998 66,646–50.

[118] Myers, A; Rosen, JC. Obesity stigmatization and coping: Relation to mental health symptoms, body image, and self-esteem. *Int. J. Obes*, 1999 23,221–30.

[119] Heinberg, L.J., & Thompson, J.K., & Matzon, J.L. Body image dissatisfaction as a motivator for healthy lifestyle change: is some distress beneficial? In: R.H. Stiegel-

Moore, & L.Smolak (Eds), Eat Disord, Washington, DC: American Psychological Association, 2001.

[120] Acevedo, P; Lopez-Ejeda, N; Alferez-Garcia, I; Martinez-Alvarez, JR; Villarino, A; Cabanas, MD; Marrodan, MD. Body mass index through self-reported data and body image perception in Spanish adults attending dietary consultation. *Nutrition*, 2014 30, 679-684.

[121] Taylor, MJ; Cooper, PJ. Experimental study of the effect of mood on body size perception. Behav Res Ther,1992 30, 53-58.

[122] Carr-Nangle, RE; et al. Body image change of the menstrual cycle in normal women. *Int. J. Eat Disord,* 1994 16,267-273.

[123] Collins, JK et al. Variability in body shape perception in anorexic, bulimic, obese and control subjects. *Int. J. Eat Disord*, 1987 6, 633-638.

[124] Gardner, RM; et al. Obesity and body image: an evaluation of sensory and non sensory components. *Psychol. Med.*, 1987 927-932.

[125] Brodie DA et al. Reliability measures in disturbing body image. *Percept Mot. Skills,* 1989 69, 723-732.

[126] Dekkers, JC; van Wier, MF; Hendriksen, IJ; Twist, JW; van Mechelen, W. Accuracy of self-reported body weight. Height and waist circumference in Dutch overweight working popolation. *Eat Weight Disord*, 2014 19,233-240.

[127] Bhanji, S; Khuwaja, AK; Siddiqui, F; Azam, I; Kazmi K. Underestimation of weight and its associated factor among overweight and obese adult in Pakistan: a cross sectional study. *BMC Public Health*, 2011 23, 363.

[128] Ettarh, R; Van de Vijver, S; Oti S, Kyobutungi C. Overweight, obesity and perception of body image among slum residents in Nairobi, Kenya, 2008-2009. *Prev. Chronic. Dis.*, 2013 19, E212.

[129] Squiers, L; Renaud, J; McCormack, L; Tzeng, J; Bann, C; Williams, P. How accurate are americans' perceptions of their own weight? *J. Health Commun.*, 2014 19, 95-812.

[130] Ter Bogt, TF; van Dorsselaer, SA; Monshouwer, K; Verdurmen, JE; Engels RC, Vollebergh, WA. Body mass index and body weight perception as risk factors for internalizing and externalizing problem behavior among adolescents. *J. Adolesc. Health*, 2006 39, 27-34.

[131] Gardner, RM. Weight status and the perception of body image in men. *Psychol. Res. Behav. Manag.,* 2014 7, 175-184.

[132] Dunkley, DM; Grilo, CM. Self-criticism, low self-estreem, depressive syntoms and over-evaluation of shape and weight in binge eating disorder patients. *Behav. Res. Ther*, 2007 45, 139-149.

[133] Hrabosky, JH; Masheb, RM; White, MA; et al. Overvaluation of shape and weight in binge eating disorder. *J. Consult. Clin. Psychol.*, 2007 75, 175-80.

[134] Grilo, CM; Masheb, RM. Correlates of body image dissatisfaction in treatment seeking men and women with binge eating disorder. *Int. J. Eat Disord*, 2005 38, 162-166.

[135] Lloyd-Richarson, EE, King, TK, Forsyth, LH, Clark MM. Body Image evaluations in obese females with binge eating disorder. *Eat Behav,* 2000 1, 161-167.

[136] De Zwaan, M; Nutzinger, DO; Schoenbeck, G. Binge eating in overweight women. *Compr. Psychiatry,* 1992 33, 256-261.

[137] Striegel-Moore, RH; Franko, DL; Thompson, D; et al. Changes in weight and body image over time on women with eating disorders. *Int. J. Eat Disord*, 2004 36, 315-327.

[138] Reas, DL; Grilo, CM; Masheb, RM; et al. Body checking and avoidance in overweight patients with binge eating disorders. *Int. J. Eat Disord*, 2005 37, 342-346.

[139] Diaz, MLB; Paredes, KF; Diaz, JMM; Rayon, GA; Aguilar, XL; Giron, T; Gonzalez, YS. Body dissatisfaction and socio-cultural factors in women with and without BED: their relation with eating psychopatology. *Eat Weight Disord,* 2012 17, 86-92.

[140] Fairburn, CG; Cooper, Z; Shafran, R. Cognitive behaviour therapy for eating disorders: a "transdiagnostic" theory and treatment. *Behav Res Ther*, 2003 41, 509-528.

[141] Digermans, AE; van Furth, EF. Binge Eating disoder psychopathology in normal-weight and obese individuals. *Int. J. Eat Disord*, 2012 45, 135-138.

[142] Fichter, MM; Quadflieg, N; Hedlund, S. Long-term course of binge eating disorder and bulimia nervosa: relevance for nosology and diadnostic criteria. *Int. J. Eat Disord*, 2008 41, 577-586.

[143] Barry, DT; Grilo, CM; Masheb, RM. Comparison of patients with bulimia nervosa, obese patients with binge eating disorder and nonobese patients with binge eating disorder. *J. Nerv. Ment. Dis.*, 2003 191, 589-594.

[144] Carrard, I; Van der Linden, M; Golay, A. Comparison of obese and nonobese individuals with binge eating disoder: delicate boundary between binge eating disorder and non-purging bulimia nervosa. *Eur. Eat Disord Rev.*, 2012 20, 350-354.

[145] Lapidoth, JM; von Yhausswolff-Juhlin Y. Eating disorder symptoms, psychiatric correlates and self-image in normal, overweight and obese eating disorder patients. *Eat Weight Disord*, 2014 19, 233-240.

In: The Different Faces of Being Overweight
Editor: Emilia Manzato
ISBN: 978-1-63483-099-7

Chapter 8

LIFESTYLES: SEDENTARY LIFESTYLE AND UNBALANCED DIET

Eleonora Roncarati
Dietitian, member of Italian Society for the Study of Eating Disorders (SISDCA), Italy

ABSTRACT

The epidemic of overweight and obesity are a well-known phenomenon affecting the world population. Mainly, the increase in adipose tissue responsible for weight gain, is related to a gap in the energy balance for which the energy intake (nutrients) are superior than the energy expenditure (Resting Metabolic Rate, thermic effect, physical activity and thermogenesis from other causes). Several studies in the literature suggest that it is more difficult to maintain the energetic balance nowadays than in the past. Urbanization, industrialization and the use of transport have lead to a general decrease in energy expenditure for physical activity that has encouraged the development of "sedentary"; furthermore, there has been an exaggerated use of industrial techniques for processing and food preparation depleting the food from its healthy components, such as fibers vitamins, minerals and enrich it of nutrients that make it hyper palatable and highly caloric (sugar, lipids, especially saturated fats, salt, preservatives and food colourings). So you get a food called "refined and manipulated" very attractive, ready for consumption, low satiety index and high-calorie that's easy to "exceed" in the amount of intake and frequency of consumption; the excess that is realized in terms of total energy (calories) and nutrients densely caloric (as lipids and sugars) determines a positive energy balance, which correlates with weight gain. Several studies have also shown that the variations of body weight appear to be more affected by a "combination" of nutrients, rather than by a single nutrient taken in excess. The analysis of dietary patterns therefore provides an opportunity to assess which food styles are more related to the development of overweight and obesity, as well as metabolic diseases, cardiovascular and oncology. The analysis of patter food has led to identify a “Healthy Patter” that has features common to the "Mediterranean Diet". Various studies have shown that the Mediterranean diet is not related to an increased risk of overweight and obesity and may play a role in the prevention of both. Instead, the food restriction in order to control body weight was unsuccessful in the long term: the imposition of a rigid control promotes the loss of control over food intake resulting in energy and nutrients unscheduled nor manageable.

Keywords: overweight, energy balance, sedentary, food refined and manipulated, dietary patterns

Introduction

Overweight is usually underestimate. In clinical practice, people who seek help to manage weight are overall obese people, not overweight individuals. Besides, also in literature the majority of the studies focuses on obesity.

However, in recent years a great number of epidemiological studies look at overweight as a growing phenomenon all over the word.

Between 1980 and 2008 mean BMI worldwide increased by 0.4 kg/m^2 per decade (95% uncertainty interval 0.2—0.6, posterior probability of being a true increase >0.999) for men and 0.5 kg/ m^2 per decade (0.3—0.7, posterior probability >0.999) for women. The USA had the highest BMI of high-income countries. In 2008, an estimated 1.46 billion adults (1.41—1.51 billion) worldwide had BMI of 25 kg/ m^2 or greater [1].

In Europe the percentage of overweight or obese people is alarming for children, adolescents and adults. Besides, every year almost 7% of the national sanitary balances all over Europe are used to treat diseases linked to overweight. Recent evidences estimate that in UE almost 2,8 million causes of death are due to overweight and obesity [2].

In Italy, 2 adults to 5 (42%) have a Body Mass Index (BMI) over 25, in particular 31% of them are overweight (25<BMI<30) and 11% of them are obese (BMI>30) [3].

According to the WHO's Childhood Obesity Surveillance Initiative (COSI) data, in 2010 in UE almost one children to three between 6-9 years old were overweight or obese. This percentage is growing compared to 2008 when the estimation was 1 to 4 [4].

For these reasons, it's important to consider overweight as a key risk factor, that indicate an imbalance in energy intake and out take.

Energy Balance

A stable body weight is the results of a precise balance between the energy intake caused by biological ossidation of the nutrients and its decrease caused by energy expenditure or vital functions or physical activity.

If a person introduces an amount of energy higher than the amount that he /she uses, energy balance become positive and it results in an increase of body weight [5].

Energy balance mechanism is extremely complex and it involves different organs and tissues.

The key principle of energy balance is the following:

Changes in energy (fat) stores= energy (calories) intake – energy expenditure.

This principle can be used to prove that body weight changes over time in response to the changes in energy intake and out-take.

When the body is in energy balance, body weight remains stable because the energy spent is replaced with an equivalent amount of energy brought by food. Thus, the energy balance is defined as the reached condition when energy intake is equivalent to energy out take [6-7].

Assessment of energy balance is usually accomplished by assessment of body weight or body composition (to estimate the total energy content).

So body weight can change when energy intake is note equal to energy expenditure over a given period of time.

Overweight develops from an alteration of energy balance that causes a discrepancy between energy intake and energy expenditure. Alteration of energy balance causes changes in body composition (percentage of fat mass and muscle) and body weight, even if the difference in time in which all this take place can explain the large variety in range concerning the individual answer to weight loss.

There are evidences that a positive energy balance determines an increase in weight in which the 60-80% of the weight gained is a consequence of the increase of fat mass [8].

If energy intake continuously exceeds energy expenditure, the excess energy ingested has to be deposited, thus increasing the body nutrient stores. The result of this hierarchy is that excess energy intake leads essentially to fat storage, mainly in subcutaneous and visceral adipose tissue [9].

According to the first thermodynamic law, energy can be transformed from one form to another, but cannot be created or destroyed: "any energy increase given by food intake, not balanced by similar increase of energy expense, cause an increase of the metabolic storage consequently in the body weight mainly concerning the fat mass gain, which appears as the principal area where fat is stored."

The basic components of energy balance include energy intake, energy expenditure, and energy storage [10].

Humans take in energy in the form of protein, carbohydrate, fat, and alcohol; these nutrients are food and beverages components.

The main activities of energy expenditure concern the basal metabolic rate or resting metabolic rate, the diet-induced thermogenesis or thermic effect (TEF), physical activity (EEact) and thermogenesis due to other causes.

The resting metabolic rate (RMR) represents the energy consumed by an individual at rest, in a neutral thermic state, fasting for at least 12-14 hours, awake and relaxed. It's the essential quantity to sustain the normal body functions and the homeostasis of physiological functions in different activity. The RMR is proportional to body mass, particularly the amount of fat-free mass, and it represents the 60-75% of the total energy expenditure [5].

The TEF refers to the energy essential to digest and absorb the food; it is proportional to the total food consumed and, in a typical mixed diet, makes up 8% to 10% of total energy ingested.

The EEact is the most variable component of energy expenditure; it involves energy expenditure due to programmed physical activity, such as sport and the N.E.A.T (Non Exercise Activity Thermogenesis) which includes all the calories burnt with everyday activities, such as walking, climbing the stairs etc. [7].

The energetic cost of EEact depends on the type, frequency and intensity of the activities done. It can vary between 15% of total energy expenditure for sedentary lifestyle to 3 to 4 times the RMR for athletes.

On average it represents the 15-30% of the total energy expenditure. L'EEact can include a variable energy consumption, between 100 and 3000 calories per day, according to one's lifestyle.

Having an active lifestyle and doing regular physical activity increases the RMR because it increases the muscles.

Thermogenesis due to other causes cover a little percentage of the energy expenditure and it can be induced by smoke, caffeine or some spices. Even cold represents an important thermogenic stimulus mediated by SNS activation and catecholamine.

The available evidence suggests that a complex physiological control system is involved in maintaining energy balance [11]. This system includes afferent signals from the periphery about the state of energy stores and efferent signals that affect energy intake and expenditure [12-15].

If energy balance were not controlled by such a system and were subject only to behavioural mechanisms controlling food intake and volitional energy expenditure, most people would routinely experience wide swings in body weight over short periods of time. The relative stability of body weight from day to day is consistent with the view that energy balance is subject to physiological control.

Factors That Influence Energy Balance in Modern Times: The Importance of Sedentary Lifestyle

There are many factors involved in the development of overweight: genetic predisposition, biological, environmental and behavioural factors. In particular, the genetic ones seems to act as predisposing factors that increase the risk to develop a positive energy balance, when a person is exposed to a certain environmental or precipitant factor. Genetic predisposition associated to environmental factors called "Obesogenic", increases the susceptibility to gain weight, but it's not the only factor involved: the chronic exposure to environmental factors alone (hyper caloric foods or sedentary lifestyle) can lead to overweight. Environmental factors have a key role in the etiopathogenesis of overweight [16].

Despite the evidence for a physiological control system of energy balance, most people in today's environment gain significant excess body weight and body fat over their adult years. This does not argue against an energy balance control system, but suggests that there may be limits to the body's ability to match intake and expenditure under the prevailing conditions in the modern environment.

Evidences suggest that it is harder to maintain the energetic balance nowadays respect to the past [5].

For example, one can develop some crude estimates of the extent to which food intake has increased and physical activity has decreased over the past decades.

Analysis of the National Health and Nutrition Examination Survey (NHANES) suggests that the average daily energy intake increased from 1971 to 2000. The average increase was 168 kcal/d for men and 335 kcal/d for women. With no active regulation or adaptation of energy balance, this increase theoretically could explain a yearly weight gain of 18 lb for men and 35 lb. for women [17].

From the point of view of the energy expenditure, Bassett et all. [18] examined physical activity patterns in an Old Order Amish population who are living an agrarian lifestyle typical of a large fraction of the population in the United States, early in the 20th century. Using pedometers, they found that Amish men walked an average of 18425 steps per day and women an average of 14196 per day. Bassett et all. [19] also reported that in 2003 the average American adult walked ≈5000 steps per day. Compared with the Amish lifestyle, this is a difference of 13000 steps per day for men and 9000 steps per day for women. Without physiological adaptation taken into account, this decline in physical activity over the past century could explain a yearly weight gain of 68 lb. for men and 47 lb. for women. Similarly Church et all. recently estimated that occupational physical activity has declined by an average of ≈142 kcal/d since 1960. This (DATA) alone could explain a substantial amount of weight gain in the population.

Another study lead in the USA highlight that the amount of time spent for physical activity in the free time has been constant since 1988, but the physical activity in terms of lifestyle, has decreased significantly [20].

Urbanization, industrialization and the use of public transports have led to a general decrease of the EEact, conducting to the develop of sedentary lifestyle. According to this decrease, there has been an increase in weight gain [7].

A very physically active person might maintain energy balance and a healthy body weight by eating and expending 3000 kcal/d. This same person, if adopting a sedentary lifestyle, could maintain energy balance and the same healthy body weight by eating and expending 2000 kcal/d. Finally, if that sedentary person failed to sufficiently reduce energy intake to match reduced energy expenditure over time, that person would gain weight and could end up achieving energy balance at 3000 kcal/d by becoming obese.

According to OMS, sedentary lifestyle is the fourth key risk factor of global mortality, provoking every year 3.2 million of deaths.

In Italy data from the system of surveillance "PASSI", reveals that 33% of the people interviewed (18-69 years old) can be classified as active (that is, doing hard work or 30 minutes of moderate physical activity for at least 5 days a week or intensive activity for more than 20 minutes for at least 3 days per week), 36% as partially active (individuals that do some physical activity in the free time, without reaching the recommended levels) and the 31% can be classified as sedentary (individuals who don't do any physical activity in the free time or at work) [21].

The total energy expended in physical activity, i.e. the period of time devoted daily to physical activity, may play a important role in determining energy balance [22].

Through which mechanisms sedentary lifestyle foster the development of overweight and obesity?

In the first Instance, during physical activity mechanical work associated with muscle contractions clearly requires energy.

The difference between the total energy expenditure and the basal energy expenditure, the suprabasal energy expenditure, includes both the thermic effect of food and physical activity. This suprabasal energy expenditure was observed to be low in obese subjects [23-24]. This finding strongly suggests that the amount of energy expended in physical activity is low in obese individuals. Whether a low physical activity exists pre-obesity, or is merely a consequence of it, remains an open question at the present time.

On the basis of many review of the energy balance literature and information about how our modern lifestyle differs from decades ago, it has been hypothesised that human physiology developed under situations that conferred an advantage for achieving energy balance at a relatively high (compared with RMR) level of energy expenditure or high energy flux [7].

Mayer and colleagues [25] in the 1950s were the firsts that proposed the idea that energy balance is best regulated at high (but not excessive) levels of physical activity.

They observed that when people were physically active energy intake was better coordinated to energy expenditure. On the contrary, physical inactivity is linked to a positive energy balance: food intake apparently does not decline when energy demand declines. This imbalance is not only due to a lower energy expenditure: this is consistent with the view that the physiology is suited to regulate energy balance best under conditions in which physical activity (energy expenditure) "pulls" appetite. Mayer et all. further hypothesized that there may be a minimum threshold of either physical activity or energy throughout above which adaptive adjustments in energy intake and expenditure to achieve balance are more sensitive to changes in the other.

This would have been necessary to maintain body weight under ancestral lifestyle conditions that undoubtedly demanded a relatively high level of physical activity for survival. Given this hypothesized system bias for optimal control under high energy throughout conditions, an individual having a low energy throughout is constantly at risk for weight gain.

Blundell et all. [26] demonstrated that at low levels of physical activity, energy intake does not adjust quickly and accurately to changes in energy expenditure, with the result being an increased propensity to gain weight. Similarly, Stubbs et all. [27] reduced physical activity from 1.8 to 1.4 times the RMR in normal-weight men studied in a whole-room calorimeter and found that there was not a compensatory reduction in energy intake. This led to positive energy balance and weight gain.

Many other studies showing that a high level of physical activity is associated with low weight gain over time and comparatively low levels of physical activity, are associated with high weight gain over time. Over the past century, the physical activity level of most of the population has declined substantially. Although it is theoretically possible to avoid weight gain in this situation, the fact that few people have accomplished this, suggests that it is difficult to maintain energy balance at a low energy throughout.

A low energy throughout is a prominent feature of sedentary American life today. The body-weight gain may therefore be seen as an adaptive change to overfeeding [28]: changes in body weight and body composition appear to be the major factors that, by increasing energy expenditure, allow energy balance to be restored.

Body composition influences human body's efficiency. Multivariate analysis shows that lean body mass is the major determinant of energy expenditure, with minor influences of fat mass, age and gender [29]. Resting metabolic rate is higher in trained individuals than in sedentary individuals of the same weight [30], but the difference can be predominantly attributed to changes in body composition, with a lower fat mass and higher lean, metabolically active, body mass in trained athletes. A higher muscle mass, as estimated through bio impedance analysis (BIA), is associated with a greater weight loss in obese patients [31].

The mechanisms responsible for this increase in energy intake, have not been extensively studied [9]. As a result of the complex network in the central nervous system, that regulates energy expenditure and the known effects of physical activity on neuro-endocrine regulations, it is very likely that the relationship between energy expended in physical activity and food intake are quite complex. However, endurance-trained athletes are characterized by a low fat mass, which may be the result of previous periods of negative energy and fat balances. They also have low leptin levels, which are essentially attributable to the low fat mass, since comparable leptin levels are observed in very lean sedentary individuals. It may indicate that a substantial decrease in fat-free mass induced by exercise is required to decrease leptin secretion before low leptin in turn increases food intake. Interestingly, this absence of effects of exercise contrasts with the effect of severe energy restriction, which rapidly decreases leptin levels before any marked changes in body composition occur [32-33]. It may indicate that exercise is more efficient than severe energy restriction in the promotion of weight loss, without undue rebound hyperphagia.

In conclusion, much of the drastic decline in daily activity (and hence daily energy expenditure) occurred during the first part of the last century as industrialization and urbanization changed typical lifestyles, and this may have been a prerequisite for enabling the increase in obesity seen over the last 30 years. In the latter part of the 20th century as food price relative to income declined [34] and access, availability [35] and convenience all increased, the physiological system had already been primed for weight gain. Under the prevailing sedentary lifestyle conditions today, gaining weight helps to increase RMR and the energy cost of physical activity, thus increasing energy throughout, which balances the higher level of energy intake. In this respect, becoming obese is simply an adaptive response to the modern environment, but it is also a trade-off for maintaining a low level of physical activity. Indeed, we speculate that becoming obese may be the only way to achieve energy balance when living a sedentary lifestyle in a food-abundant environment.

Overweight: Nourishing and Eating Behaviour Alterations

Eating represents a key factor in the energetic balance and the nutritional state as well.

It's important to distinguish between nourishing and eating behaviour.

The nourishing behaviour is the combination of processes thanks to which the organism receives, transforms and uses chemical substances contained in food; the eating behaviour consist in the form and modality with which this food is given to the organism and it's the consequence of voluntary and aware activities with which the individual choose the food, free them from the waste, transform and ingest them.

After ingestion nourishing behaviour begins: food is digest in the gastro enteric tube, nutrients are absorbed e then lead to the liver and peripheral tissues, where they are used. This process is involuntary and unaware [36].

So there are different ways to eat, but just one way to nourish the body.

From all this we can resume that human nutrition depends essentially from his eating behaviour: the organism uses all that it receive and, since nutrition is voluntary, it's also susceptible to different factors' influence (individual, cultural, familiar factors...).

It's very important to have an eating behaviour seek to balanced and varied absorption of nutrients, to maintain a good health and wellbeing.

In fact, different pathological conditions in our society are linked to a dysfunctional eating behaviour, for example overweight.

REFINED AND MANIPULATED FOODS: FOOD ADDICTION AND OVERWEIGHT

Another factor related to lifestyle and modern consumption linked to weight gain, is the increase in number of fast foods together with the increase of number of overweight and obese individuals [37]. It has been estimated that in the USA from 1958 to 2010, the number of fast foods has increased from 600 up to 222000; on average, every American pay the 48% of the money reserved for his nutrition in these structures [38].

There are different aspects that influence the success of this form of distribution: they are cheap, you can find them in poorer and rural areas or near the schools [39]. In this sense, they have been pointed as a threat to kids and adolescents wellbeing and health.

The modern age is characterized by an exaggerated use of industrial techniques for the preparation of food. These processing impoverish the food from its healthy components, such as vitamins, fibres and minerals and enrich it of nutrients that make it hyper palatable and highly caloric (sugar, lipids, salt, preservatives..).

With these processes we obtain a refined and manipulated food, very palatable, ready to be consumed, with a low index of satiety and with high caloric content. With these type of foods it's easy to exceed in the amount and frequency of consumption. The excess in terms of total energy (calories) and highly caloric nutrients (such as lipids and sugars) determines a positive energy balance that is correlated to weight gain.

As reported in chapter 5 (part I), recent evidences have highlighted that people are pushed to exceed in the consumption of refined and manipulated foods, even if they are aware of the negative consequences. This is not due only to the cost of the food, the fast serving or their taste.

Animal and neuroimaging studies on humans have focused the attention on reward system in relation to food consumption [40]. These studies have appreciated that palatable macronutrient can be linked to addiction mechanisms [41].

As concern environmental factors, hyper palatability (quite extended peculiarity in "obesogene" environment, nowadays, where Food Production play an important role) is mainly linked to the risk of addiction.

A set of investigations have assessed which palatable macronutrients could be linked to addiction.

Sugar is made of a collection of molecules that are linked to addiction: in animal studies, we can observe binge eating for sugared foods, withdrawal symptoms and craving when the rodent can't consume them. A key role is played by the intermittent administration of the sugary substance. In the same way, individuals show irritability and discomfort when they can't have sweets food and they tend to consume it to alleviate discomfort [42].

The second category is fat, towards which rodents show binge eating behaviours in intermittent assumption conditions [42].

In fast food we can find different combinations of macronutrients: they add sugary components to fat foods and this seems to lead to an increased addiction compared to fat foods alone [43-44]. The absence of withdrawal symptoms in rodents in fat deprivation compared to sugary food deprivation, lead to the hypothesis that there could be different mechanisms activated by different food [45].

The result of a nutrition rich in refined and manipulates food is eating more than needed. This produce an energetic imbalance in which caloric intake is greater compared to the out-take.

Another aspect very present in the Industrial Products that we don't see in nature and that is linked to overweight, is MSG – monosodium glutamate. Monosodium glutamate represents the salt of glutamate acid. Nowadays it's an industrial product; it's made from yeast cultivation made to leaven on beetroot molasses. Glutamic acid is one of the most common amino acids and is known as the physiologic ligand of the taste receptor umami, which is responsible for the immediate sensory effect of MSG on the palatability of food.

Glutamate is part of molecules defined exotoxins that can cause very severe problems in individuals with allergies, specific diseases or intolerances.

Monosodium glutamate (MSG), also called umami, has been used for 100 y in household food preparation and commercially processed foods. For long time, it was supposed that MSG was only used in Asian cuisine. It is generally believed that Asians have higher MSG consumption because MSG is more popular in Asian cuisine; in particular, many more Asians than Westerners add MSG in food preparation. However, people in Western countries may also consume substantial amount of MSG by adding seasonings and other condiments with hidden MSG.

Today, MSG has become one of the world's most widely used food additives. It exists in most processed foods, but may be hidden on ingredient labels and listed under other names [46-47].

Humans are five times more responsive to glutamate toxicity compared to animals and kids are 4 times more sensitive than adults. According to some Authors, for new generations, the first exposure to glutamate is one of the causes of the increase of obesity.

Data from both animal models [48-51] and human studies [52-53] propose a possible association between MSG and overweight/obesity.

In 1969 Dr John Onley found out that young rodents fed with monosodic glutamate gained weight rapidly (as a consequence of the increase of adipose tissue).

Potential mechanisms for the MSG-obesity link include the possible influence of MSG on energy balance by increasing palatability [54] and by disrupting the hypothalamic signalling cascade of leptin action [55].

The mechanisms are not completely understood, a hypothesis has been made that chronic MSG intake may induce pathologic changes of the arcuate nucleus neurons and disrupt the hypothalamic signalling cascade of leptin action, causing leptin resistance related to overweight and obesity [55]. The arcuate nucleus is the major site of glutamic acid–induced neuronal damage in the hypothalamus [56]. In addition, leptin is produced in the adipose tissue, crosses the blood-brain barrier by active transport systems, and stimulates a specific signalling cascade [57]. The hypothalamic arcuate nucleus is essential for mediating the anorectic effects of leptin influencing energy balance. Studies suggest that MSG may cause leptin resistance. For instance, leptin production is increased in animal models of obesity associated with experimentally induced hypothalamic damage, including the MSG-treated model. Also, it was reported that leptin suppressed body weight gain in controls but did not suppress weight gain in MSG-treated rats, and that leptin significantly inhibited food intake and caused weight loss in control rats, whereas MSG-treated rats were unresponsive to leptin treatment.

Some studies have examined the effects of orally administered MSG and found that oral MSG use at a level similar to the amount typically added to food had significant potential of damaging the hypothalamic regulation of appetite.

An interesting longitudinal study [58-59] have examined MSG intake in relation to incidence of overweight and change in body mass index (BMI) in 10095 apparently healthy Chinese adults from the China Health and Nutrition Survey (CHNS)—a longitudinal open-cohort, on-going, nationwide survey that has available MSG data. He found that MSG intake was positively, longitudinally associated with BMI and incidence of overweight independent of baseline BMI, physical activity, total energy intake, and other potential confounders among apparently healthy Chinese adults. Although the magnitude of weight gain in MSG users compared with nonusers is modest, it is of great public health significance if the weight gain is solely caused by MSG intake given that MSG is increasingly used worldwide.

Glutamate is always present in industry product, often with other additives with the same effect. It's a sapidity magnifier: it gives a taste to food that doesn't have it anymore, because of the processing and manipulations. It's easy to find it, for example, in snacks, sauces, vegetable conserves, but overall in stock cubes and soup preparations.

Fresh food, non manipulated or processed food, does not contain glutamate.

Nutritional Models That Promote Overweight

As reported in the previous paragraph, it has been proved that some nutrients or food are more correlated with behavioural and/or biological mechanisms responsible for gain weight.

However, dietary determinants of weight gain remain controversial [60]. Inconsistent findings may be explained in part by limitations in the single-nutrient approach (which is commonly used in nutritional epidemiologic research) and by an inability to detect small effects from single nutrients [61-63].

A recent review of intervention trials found that minor weight loss was greater in studies in which subjects consumed a high-fibre diet compared with a low-fibre diet, than in studies in which subjects consumed a low-fat diet compared with a high-fat diet. However, weight loss was more than 3 times as great in those studies in which subjects consumed a combination low-fat, high-fibre diet (3.4 kg over 6 mo.) compared with a low-fat diet alone (1.0 kg over 6 mo.), which suggests additive effects of fat and fibre in weight loss [64].

Weight swings are more influenced by a combination of nutrients rather than by a single nutrient in excess or in fault.

So it's very important to evaluate the energy intake and the nutrients also in terms of nutritional style and identify which combination of nutrients or foods can be more associated to overweight.

In comparison to individual foods or nutrients, dietary patterns are more realistic in describing the relation of diet to health and disease, because neither one nutrient nor one food adequately describes dietary behaviour. Identification of a good or bad food or nutrient is less helpful than describing healthy dietary or food patterns, which assist people to understand the totality of diet while selecting foods that meet their tastes and life styles.

In literature it has been demonstrated that a factor analysis approach to describing dietary patterns, reduces the complexity of diets to a few important foods, which describe a dietary behaviour.

Factor analysis has been shown to have good reproducibility and validity [65] and has been used to describe dietary patterns of populations.

In nutritional epidemiology, there is increased interest in the analysis of dietary pattern, a comprehensive variable that integrates consumption of several food or food groups [66]. Understanding how people actually eat in natural settings through the use of eating pattern methods provides an advantage over single nutrient approach. Such analyses are limited by biologic interactions and co-linearity among nutrients, as well as by the inability to detect small effects from single nutrients.

The effect of a single nutrient, food, or food group on disease risk and morbid conditions is difficult to assess in observational studies, because food and nutrients are consumed in combination and their complex effects are likely to be interactive or synergistic [67]. Therefore, analysis using dietary pattern could be used as a complementary approach in nutritional epidemiology.

Nutritional models analysis offers the chance to investigate the relations between nutrition and health in the nutritional epidemiology; it allows to identify which nutritional styles can be more liked to the development of obesity and overweight or other metabolic, cardiovascular or oncological diseases [68-70].

A nutritional model can be defined as the combination of foods and eating habits that characterizes a population or a group of population. It refers to an "eating pattern" that has common characteristics within the population.

Every specific model can influence the health of the population in virtue of the nutrients mainly present in food. Besides the components of the diet contain an ample source of molecules with antioxidant and anti-inflammatory actions, among which omega-3 fatty acids, oleic acid, and phenolic compounds hold a prominent place. This molecules seem to have a pharmacological activity within the human body and for this reason they play a key role in the prevention of many chronic diseases and in the maintenance of a good health.

Dietary patterns may differ with regard not only to age and sex but also resident area, ethnic group, and culture [71-73].

To date, several studies have examined the reproducibility and validity of dietary patterns.

Cluster and factor analyses have emerged as methods to empirically derive dietary (or food) patterns and possibly explain nutrient-disease relations.

Factor analysis is statistically quite different from cluster analysis. Whereas cluster analysis separates people into mutually exclusive groups based on differences in mean food intakes (clusters), factor analysis separates foods into groups based on correlations between food (factors), and people receive a factor score for each of the derived factors. With the use of the factor analysis procedure, a person's dietary pattern would be best represented by looking at his or her factor scores for each of the derived vectors.

In literature we find different longitudinal studies that highlight a relationship between some specific nutritional models and the weight variations (in term of overweight or obesity) and/or metabolic, cardiovascular, oncological diseases [74-76].

Many studies that have used factor or principal components analysis have empirically derived a "healthy or prudent food pattern" characterized by the presence of nutrients and food found in different populations; healthy pattern in fact is high in fruit, vegetables, seafood, fibre. Every population have other "healthy" food [77-78] that are typical of the population itself. For example most studies in Japan have identified "a prudent Japanese pattern" that is characterized by high intakes of not only vegetables and fruit, but also typical Japanese foods, including soy products, seaweed, mushrooms, fish, and green tea.

Patterns may therefore be difficult to reproduce and compare across studies, especially between populations in whom diet differs. However, there does seem to be homogeneity of dietary patterns across populations. With the use of cluster or factor analysis, several studies have identified healthy and meat-based patterns [79-82], a white-bread pattern [83-85], a sweets pattern [86-87], and an alcohol pattern [88] in which food intakes were similar to those of the same-named patterns observed in this study. The consistency of patterns across studies derived from either cluster or factor analysis suggests that dietary patterns are reasonably reproducible.

We report important results of some studies that have investigated the relations between specific nutritional patterns and body weight's swings in terms of Body Mass Index (BMI) or waist circumference.

The BMI is an important marker of the nutritional state (underweight, normal weight, overweight and obesity) but it can't discriminate the swings of body composition (fat mass, muscle and liquids).

Instead, measuring of waist circumference is important to identify the amount of visceral fat.

An interesting longitudinal study has been done to examine the relationship between eating habits and the swings of body composition in 459 healthy men and women participating in the Baltimore Longitudinal Study of Aging (BLSA) [89].

In the first edition of the study [90], it has been noted that patterns derived by using cluster analysis, were significantly related to longitudinal changes in anthropometric measures.

To perform a dietary pattern analysis with the use of cluster analysis, individual food and food ingredients from the dietary records, must be aggregated into groups. They formed 41 food groups, mainly according to macronutrient composition (e.g., fat or fiber content) and culinary use; several foods (e.g., pizza, eggs) composed their own groups. Where possible, foods were separated into full- and reduced-fat groups (e.g., high-fat dairy and low-fat dairy). Cereals were divided into those that were a good source of fiber ($\geq$ 2.5 g/serving) and those that were low in fiber (< 2.5 g/serving) [91]. For entry into the cluster analysis, food groups may be measured by absolute weight in grams, the number of servings, or the percentage of energy intake from each food group [92]. Their chose to consider the food group variables in terms of the percentage of energy contributed by each of the 41 groups, and their calculated those values for each subject from the average of diet records. The percentage contribution from each food group for each subject was then entered into the cluster analysis.

Specifically, five dietary patterns were derived, which their labelled healthy, white bread, alcohol, sweets, and meat and potatoes, on the basis of the food that contributed relatively greater proportions of energy to each cluster. Differences in energy intake from food groups were seen across patterns. Energy intakes in the white-bread, alcohol, and sweets patterns were greatest from these respective food sources. The healthy pattern contained relatively greater contributions from "healthy" foods, including fruit, high-fibre cereal, and reduced-fat dairy, and relatively smaller contributions from fast food, non-diet soda, and salty snacks.

A significantly higher percentage of energy from carbohydrate and a higher intake of fibre was seen in the healthy pattern than in all other clusters; no significant differences were seen in protein or total energy intake across patterns. Subjects in the healthy pattern had the smallest waist circumference ($P < 0.05$) at baseline, but there were no significant differences in baseline BMI ($P > 0.05$).

Regression results associating change in BMI and change in waist circumference for all clusters compared with the healthy pattern. There was a significantly greater annual increase in BMI among subjects in the meat-and-potatoes pattern ($\beta = 0.25$; 95% CI: 0.07, 0.43; $P < 0.05$) and in waist circumference among subjects in the white-bread pattern ($\beta = 0.90$ cm; 95% CI: 0.12, 1.68; $P < 0.05$) than among subjects in the healthy cluster.

In conclusion the "healthy dietary pattern" showed smaller gains in both BMI and waist circumference than did the other dietary patterns (white bread, sweets, alcohol, and meat and potatoes). Consuming a diet high in fruit, vegetables, reduced-fat dairy, and whole grains and low in red and processed meat, fast food, and soda was associated with smaller gains in BMI and waist circumference.

In the second edition of the same study [93], Authors continue to examine prospectively whether eating patterns are related to anthropometric changes in women and men participating in the Baltimore Longitudinal Study of Aging (BLSA) by using a distinctly different patterning method-factor analysis. Specifically, their used principal components to extract factors, in which a given set of variables is transformed into a reduced set of correlated variables [94].

The objective of the study was to examine whether food patterns derived from exploratory factor analysis specifically, principal components analysis, are related to anthropometric changes in BMI and waist circumference.

It have been used dietary patterning methods to clarify the nutritional aetiology of the adiposity variations over time. Diet was assessed by using 7-day dietary records, from which 40 food groups were formed and entered into a factor analysis.

It has been hypothesized that adopting and healthy food pattern could lead to lower changes in the BMI and waist circumference over lifetime, than would other food patterns in models adjusted for baseline anthropometric measures.

Six food patterns were derived: healthy (1), protein and alcohol (2), sweets (3), vegetables fat and vegetables (4), fatty meats (5), eggs bread and soup (6). Factor 1 or "healthy pattern" (reduced-fat dairy products, fruit, and fibre) was most strongly associated with fibre ($r = 0.39$) and had high positive loadings for reduced fat dairy products, cereal, fruit, fruit juice, non-white bread, nuts and seeds, whole grains, beans and legumes and high negative loadings for white bread and refined grains, processed meat, potatoes, meat, and non-diet soda.

Factor 1 was inversely associated with annual change in BMI ($\beta = -0.51$; 95% CI: −0.82, −0.20; $P < 0.05$; P for trend < 0.01) in women and inversely associated with annual change in waist circumference ($\beta = -1.06$ cm; 95% CI: −1.88, −0.24 cm; $P < 0.05$; P for trend $= 0.04$) in both sexes.

The results of this study suggest again that a pattern rich in reduced-fat dairy products and high-fibre foods (cereal, fruit, fruit juice, non-white bread, nuts and seed, whole grains, and beans and legumes) may lead to smaller gains in BMI in women and smaller gains in waist circumference in both women and men.

Research from the Health Professionals Follow-Up Study (HPFS) and the Nurses' Health Study cohorts have highlight that a "western" eating pattern, characterized by high consumption of refined cereals, red meat, sweet and high fat dairy products is associated to overweight and obesity and it's a risk factor for chronic illness (coronary illness, colon cancer and diabetes) [95-97].

On the contrary, nutritional pattern characterized by an high consumption of fruit, vegetables, cereals, legumes and poultry (defined prudent pattern) is associated with an healthy weight, a lower risk of coronary illness, a lower insulin resistance and a decrease of the risk to develop the metabolic syndrome [98-101].

A longitudinal study conducted by Medical Research Council (MRC) National Survey of Health and Development (NSHD, also known as the 1946 British Birth Cohort) [102] to identify the relations between dietary patterns during adult life and risk factors for chronic disease, has revealed that whiten women, the animals "prudent" eating pattern – characterized by regular assumption of fruit, vegetables and low fat products – is inversely proportional to BMI and waist circumference. However in men, fewer significant associations were observed.

In 2 cross-sectional studies, people with type 1 diabetes (n = 2868) who consumed a diet high in carbohydrates, cereal fibre and low-glycaemic-index foods had a significantly smaller waist circumference and BMI, and healthy adults (n = 2110) participating in the original and offspring US Framingham Heart Study and European SENECA studies who were in the "meat and fat cluster" had a larger waist circumference and BMI than did those who were in the "fish and grain cluster" [103].

A recent crossover study among 11 healthy men who consumed a high-glycaemic-index diet and a low-glycaemic-index diet for 5 weeks each, found that the low-glycaemic-index diet led to a decrease in trunk mass and an increase in lean body mass with no change in body weight [104].

The assumption of low glycaemic index food has determined an improvement in body composition: fat mass decrease and fat free mass increase. Body weight has been maintained thanks to the development of a new energy balance, more functional compared to the previous condition, due to an improvement of body composition.

Authors suggest several possible mechanisms, including shifts in substrate utilization, decreases in the proteolytic counter regulatory hormones and a reduction in lipoprotein lipase activity, which could explain the change in fat mass.

Other studies have proved an association between eating pattern and systemic inflammatory markers [105-106]. It has been seen that an animal's eating pattern is inversely correlated with C-reactive protein (CRP), while a western eating pattern is positively correlated with CRP in different populations [107].

Mechanisms underlying these associations are still to be clarified. Intestinal flora seems to play an important role in this sense; it's seen as a key actor that links external macro-environmental changes to internal biology, in particular for what concern inflammatory mechanisms, metabolism and homeostasis of body weight.

In conclusion, dietary patterns are important precursors of disease and good health. Dietary patterns are related to changes in body mass index (BMI) and plasma micronutrients levels [108] and predict overweight, obesity, cardiovascular disease and colon cancer [109].

Given that foods are not consumed in isolation, dietary pattern research based on natural eating behaviour may be useful in understanding dietary causes of overweight and in helping individuals trying to control their weight.

These studies cannot conclude whether one of these mechanisms or another, as yet unknown mechanism was responsible for the gains in BMI and waist circumference, but it is likely, rather, that there are multiple pathways through which food intake, including both dietary composition and total food volume, affects energy balance.

The inverse relation seen in these studies between "healthy or prudent pattern" and anthropometric changes may be explained by the roles of fibre [110], glycaemic index [111], and energy density [112-113] on food intake and appetite.

Subjects consuming the healthy dietary pattern had the highest intake of foods such as high-fibre cereal, reduced-fat dairy, fruit, non-white bread, whole grains, beans and legumes, and vegetables and the smallest gains in BMI and waist circumference. Several mechanisms may be responsible for this effect. These high-fiber foods may affect weight by increasing satiety and satiation through decreased gastric emptying, increased colonic transit, and decreased insulin response [110]. This hypothesis with regard to the role of fibre may be extended to the role of the glycaemic index [111]. Many of the foods in the healthy pattern are low in glycaemic load, which evokes a decreased insulin response and therefore decreases hunger and energy intake [114]. The healthy dietary pattern also contained food that are low in energy density (e.g., fruit and vegetables), which may be responsible for mediating energy intake rather than dietary composition in itself [112].

Compared with subjects in the healthy pattern, those in the meat-and-potatoes pattern had relatively higher intakes of meat, potatoes, fast food, pizza, and nondiet soda—foods that are low in fibre and high in energy density and glycaemic load—whereas those in the white-bread pattern received almost 16% of their daily energy intake from white bread—the food with the highest glycaemic index value [115].

Mediterranean Diet versus Overweight

The healthy eating pattern is similar to Mediterranean diet. Indeed, the Mediterranean pattern is characterized by: a high consumption of vegetables, fruits and legumes; the presence of integral complex carbohydrates; extra virgin olive oil as main source of lipids; adequate sources of protein with preference to fish rather than meat; consumption of moderate amounts of red wine, preferably during meals [116-117].

Different studies has demonstrated that Mediterranean Diet is not correlated to an increase of the risk to develop overweight or obesity and that it might have a role in the prevention of both, since some physiological mechanisms might explain this protective role [118]. However, more long term studies are needed to prove the efficacy of the Mediterranean Diet in the promotion and the prevention of overweight and obesity (Level I, Strength of the Recommendation B) [119-122].

An interesting study [123] has systematically reviewed and analysed the epidemiological evidence on the Mediterranean diet and overweight/obesity. It has identified 21 epidemiological studies that explored the relationship between the Mediterranean diet and weight. Of these, 13 studies reported that Mediterranean diet adherence was significantly related to less overweight/obesity or more weight loss.

Exploring the relationship between the Mediterranean diet and overweight/obesity is complex, and there are important methodological differences and limitations in the studies that make it difficult to compare results. Although the results are inconsistent, the evidence points towards a possible role of the Mediterranean diet in preventing overweight/obesity, and physiological mechanisms can explain this protective effect.

RESTRICTIVE DIETS AND OVERWEIGHT

Food restriction is a common strategy for treating overweight and obesity [124].

Food restriction produces weight loss, but it also produces compensatory decreases in other components of energy balance, i.e. , decreases in energy expenditure and body energy stores [125-126] [10] and an increase in hunger [127].

Because energy requirements fall with weight loss, a common strategy for weight loss maintenance is trying to match a lower level of energy expenditure with a lower energy intake.

RMR declines with loss of body mass (1 component of energy balance affects another) [128-129], so energy requirements are greatly reduced after intentional weight loss. The reductions can be from 170 to 250 kcal/d for a 10% weight loss and from 325 to 480 for a 20% weight loss [130-131].

The aspect of hunger is the effect of disinhibition that derives from dietary restraint.

It is thought that in order to maintain weight loss, people must avoid disinhibited eating, which describes loss of control over eating in response to emotional, cognitive, or social cues.

Loss of control with food is also a consequence of physiological mechanisms: dietary restraint causes a condition of energy and nutrient deprivation; this is the reason why hungry body produces hormones and neurotransmitters that lead the individual search for food as a defence and surviving mechanism.

Similarly, individuals would need to exercise dietary restraint or be vigilant about monitoring their intake and consciously limit what they eat in order to avoid regaining weight [132].

Restrictive diets paradox is that they are fattening in the long term: a rigid control furthers loss of control with food with a resulting non-programmed and non-manageable assumption of food [133].

An interesting review [134] in which five quantitative studies were identified, examined the relationship of these factors to weight loss maintenance. It's very important to examine factors involved in the maintenance of weight loss to evaluate behavioural and cognitive mechanisms that can promote weight gain, overweight and obesity.

The Maastricht Weight Maintenance Study is a longitudinal study about 91 men and women living in The Netherlands who participated in a very low-calorie diet to lose weight [135].

Dietary restraint and disinhibition were among the variables measured as possibly predisposing to weight regain. Measures were performed at baseline, following the diet, and at 2–8 years. Findings showed a significant negative correlation ($r = -0.47$) between increased dietary restraint and BMI regain ($p < 0.05$). In other words, an early increase in dietary restraint during the weight loss phase, was associated with less regain in the maintenance phase. A second study by Vogels and Westerterp-Plantenga (2007) [136] also measured disinhibition and dietary restraint as part of their effort to find factors associated with successful weight maintenance. Subjects (n = 103) completed a 6-week very low-calorie diet and 2-year weight maintenance program. Ninety subjects regained >10% of their weight and were classified as unsuccessful at weight loss maintenance. Thirteen subjects regained <10% of their weight and were classified as successful. The successful subjects increased their dietary restraint significantly more than the unsuccessful subjects ($p < 0.05$) over the course of the study. Dietary restraint was inversely correlated with disinhibition for the entire study period ($p < 0.001$). Thus, the combination of high dietary restraint maintained over time and low disinhibition were associated with successful weight maintenance. A third study examined the disinhibition section of the Eating Inventory to determine how its factors relate to weight loss maintenance (Niemeier et all., 2007) [137]. The researchers found that the disinhibition scale represents two types of factors including external cues—such as parties and social influence; or internal cues—thoughts, feelings, and emotional responses. Data were collected from 202 participants in a behavioural weight loss trial (TRIM) and 2765 members of the National Weight Control Registry (NWCR). The NWCR is a registry of self-selected people who have lost a minimum of 30 lbs. and kept it off for at least 1 year. Registry members report how they have lost and maintained their weight and are periodically surveyed to determine what factors are related to continued success with weight loss maintenance. In the TRIM group, disinhibited eating in response to internal cues was a marginally significant predictor ($p < 0.06$) of weight regain at 18-month follow-up. In the NWCR group, internal disinhibition was a significant predictor ($p = 0.0001$) of weight regain in the first year of membership. Disinhibited eating in response to external cues was not predictive of weight regain in either group. The fourth study was also a descriptive report of data collected from the NWCR (Wing & Phelan, 2005) [138]. One of the variables related to successful weight loss maintenance, was a lower level of dietary disinhibition, meaning individuals experienced less loss of control over eating. NCWR members who had lower disinhibition scores or who had less loss of control over eating, were 60% more likely to maintain their weight over 1 year. Members who experienced diminished dietary restraint, or were less vigilant about monitoring intake, regained weight. No information was provided on the number of subjects surveyed. A fifth study by Wing et al. (2008) [139] examined predictors of weight regain by evaluating behavioural and psychological variables at baseline, 6 months, 12 months, and 18 months on 261 individuals. Subjects had lost at least 10% of their body weight in an 18-month controlled trial (STOP Regain) during which they were taught self-regulation behaviours to control weight. Baseline measures of dietary restraint and disinhibition were not predictive of weight maintenance outcomes at any point. However, an increase in disinhibition over time was significantly related to weight regain ($p < 0.0001$). Decreases in dietary restraint were likewise associated with weight regain ($p < 0.0011$).

Results of this review overall showed the ability to maintain control over eating, low disinhibition, and exercising dietary restraint or consciously restricting intake played a significant role in maintaining weight loss. Also, disinhibited eating in response to internal cues such as thoughts, feelings, and emotions seemed to play a significant role in weight regain.

CONCLUSION

In conclusion, substantial weight loss and subsequent maintenance, require substantial and permanent behaviour change. The lack of success in long-term weight loss maintenance [140] suggests that food restriction may not be an optimum strategy: most people are not able to sustain the degree of behaviour change they need to keep weight off. Lowering energy intake is opposed by biology [10] and the environment [141].

On the other hand, increasing physical activity serves to increase total energy expenditure, allowing a higher energy intake for a given level of body weight and requiring less food restriction. In fact, individuals who are successful in long-term weight loss maintenance report engaging in high amounts of physical activity [142]. Just as restricting food intake is difficult, it is not easy to produce sustained increases in physical activity, but from an energy balance point of view, including physical activity in the strategy, would improve the likelihood of successfully matching energy intake and expenditure at a lower body weight.

However, simply preventing positive energy balance should not produce significant compensation through increased energy intake or a reduction in RMR. A reasonable starting point in addressing overweight and obesity is to developed behaviour goals for primary prevention of weight gain. In energy balance terms, this would require less change than producing and maintaining weight loss, because the degree of positive energy balance producing this gradual weight gain, seems to be relatively small.

REFERENCES

[1] Finucane, MM; Stevens, GA; Cowan, MJ; Danaei, G; Lin, JK; Paciorek, CJ; Singh, GM; Gutierrez, HR; Lu, Y; Bahalim, AN; Farzadfar, F; Riley, LM; Ezzati, M. National, regional, and global trends in body-mass index since 1980: systematic analysis of health examination surveys and epidemiological studies with 960 country-years and 9·1 million participants. *The Lancet*, 2011 377, 557 – 567.

[2] World Health Organisation. Global Status Report on Non-Communicable Diseases. 2010. Available from: http://www.who.int /nmh/publications/ncd_report2010/en/

[3] National Center for Epidemiology, Surveillance and Health Promotion - Institute of Health, EpiCentro CCM - Ministry of Health. Overweight and obesity in Italy: Data "PASSI" (2010-2013) and "PASSI D'ARGENTO". 2012. Available from: http://www.epicentro.iss.it/passi /dati/sovrappeso.asp

[4] World Health Organization, US Centers for Disease Control and Prevention. Global School-based Student Health Survey. 2012. Available from: http://www.who.int /chp/gshs/en/

[5] O Hill, J; Wyatt, HR; Peters, JC. The Importance of Energy Balance. *Obesity*, 2012, 27-31.

[6] Hafekost, K; Lawrence, D; Mitrou, F et all. Tackling overweight and obesity: does the public health message match the science?. *BMC Med*, 2013 11-41.

[7] Hill, JO; Wyatt, HR; Peters, JC. Energy balance and obesity. *Circulation*, 2012 126, 126–132

[8] Hill, JO; Commerford, R. Physical activity, fat balance, and energy balance. *Int J Sport Nutr*, 1996 6, 80–92

[9] Tappy, L; Binnert, C; Schneiter, P. Energy expenditure, physical activity and body-weight control. *Proc Nutr Soc*, 2003 62(3), 663-6.

[10] Hill, JO; Levine, JS; Saris, WHM. Energy expenditure and physical activity. In: Bray G, Bouchard C eds. *Handbook of Obesity. 2nd ed.* New York, NY: Marcel Dekker, Inc; 2003; 631– 654.

[11] Sandoval, D; Cota, D; Seeley, RJ. The integrative role of CNS fuel-sensing mechanisms in energy balance and glucose regulation. *Ann Rev Physiol*, 2008 70, 513–535.

[12] Horton, TJ; Drougas, H; Brachey, A; Reed, GW; Peters, JC; Hill, JO. Fat and carbohydrate overfeeding in humans: different effects on energy storage. *Am Clin Nutr,* 1995 62, 19–29.

[13] Blundell, JE; Stubbs, RJ; Hughes, DA; Whybrow, S; King, NA. Cross talk between physical activity and appetite control: does physical activity stimulate appetite? *Proc Nutr Soc,* 2003 62, 651–661.

[14] Diaz, EO; Prentice, AM; Goldberg, GR; Murgatroyd, PR; Coward, WA. Metabolic response to experimental overfeeding in lean and overweight healthy volunteers. *Am J Clin Nutr,* 1992 56, 641–55.

[15] Leibel, RL; Rosenbaum, M; Hirsch, J. Changes in energy expenditure resulting from altered body weight. *N Engl Med,* 1995 332, 621–628.

[16] Martinez, JA. Body-weight regulation: causes of obesity. *Proceedings of the Nutrition Society,* 2000 59(3), 337-345.

[17] Centers for Disease Control and Prevention. National Health and Nutrition Examination Survey. January 31, 2012. Available from: http://www.cdc.gov/nchs/nhanes.htm.

[18] Bassett, DR; Schneider, PL; Huntington, GE. Physical activity in an Old Order Amish community. *Med Sci Sports Exerc*, 2004 36, 79–85.

[19] Bassett, DR Jr; Wyatt, HR; Thompson, H; Peters, JC; Hill, JO. Pedometer-measured physical activity and health behaviors in U.S. adults. *Med Sci Sports Exerc,* 2010 42, 1819–1825.

[20] Ham, SA; Kruger, J; Tudor-Locke, C. Participation by US adults in sports, exercise, and recreational physical activities. *J Phys Act Health*, 2009 6, 6–14.

[21] Sistema di sorveglianza "PASSI- Progressi delle Aziende Sanitarie per la Salute in Italia". 2012. Availabre from: http://www.salute.gov.it/

[22] National Center for Epidemiology, Surveillance and Health Promotion Institute of Health. Available from: http://www.epicentro.iss.it/passi/dati /sovrappeso.asp

[23] Schoeller, DA; Fjeld, CR. Human energy metabolism: what have we learned from the doubly labeled water method? *Annual Review of Nutrition*, 1992 11, 355–373.

[24] Barsh, GS; Farooqi, IS; O'Rahilly, S. Genetics of body weight regulation. *Nature*, 2000 404, 644–651.

[25] Mayer, J; Purnima, R; Mitra KP. Relation between caloric intake, body weight and physical work: studies in an industrial male population in West Bengal. *Am J Clin Nutr,* 1956 4, 169–175

[26] Blundell, JE; King, NA. Physical activity and regulation of food intake: current evidence. *Med Sci Sports Exerc,* 1999 31, S573–S583.

[27] Stubbs, RJ; Hughes, DA; Johnstone, AM; Horgan, GW; King, N; Blundell JE. A decrease in physical activity affects appetite, energy, and nutrient balance in lean men feeding ad libitum. *Am J Clin Nutr,* 2004 79, 62–69.

[28] Jéquier, E; Tappy, L. Regulation of body weight in humans. *Physiological Review,* 1999 79, 451–480.

[29] Ravusin, E; Burnand, B; Schutz, Y; Jèquier, E. Twenty-fourhour energy expenditure and resting metabolic rate in obese, moderately obese and control subjects. *The American Journal of Clinical Nutriton,* 1982 35, 56-573.

[30] Matzinger, O; Schneiter, P; Tappy, L. Effects of fatty acids on exercise plus insulin-induced glucose utilization in trained and sedentary subjects. *American Journal of Physiology Endocrinology and Metabolism,* 2002 282, E125–E131.

[31] Dicembrini, I; Pala, L; Cresci, B; Cremasco, F; Rotella, CM. Predictors of weight loss in the clinical management of obese patients: the relevance of body composition. *Obes Metab*, 2010 6,29–33

[32] Sacks, MF; Bray, GA; Carey, VJ; Smith, V; Ryan, DH; Anton, SD; McManus, K; Champagne, CM; Bishop, LM; Laranjo, RDN; Meryl BA; Leboff, MF; Rood, JC; de Jonge, L; Greenway, FL; Loria, CM; Obarzanek, E; Williamson, DA. Comparison of Weight-Loss Diets with Different Compositions of Fat, Protein, and Carbohydrates. *N Engl J Med*, 2009 360, 859-873.

[33] Boden, G; Chen, X; Mozzoli, M; Ryan, I. Effect of fasting on serum leptin in normal human subjects. *Journal of Clinical and Endocrinological Metabolism*, 1996 81, 3419–3423.

[34] Christian, T; Rashad, I. Trends in U.S. food prices, 1950–2007. *Econ Hum Biol,* 2009 7, 113–120.

[35] US Department of Agriculture. Loss-adjusted food availability: spreadsheets. January 31, 2012 Avaible from: http://www.ers.usda.gov /Data/FoodConsumption/FoodGuide Spreadsheets.htm.

[36] Binetti, P; Marcelli, M; Baisi, R. *Manuale della nutrizione clinica e scienze dietetiche applicate*, Società Editrice Universo, Roma, 2007.

[37] Fortuna, JL. The obesity epidemic and food addiction: clinical similarities to drug dependence. *J Psychoactive Drugs*, 2012 44(1), 56-63.

[38] National Restaurant Association. Restaurant Industry Forecast 2014. 2014. Available from: https://www.restaurant.org

[39] Alsiö, J et al. Feed-forward mechanisms: addiction-like behavioral and molecular adaptations in overeating. *Front Neuroendocrinol,* 2012 33(2), 127-39.

[40] Avena, NM. Binge eating: neurochemical insights from animal models. *Eat Disord,* 2009 17(1), 89-92.

[41] Wang, GJ et all. The role of dopamine in motivation for food in humans: implications for obesity. *Expert Opin Ther Targets*, 2002 6(5), 601-9.

[42] Avena, NM et all. Overlaps in the nosology of substance abuse and overeating: the translational implications of "food addiction". *Curr Drug Abuse Rev,* 2011 4(3), 133-9.

[43] Garber, AK; Lustig RH. Is fast food addictive? *Curr Drug Abuse Rev*, 2011 4(3), 146-62.

[44] Ludwig, DS; Majzoub, JA; Al-Zahrani, A; Dallal, GE; Blanco, I; Roberts, SB. High glycemic index foods, overeating, and obesity. *Pediatrics*. 1999 103, E261–E266.

[45] Avena, NM et all. Further developments in the neurobiology of food and addiction: update on the state of the science. *Nutrition,* 2012 28(4), 341-3.

[46] Ito, M. Domestic and overseas food products business FY 2008-2010 medium term plan. Cited 12 September 2009. Available from: http://www.ajinomoto.com/ir/pdf /08July02-food-E.pdf

[47] Erb, JE; Erb, TM. *The slow poisoning of America*. Paladins Press, Virginia Beach, 2003.

[48] Lney, JW. Brain lesions, obesity, and other disturbances in mice treated with monosodium glutamate. *Science,* 1969 164, 719–21.

[49] Dawson, R; Pelleymounter, MA; Millard, WJ; Liu, S; Eppler, B. Attenuation of leptin-mediated effects by monosodium glutamate-induced arcuate nucleus damage. *Am J Physiol*, 1997 273, E202–6.

[50] Tang-Christensen, M; Holst, JJ; Hartmann, B; Vrang, N. The arcuate nucleus is pivotal in mediating the anorectic effects of centrally administered leptin. *Neuroreport,* 1999 10, 1183–7.

[51] Bergen, HT; Mizuno, TM; Taylor, J; Mobbs, CV. Hyperphagia and weight gain after gold-thioglucose: relation to hypothalamic neuropeptide Y and proopiomelanocortin. *Endocrinology*, 1998 139, 4483–8.

[52] He, K; Zhao, L; Daviglus, ML et all. Association of monosodium glutamate intake with overweight in Chinese adults: the INTERMAP Study. *Obesity (Silver Spring),* 2008 16, 1875–80.

[53] Yeomans, MR; Gould, NJ; Mobini, S; Prescott J. Acquired flavor acceptance and intake facilitated by monosodium glutamate in humans. *Physiol Behav*, 2008 93, 958–66.

[54] Hermanussen, M; Garcia, AP; Sunder, M; Voigt, M; Salazar, V; Tresguerres, JA. Obesity, voracity, and short stature: the impact of glutamate on the regulation of appetite. *Eur J Clin Nutr,* 2006 60, 25–31.

[55] Hermanussen, M; Tresguerres, JA. Does high glutamate intake cause obesity? *J Pediatr Endocrinol Metab*, 2003 16, 965–8.

[56] Lney, JW; Ho, OL; Rhee, V. Brain-damaging potential of protein hydrolysates. *N Engl J Med*, 1973 289, 391–5

[57] Jequier, E. Leptin signaling, adiposity, and energy balance. *Ann N Y Acad Sci*, 2002 967, 379–88.

[58] He, K1; Du, S; Xun, P; Sharma, S; Wang, H; Zhai, F; Popkin, B. Consumption of monosodium glutamate in relation to incidence of overweight in Chinese adults: China Health and Nutrition Survey (CHNS). *Am J Clin Nutr,* 2011 93(6), 1328-36.

[59] Fernandez-Tresguerres Hernandez, JA. Effect of monosodium glutamate given orally on appetite control (a new theory for the obesity epidemic). *An R Acad Nac Med (Madr)*, 2005 122(2), 341–55; discussion 55–60 (in Spanish).

[60] Bray, GA; Popkin, BM. Dietary fat intake does affect obesity. *Am J Clin Nutr*, 1998 68, 1157–73.

[61] Wirfalt, AK; Jeffery, RW. Using cluster analysis to examine dietary patterns: nutrient intakes, gender, and weight status differ across food pattern clusters. *J Am Diet Assoc,* 1997 97, 22–9.

[62] Sacks, F; Obarzanek, E; Windhauser, M. Rationale and design of the Dietary Approaches to Stop Hyptertension Trial (DASH): a multicenter controlled feeding study of dietary patterns to lower blood pressures. *Ann Epidemiol*, 1994 5, 108–18.

[63] Vollmer, WM; Svetkey, LP; Appel, LJ et al. Recruitment and retention of minority participants in the DASH controlled feeding trial. *Ethnicity Dis*, 1998 8, 198- 208.

[64] Roberts, SB; McCrory, MA; Saltzman, E. The influence of dietary composition on energy intake and body weight. *J Am Coll Nutr,* 2002 21, 140S–5S.

[65] Hu, FB; Rimm, E; Smith-Warner, SA; Feskanich, D; Stampfer, MJ; Ascherio, A; Sampson, L; Willett, WC. Reproducibility and validity of dietary patterns assessed with a food-frequency questionnaire. *Am. J. Clin. Nutr*, 1999 69, 243–249.

[66] Nanri, A; Shimazu, T; Ishihara, J; Takachi, R; Mizoue, T; Inoue, M; Tsugane, S. JPHC FFQ Validation Study Group. Reproducibility and validity of dietary patterns assessed by a food frequency questionnaire used in the 5-year follow up survey of the Japan Public Health Center-Based Prospective Study. *J Epidemiol,* 2012 22(3), 205-15.

[67] Hu FB Dietary pattern analysis: a new direction in nutritional epidemiology. Curr Opin Lipidol. 2002;13:3–9 10.1097/00041433-200202000-00002

[68] Schulze, MB; Hoffmann, K; Kroke, A; Boeing, H. Dietary patterns and their association with food and nutrient intake in the European Prospective Investigation into Cancer and Nutrition (EPIC)-Potsdam study. *Br J Nutr,* 2001 85, 363–73

[69] Costacou, T; Bamia, C; Ferrari, P; Riboli, E; Trichopoulos, D et all. Tracing the Mediterranean diet through principal components and cluster analyses in the Greek population. *Eur J Clin Nutr*, 2003 57, 1378–85.

[70] Kant, AK. Dietary patterns and health outcomes. *J Am Diet Assoc*, 2004 104, 615–35.

[71] Borland, SE; Robinson, SM; Crozier, SR; Inskip, HM. SWS Study Group Stability of dietary patterns in young women over a 2-year period. *Eur J Clin Nutr,* 2008 62, 119–26.

[72] Hu, FB; Rimm, E; Smith-Warner, SA; Feskanich, D; Stampfer, MJ; Ascherio, A et all. Reproducibility and validity of dietary patterns assessed with a food-frequency questionnaire. *Am J Clin Nutr,* 1999 69, 243–9

[73] Togo, P; Heitmann, BL; Sørensen, TI; Osler, M. Consistency of food intake factors by different dietary assessment methods and population groups. *Br J Nutr,* 2003 90, 667–78.

[74] Newby, PK; Weismayer, C; Akesson, A; Tucker, KL; Wolk, A. Longitudinal changes in food patterns predict changes in weight and body mass index and the effects are greatest in obese women. *J Nutr*, 2006 136, 2580–7.

[75] Schulze, MB; Fung, TT; Manson, JE; Willett, WC; Hu, FB. Dietary patterns and changes in body weight in women. *Obesity (Silver Spring)*, 2006 14, 1444–53.

[76] McNaughton, SA; Mishra, GD; Stephen, AM; Wadsworth ME. Dietary patterns throughout adult life are associated with body mass index, waist circumference, blood pressure, and red cell folate. *J Nutr*, 2007 137, 99–105.

[77] Hu, FB; Rimm, E; Smith-Warner SA et all. Reproducibility and validity of dietary patterns assessed with a food- frequency questionnaire. *Am J Clin Nutr,* 1999 69, 243–9.

[78] Nolan, CC; Gray-Donald, K; Shatenstein, B; O'Loughlin J. Dietary patterns leading to high fat intake. *Can J Public Health*, 1995 86, 389–91.

[79] Haveman-Nies, A; Tucker, KL; de Groot, LC; Wilson, PW; van Staveren, WA. Evaluation of dietary quality in relationship to nutritional and lifestyle factors in elderly people of the US Framingham Heart Study and the European SENECA study. *Eur J Clin Nutr,* 2001 5, 870–80.

[80] Pryer, JA; Nichols, R; Elliott, P; Thakrar, B; Brunner, E; Marmot, M. Dietary patterns among a national random sample of British adults. *J Epidemiol Community Health,* 2001 55, 29–37.

[81] Pryer, JA; Cook, A; Shetty, P. Identification of groups who report similar patterns of diet among a representative national sample of British adults aged 65 years of age or more. *Public Health Nutr*, 2001 4, 787–95.

[82] Millen, BE; Quatromoni, PA; Gagnon, DR; Cupples, LA; Franz, MM,; D'Agostino RB. Dietary patterns of men and women suggest targets for health promotion: the Framingham Nutrition Studies. *Am J Health Promot,* 1996 11, 42–52.

[83] Wirfalt, AK; Jeffery, RW. Using cluster analysis to examine dietary patterns: nutrient intakes, gender, and weight status differ across food pattern clusters. *J Am Diet Assoc,* 1997 97, 272–9

[84] Wirfalt, E; Mattisson, I; Gullberg, B; Berglund, G. Food patterns defined by cluster analysis and their utility as dietary exposure variables: a report from the Malmo Diet and Cancer Study. *Public Health Nutr,* 2000 3, 159–73.

[85] Speck, BJ; Bradley, CB; Harrell, JS; Belyea, MJ. A food frequency questionnaire for youth: psychometric analysis and summary of eating habits in adolescents. *J Adolesc Health,* 2001 28, 16–25.

[86] Haveman-Nies, A; Tucker, KL; de Groot, LC; Wilson, PW; van Staveren, WA. Evaluation of dietary quality in relationship to nutritional and lifestyle factors in elderly people of the US Framingham Heart Study and the European SENECA study. *Eur J Clin Nutr*, 2001 55, 870–80.

[87] Wirfalt, E; Mattisson, I; Gullberg, B; Berglund, G. Food patterns defined by cluster analysis and their utility as dietary exposure variables: a report from the Malmo Diet and Cancer Study. *Public Health Nutr*, 2000 3, 159–73.

[88] Randall, E; Marshall, JR; Graham, S; Brasure, J. Patterns in food use and their associations with nutrient intakes. *Am J Clin Nutr*, 1990 52, 739–45.

[89] Shock, N; Greulich, R; Andres, R et all. *Normal human aging: the Baltimore Longitudinal Study of Aging. National Institutes of Health.* Washington, DC: Government Printing Office, 1984.

[90] Newby, PK; Muller, D; Hallfrisch, J; Qiao, N; Andres, R; Tucker, K. Dietary patterns and changes in body mass index and waist circumference in adults. *Am J Clin Nutr*, 2003 77, 1417–25.

[91] Center for Food Safety and Applied Nutrition. US Food and Drug Administration. A food labeling guide. September 1994. Available from: http://www.cfsan.fda.gov/%7Edms/flg-6b.html (accessed 30 January 2002).

[92] Schwerin, HS; Stanton, JL; Smith, JL; Riley, AM Jr; Brett, BE. Food, eating habits, and health: a further examination of the relationship between food eating patterns and nutritional health. *Am J Clin Nutr*, 1982 35, 1319–25.

[93] Newby, PK; Muller, D; Hallfrisch, J; Andres, R; Tucker, KL. Food patterns measured by factor analysis and anthropometric changes in adults. *Am J Clin Nutr,* 2004 80, 504–13.

[94] Kim, J-O; Mueller, C. *Factor analysis: statistical methods and practical issues.* Newbury Park, CA. Sage Publications, Inc, 1978.

[95] James, PT; Leach, R; Kalamara, E; Shayeghi, M. The worldwide obesity epidemic. *Obes Res,* 2001 9(suppl), 228S–33S.

[96] Van Dam, RM; Rimm, EB; Willett, WC; Stampfer, MJ; Hu FB. Dietary patterns and risk for type 2 diabetes mellitus in U.S. men. *Ann Intern Med*, 2002 136, 201–9.

[97] Fung, T; Hu, FB; Fuchs, C; Giovannucci, E; Hunter, DJ; Stampfer, MJ; Colditz, GA; Willett, WC. Major dietary patterns and the risk of colorectal cancer in women. *Arch Intern Med*, 2003 163, 309–14.

[98] Hu, FB; Rimm, EB; Stampfer, MJ; Ascherio, A; Spiegelman, D; Willett, WC. Prospective study of major dietary patterns and risk of coronary heart disease in men. *Am J Clin Nutr*, 2000 72, 912–021.

[99] Fung, TT; Willett, WC; Stampfer, MJ; Manson, JE; Hu, FB. Dietary patterns and the risk of coronary heart disease in women. *Arch Intern Med*, 2001 161, 1857–62.

[100] Anderson, AL; Harris, TB; Tylavsky, FA; Perry, SE; Houston, DK et all. Dietary patterns, insulin sensitivity and inflammation in older adults. *Eur J Clin Nutr*, 2012 66, 18–24.

[101] Kesse-Guyot, E; Ahluwalia, N; Lassale, C; Hercberg, S; Fezeu, L. Adherence to Mediterranean diet reduces the risk of metabolic syndrome: a 6-year prospective study. *Nutr Metab Cardiovasc Dis*, 2014 23, 677–83.

[102] Stark, O; Atkins, E; Wolff, OH; Douglas, JW. Longitudinal study of obesity in the National Survey of Health and Development. *Br Med J (Clin Res Ed),* 1981 283 (6283), 13-17.

[103] Toeller, M; Buyken, AE; Heitkamp, G; Cathelineau, G; Ferriss, B; Michel, G. Nutrient intakes as predictors of body weight in European people with type 1 diabetes. *Int J Obes Relat Metab Disord*, 2001 25, 1815–22.
[104] Bouche, C; Rizkalla, SW; Luo, J et all. Five-week, low-glycemic index diet decreases total fat mass and improves plasma lipid profile in moderately overweight nondiabetic men. *Diabetes Care,* 2002 25, 822–8.
[105] Esmaillzadeh, A,; Kimiagar, M; Mehrabi, Y; Azadbakht, L; Hu, FB et all. Dietary patterns and markers of systemic inflammation among Iranian women. *J Nutr*, 2007 137, 992–8.
[106] Ahluwalia, N; Andreeva, VA; Kesse-Guyot, E; Hercberg, S. Dietary patterns, inflammation and the metabolic syndrome. , 2013 39, 99–110.
[107] Griep, L; Wang, H; Chan, Q. Empirically Derived Dietary Patterns, Diet Quality Scores, and Markers of Inflammation and Endothelial Dysfunction. *Current Nutrition Reports,* 2013 2, 97–104.
[108] Haveman-Nies, A; de Groot, LP; van Staveren, WA. Snack patterns of older Europeans. *J. Am. Diet. Assoc.*, 1998 98, 1297–1302.
[109] Slattery, ML; Boucher, KM; Caan, BJ; Potter, JD; Ma, KN. Eating patterns and risk of colon cancer. *Am. J. Epidemiol.*, 1998 148, 4–16.
[110] Kimm, SY. The role of dietary fiber in the development and treatment of childhood obesity. *Pediatrics,* 1995 96, 1010–4.
[111] Jenkins, DJ; Kendall, CW; Augustin, LS et all. Glycemic index: overview of implications in health and disease. *Am J Clin Nutr,* 2002 76(suppl), 266S–73S.
[112] Prentice, AM. Manipulation of dietary fat and energy density and subsequent effects on substrate flux and food intake. *Am J Clin Nutr,* 1998 67(suppl), 535S–41S.
[113] Rolls, BJ; Bell, EA. Intake of fat and carbohydrate: role of energy density. *Eur J Clin Nutr*, 1999 53(suppl), 166–73.
[114] Ludwig, DS. The glycemic index: physiological mechanisms relating to obesity, diabetes, and cardiovascular disease. *JAMA*, 2002 287, 2414–23.
[115] Wolever, TM. The glycemic index. *World Rev Nutr Diet,* 1990 62, 120–85.
[116] Center for Genetics, Nutrition and Health, Washington, DC, USA. The Mediterranean diets: What is so special about the diet of Greece? The scientific evidence. Simopoulos AP. *The J Nutr*, 2001 131(11 Suppl), 3065S-73S.
[117] Trichopoulou, A; Lagiou, P; Kuper, H; Trichopoulos, D. Cancer and Mediterranean dietary traditions. *Cancer Epidemiol. Biomarkers Prev.,* 2009 9, 869–873.
[118] Busetto, L; Cresci, B; Cuzzolaro, M; Donini, LM; De Feo, P; Lapolla, A; Lucchin, L; Maffeis, C; Nisoli, E; Pasanisi, F; Rotella, C; Zamboni, M. Standard Italiani per la cura dell'obesità. SIO, ADI. 2012-2013.
[119] Issa, C; Darmon, N; Salameh, P; Maillot, M; Batal, M; Lairon D. A Mediterranean diet pattern with low consumption of liquid sweets and refined cereals is negatively associated with adiposity in adults from rural Lebanon. *Int J Obes (Lond)*, 2011 35(2), 251-8.
[120] Razquin, C; Martinez, JA; Martinez-Gonzalez, MA; Bes-Rastrollo, M; Fernandez-Crehuet, J; Marti, A. A 3-year intervention with a Mediterranean diet modified the association between the rs9939609 gene variant in FTO and body weight changes. *Int J Obes (Lond)*, 2010 34(2), 266-72.
[121] Sofi, F; Cesari, F; Abbate, R; Gensini, GF; Casini, A. Adherence to Mediterranean diet and health status: meta-analysis. *BMJ*, 2008 11, 337-1344.
[122] Buckland, G; Bach, A; Serra-Majem, L. Obesity and the Mediterranean diet: a systematic review of observational and intervention studies. *Obes Rev*, 2008 9(6), 582-93.

[123] Wadden, TA. Treatment of obesity by moderate and severe caloric restriction: results of clinical research trials. *Ann Intern Med*, 1993 13 (suppl 2), 91– 93.

[124] Jebb, SA; Prentice, AM; Goldberg, GR; Murgatroyd, PR; Black, AE; Coward, WA. Changes in macronutrient balance during over- and underfeeding assessed by 12-d continuous whole-body calorimetry. *Am J Clin Nutr*, 1996 64, 259-266.

[125] Dulloo, AG; Jacquet, J. Adaptive reduction in basal metabolic rate in response to food deprivation in humans: a role for feedback signals from fat stores. *Am J Clin Nutr,* 1998 68, 599–606.

[126] Schwartz, MW; Woods, SC; Porte, D Jr; Seeley, RJ; Baskin, DG. Central nervous system control of food intake. *Nature,* 2000 404, 661–671.

[127] Heyman, MB; Young, VR; Fuss, P; Tsay, R; Joseph, L; Roberts, SB. Underfeeding and body weight regulation in normal-weight young men. *Am J Physiol,* 1992 263, R250–R257.

[128] Jebb, SA; Prentice, AM; Goldberg, GR; Murgatroyd, PR; Black, AE; Coward, WA. Changes in macronutrient balance during over- and underfeeding assessed by 12-d continuous whole-body calorimetry. *Am J Clin Nutr*, 1996 64, 259 –266.

[129] Hill, JO; Wyatt, HR; Peters, JC. Using the energy gap to address obesity: a commentary. *J Am Diet Assoc*, 2009 109, 1848 –1854.

[130] Hill, JO. Can a small changes approach help address the obesity epidemic? A report of the Joint Taskforce of the America Society for Nutrition (ASN), Institute of Food Technologists (IFT), and the International Food Information Council (IFIC). *Am J Clin Nutr*, 2009 89, 477– 484.

[131] Niemeier, HM; Phelan, S; Fava, JL; Wing, RR. Internal disinhibition predicts weight regain following weight loss and weight loss maintenance. *Obesity*, 2007 15(10), 2485–2494.

[132] Oliva, L. (2010) *Corpi uguali, Storie diverse*, Mestre: Litostampa Veneta srl di Mestre Venezia

[133] Ohsiek, S; Williams, M. Psychological factors influencing weight loss maintenance: An integrative literature review. *Journal of the American Academy of Nurse Practitioner,* 2011 23(11), 592–601.

[134] Vogels, N; Diepvens, K; Westerterp-Plantenga, MS. Predictors of long-term weight maintenance. *Obesity Research*, 2005 13(12), 2162– 2168.

[135] Vogels, N; Westerterp-Plantenga, M. Successful long-term weight maintenance: A 2-year follow-up. *Obesity (Silver Spring, Md.),* 2007 15(5), 1258–1266.

[136] Niemeier, HM; Phelan, S; Fava, JL; Wing, RR. Internal disinhibition predicts weight regain following weight loss and weight loss maintenance. *Obesity*, 2007 15(10), 2485–2494.

[137] Wing, RR; Phelan, S. Long-term weight loss maintenance. *American Journal of Clinical Nutrition*, 2005 82(Suppl.), 222S–225S.

[138] Wing, RR; Papandonatos, G; Fava, JL; Gorin, AA; Phelan, S; McCaffery, J et all. Maintaining large weight losses: The role of behavioral and psychological factors. *Journal of Consulting and Clinical Psychology*, 2008 76(6), 1015–1021.

[139] Kraschnewski, JL; Boan, J; Esposito, J; Sherwood, NE; Lehman, EB; Kephart, DK; Sciamanna, CN. Long-term weight loss maintenance in the United States. *Int J Obes (Lond)*, 2010 34,1644 –1654.

[140] Dulloo, AG; Jacquet, J. Adaptive reduction in basal metabolic rate in response to food deprivation in humans: a role for feedback signals from fat stores. *Am J Clin Nutr*, 1998 68, 599–606.

[141] Brownell, KD. Public policy and the prevention of obesity. In: Fairburn CG and Brownell, eds. *Eating Disorders and Obesity*. New York, NY: The Guilford Press; 2001; 619–624.

[142] Wing, RR; Hill, JO. Successful weight loss maintenance. *Ann Rev Nutr*, 2001 21, 323–341.

In: The Different Faces of Being Overweight
Editor: Emilia Manzato

ISBN: 978-1-63483-099-7

Chapter 9

Overweight and Obesity in Internal Medicine

Lorenzo M. Donini*, MD
Experimental Medicine Department, Medical Pathophysiology,
Food Science and Endocrinology Section,
Food Science and Human Nutrition Research Unit,
Sapienza University of Rome, Italy
National Council Member,
Italian Society for the Study of Eating Disorder (SISDCA), Italy

Abstract

Obesity may be secondary to other diseases due to genetic or acquired conditions that are characterized by alterations in the control of systems regulating hunger-satiety and / or weight, in the gastrointestinal system and the intestinal microbiota, in endocrine pathways. Secondary obesity may be due to maternal metabolic conditions, to neurobiological and psychological determinants, to sleep debt and smoking cessation, to disability and to various medications.

Keywords: obesity, secondary obesity

Introduction

The obesity epidemic is considered one of the biggest public health concerns facing across the globe not only developed countries. An imbalance between energy intake and energy expenditure is always necessary to result in increased fat mass. However the obesogenic environment is not always necessary or sufficient to cause obesity: an individual can become obese in the absence of an obesogenic environment, and does not necessarily become obese in an obesogenic environment. Other factors may play a role and contribute to obesity. In fact the etiology of obesity is based on the interaction of several genes,

* Email: Lorenzomaria.donini@uniroma1.it.

environmental factors and individual behavior. Obesity may be secondary to other diseases due to genetic or acquired conditions that are characterized by alterations in the control of systems regulating hunger-satiety and / or weight, in the gastrointestinal system and the intestinal microbiota, in endocrine pathways. Moreover some drugs can cause directly or indirectly an increase of fat mass (1-3).

Genetic Syndromes

Obesity is a manifestation of several genetic syndromes. The hypothalamus plays a key role in the regulation of body weight by balancing the intake of food, energy expenditure, and body fat stores. Most monogenic syndromes of morbid obesity result from mutations in genes expressed in the hypothalamus. Hypothalamic obesity is a result of impairment in the hypothalamic regulatory centers, and may be caused by structural damage to the hypothalamus, radiotherapy, and mutations in some genes (*LEP*, *LEPR*, *POMC*, *MC4R* and *CART)*. The pathophysiology includes loss of sensitivity to afferent peripheral humoral signals, dysregulated insulin secretion, and impaired activity of the sympathetic nervous system.

Other rare single gene defects where obesity is the specific abnormality are represented by:

- syndromes related to the leptin signaling pathway (e.g. animal models of ciliopathies like Bardet-Biedl and Alstrom syndromes);
- Prader-Willi syndrome which is associated with hyperghrelinaemia (the mechanism of hyperphagia remains unclear);
- haploinsufficiency of BDNF (the *brain-derived neurotrophic factor is* a downstream mediator of leptin action) which is associated with hyperphagia and obesity in children with WAGR syndrome (where Wilms tumor, Aniridia, Genitourinary anomalies, and Retardation are associated) [4-10].

Neurobiological and Psychological Determinants

A growing body of evidence studying neurotransmitter regulation, neuronal projection pathways, clinical comorbidities, and behavioral studies considers that overeating and obesity are tightly linked to neurobiological and psychological aspects such as mood status, addictive behavior, motivation and reward processing as well as coping with psychosocial stress. The involvement of neuronal pathways that include brain areas assigned to reward, motivation, learning, memory, and cortical inhibitory control is more and more evident. Some Authors consider that, at minimum, obesity is a brain disease that is mediated by the interaction between energy homeostasis, detrimental hyperactivity of the stress systems, and activation of dopaminergic reward pathways. Chronic consumption of comfort foods alters brain functions (mesolimbic circuitry), and overeating may depend on reinforced reactivity to stimuli associated with palatable high calorie foods.

Stress may contribute to neurobiological pathogenesis of obesity: the neurobiology of stress overlaps significantly with that of appetite and energy regulation. Stress is a key risk factor in the development of addiction and in addiction relapse. High levels of stress change eating patterns in particular towards an increased consumption of highly palatable (HP) foods. With overconsumption of these foods, there are adaptations in stress and reward circuits that promote stress-related and HP food-related motivation as well as concomitant metabolic adaptations (alterations in glucose metabolism, insulin sensitivity, and other hormones related to energy homeostasis). These metabolic changes in turn might also affect dopaminergic activity to influence food motivation and intake of HP foods.

Therefore psychotherapeutic approaches (conventionally applied treatments for addiction, methods of conditioning to disconnect feelings of stress and reward from food intake behavior, learning stress coping strategies) together with psychopharmacological strategies (targeting neurotransmitter and neurohumoral circuits involved in mood regulation, reward perception, or addictive behavior such as serotonin, dopamine, or glutamate systems) may be appropriate to overcome the neuropsychological problem of obesity [11-16].

SLEEP DEBT

Over the past 50 years decrease in sleep duration (both in adults and children) was accompanied by an increase in obesity prevalence. Sleep quality and duration affect biological mediators of appetite and energy homeostasis. Therefore sleep deprivation in animal models tends to cause an increased food intake.

Different hormones and peptides regulating food intake and energy expenditure (ghrelin, leptin, galanin, orexin) may play a role in sleep-deprivation related increase of food intake, energy storage, and weight gain. Sleep-deprived subjects tend to have significantly increased appetite for energy-dense, high-carbohydrate foods and decreased activity caused by increased tiredness. Chronic, non-severe sleep deprivation may therefore affect glucose and insulin metabolism.

These data may be, at least partially, explained by the anti-obesogen and the weight-reducing effects of melatonin. Melatonin is a powerful chronobiotic being responsible, in part, by the daily distribution of metabolic processes. Experimental evidence demonstrates that melatonin is necessary for the proper synthesis, secretion, and action of insulin; it acts by regulating GLUT4 expression and/or triggering, via its G-protein-coupled membrane receptors, the phosphorylation of the insulin receptor and its intracellular substrates mobilizing the insulin signaling pathway. Furthermore, melatonin contributes to the control of energy balance mainly by regulating the energy flow to and from the stores, directly controlling the energy expenditure through the activation of brown adipose tissue and participating in the browning process of white adipose tissue [17-24].

ENDOCRINE DISORDERS

Among the endocrine abnormalities that may cause obesity we can find:

- Cushing's disease (characterized by an overproduction of adrenocorticotropic hormone ACTH). The distribution of fat mass is typically centripetal and it involves the face, the neck, the abdomen and the trunk, while arms and legs can be particularly thin due to sarcopenia;
- reduced secretion or action of GH (growth hormone). Also the overproduction of GH, as it happens in acromegaly and pituitary gigantism, may be accompanied (in approximately 30% of cases) to central obesity;
- hyperprolactinemia;
- primary hypothyroidism (reduced ability of the thyroid to synthesize a sufficient amount of thyroid hormones T3 and T4) or secondary (reduced secretion of thyroid stimulating hormone TSH);
- hypogonadotropic hypogonadism (decreased androgen production resulting from alterations that compromise the pituitary gonadotropin secretion);
- hypopituitarism with decreased secretion of all pituitary hormones;
- insulinoma;
- polycystic ovarian syndrome (characterized by oligo-anovulation, hyperandrogenism and multiple ovarian cysts) which is a consequence of but also a possible contributor to obesity;
- primary hypogonadism.

Finally it has to be considered that endocrine disorders are in most cases a consequence rather a cause of obesity. For example there is controversy concerning whether the changes in the levels of thyroid hormones and TSH in obesity are causes or consequences of weight status and whether these differences, that are normally slight, merit treatment with thyroxine. In a recent review it was found that the elevated TSH levels in obesity seem a consequence rather than a cause of obesity. The alterations in hormone levels seem to be an adaptive response designed to reduce the availability of energy for conversion into fat.

Chemicals that can disrupt endocrine functions are recently considered among the possible causes of obesity. Endocrine disruptors (EDs) may mimic the effect of hormones. Different chemicals have been studied as possible contributors to obesity: pesticides such as tributylin (TBT) and organophosphate or organochloride containing compounds (dichlorodiphenyltrichloroethane -DDT)), flame retardants such as polybrominated diphenyl ether (PBDE), plasticizers such as Bisphenol A (BPA) and phthalates, compounds used in non-stick coatings such as perflouroalkyl sulfonate and perfluorooctanoic acid (PFOA), and polychlorinated bisphenols (PCBs) used in electronics.

Some of these substances (e.g.: PCPs, PBDE, and DDT) are persistent organic pollutants with a high bioaccumulation while other chemicals (e.g.: BPA, phthalates, and PBDE) are produced in high volumes and, although they are less persistent in the environment, the exposure is nearly ubiquitous.

EDs may act in different ways depending on the chemical: some of them may directly induce adipogenesis, other will modify sex hormone metabolism or foetal development. The exposure during critical developmental stages may be important for the induction of obesity. Studies on animal models in particular have shown that perinatal PCB and TBT exposure causes obesity in rodent models.

Data on epidemiological association between ED exposure and obesity in humans have been reported but the consistency of the association is not constant and seems to depend on dose, developmental stage of exposure, and follow-up time [25-32].

ADIPOSE DISORDERS

Lipodystrophies or fat redistribution syndromes involve a primary lack/loss of subcutaneous adipose tissue (SAT) or an increase of it that can be confused with lifestyle-induced obesity.

1. HIV-and highly active antiretroviral treatment (HAART)-associated lipodystrophy includes loss of SAT from the face buttocks, arms, and legs. In men with lipodystrophy, SAT can be increased on the abdomen and chest (gynecomastia), and as a dorsocervical fat pad or "buffalo hump". In HIV+ women more frequently we may have increased intermuscular fat and SAT on the legs and on the upper part of the arm, large breasts (in particular in Black women and other non-Caucasian ethnicities);
2. acquired partial lipodystrophy (APL; Barraquer-Simons syndrome) is characterized by a regional loss of SAT starting at the face and extending to the waist. SAT may be increased on the legs. APL is thought to be autoimmune occurring after a viral illness with low levels of complement factor 3 and the presence of a circulating autoantibody called complement 3-nephritic factor;
3. familial partial lipodystrophies (FPLD):
   a) FPLD Type 1 (Köbberling lipodystrophy). It is a partial lipodystrophy primarily found in women causing a lipodystrophy of the arms, legs, and sometimes breasts, with an increase in fat on the abdomen and of the trunk;
   b) FPLD Type 2 (Dunnigan lipodystrophy). In FPLD2, SAT is lost during the puberty from the legs, arms, buttocks, abdomen and chest; areas of remaining SAT deposits are on the back, face and chin, giving a Cushingoid appearance; fat is increased in the labia majora in women;
4. rare adipose disorders (RADs) including multiple symmetric lipomatosis (MSL), lipedema and Dercum's disease (DD) may be misdiagnosed as obesity. RAD likely results from the growth of a brown stem cell population with secondary lymphatic dysfunction in MSL, or by primary vascular and lymphatic dysfunction in lipedema and DD [33-34].

MATERNAL METABOLIC CONDITIONS

The intrauterine environment influences the development of the foetus. The energy availability together with the foetus plasticity during gestational development are crucial not only for adapting it to its anticipated environment but also for the development of obesity.

Mother's under-nutrition may influence offspring body fatness in different ways. Children of nutrient-deprived mothers have greater preference for high fat diets, are more sedentary and the adipogenesis may be overstated if the offspring are exposed to a high-fat diet post-weaning. Maternal leptin levels seem be a key factor regulating this response.

Maternal over nutrition may influence too offspring outcomes. Animal and human studies suggest that maternal high fat diet and/or obesity, produces hyperphagic offspring with greater fat mass, and reduced activity levels. In this case the regulation depends on the effect of insulin, since maternal gestational diabetes may result in giving birth to large for gestational age offspring.

Maternal obesity and dysmetabolic syndromes may influence offspring outcomes and may induce obesity in them due to energy supply to the foetus, to changes in insulin resistance or to other metabolic factors that are present in the obese maternal environment. Studies comparing obesity in children whose mothers had undergone bariatric surgery for extreme morbid obesity showed that siblings born before surgery were more obese than were siblings born after weight loss in response to surgery.

Moreover in populations at high risk of obesity and diabetes (eg, Pima Indians), exposure to gestational diabetes is associated with increased risk of childhood and early adult obesity in offspring [35-44].

Calcium and Vit D

Low intakes of calcium and inadequate vitamin D status are associated with higher prevalence rates of obesity. There is consistent evidence that calcium and vitamin D increase whole body fat oxidation after single and multiple meals, and that calcium promotes a modest energy loss through increased faecal fat excretion. Calcium and vitamin D seem to be related to a greater diet-induced thermogenesis, to an increased lipolysis, to the suppression of key lipogenic enzymes, to decreased hunger ratings or reduced energy/macronutrient intake.

Moreover some studies found a potential improvement in insulin sensitivity following vitamin D supplementation that would suggest an effect on food intake and substrate oxidation [45-48].

Systemic Infections and Intestinal Microbiota

Pathogenic and symbiotic microorganisms, may influence metabolism and body fatness. Some infections alter hypothalamic regulation of energy balance, while others increase adipogenesis. The ability of pathogens to cause obesity is pathogen-specific and not a general result of infection, and the effect may be mediated, in most cases, through inflammatory processes. Different microorganisms linked, in particular, to common infections (adenoviruses SMAN-1 and Ad-36) and to pneumonia (Chlamidia) have been associated with obesity pathogenesis.

Gut microbiota also plays a role in the control of fat storage. Gut hormones seem to communicate information from the gastrointestinal tract to the regulatory appetite centers within the central nervous system via the so-called 'Gut-Brain-Axis'. Such information may be transferred to the CNS either via vagal or non-vagal afferent nerve signaling or directly via blood circulation. Complex neural networks, distributed throughout the forebrain and brainstem, control feeding and energy homoeostasis. Indigenous gut microbiota is implicated in the aetiopathogenesis of obesity and obesity-related disorders and has been shown to contribute to the low grade inflammation that characterises obesity. The microbiota and its metabolites mediate some of the alterations of the microbiota-gut-brain axis, the endocannabinoid system, and the bile acid metabolism, found in obesity-related disorders.

In animal and human studies, a high ratio of Firmicutes to Bacteriodetes is associated with greater energy harvest and a genetic predisposition to obesity. The introduction of gut microbiota from genetically obese mice into germ-free mice induces greater adiposity than microbiota from genetically lean mice. The reduction of the Firmicutes to Bacteriodetes ratio, through prebiotic treatment, decreases the fat mass and increases the muscle mass. It is not clear weather obesity precedes or follows changes in intestinal microbiota, animal models and human epidemiology demonstrate the ability of microorganisms to play a causative role in obesity [49-57].

Smoking Cessation

The prevalence of obesity and of smoking habits have had an opposite trend in recent decades. Smoking reduction is important from the point of view of public health and has been fostered through effective policies from health care institutions. However smoking cessation has been implicated as a contributor to increased obesity rates in several epidemiological studies. Nicotine is a thermogenic agent and may impact peptides involved in eating behaviours promoting elevated caloric intake. Smoke has metabolic effects which are known to decrease appetite while smoking cessation will be accompanied by an improved digestive function. Finally nicotine dependence may be substituted by a crazing behavior at the cessation of smoking [58-61].

Disability

People with disabilities (physical or cognitive) are more likely to experience more nutrition-related problems and are disproportionately more likely to be overweight or obese. Moreover obesity contributes to a variety of major medical concerns that may lead to further disability.

People with disabilities may experience functional limitations and/or they may have limited time or energy that may impact their ability to perform many tasks essential to proper nutrition: shopping for groceries, cooking, or even prepare meals. Additionally, people with disabilities are more likely to have lower incomes limiting their ability to afford healthier foods and often take medications that can complicate nutrient absorption or cause weight gain [62-64].

Iatrogenic Obesity

Various medications, such as psychotropics, antihypertensives, antidiabetics, steroid hormones and contraceptives, protease inhibitors, and antihistamines have been associated with weight gain:

1. antipsychotics (tricyclic antidepressants, selective serotonin reuptake inhibitors (SSRIs), such as paroxetine), are associated with increased appetite, weight gain, and metabolic abnormalities with significant weight gain;
2. antidiabetic medications, including thiazolidinediones, sulfonylureas, and insulin, can induce significant weight gain;
3. anti-inflammatory drugs (corticosteroid hormones) have been shown to cause weight gain due to increased visceral and truncal fat deposition (visceral adiposity) and appetite stimulation;
4. H1 antihistamines users have a significantly higher weight, waist circumference, and insulin concentration probably related to sedation side effect. that resulted in decreased energy expenditure and to disruption of H1 receptor expression and binding, leading to impaired insulin and leptin signaling [65-69].

References

[1] Dhurandhar, EJ; Keith, SW. The aetiology of obesity beyond eating more and exercising less. *Best Pract. Res. Clin. Gastroenterol.,* 2014 28, 533-544.

[2] Han, JC; Lawlor, DA; Kimm, SYS. Childhood obesity. *Lancet* 2010 375, 1737–48.

[3] Reinehr, T; Hinney, A; de Sousa, G; Austrup, F; Hebebrand, J; Andler, W. Definable Somatic Disorders in Overweight Children and Adolescents. *J. Pediatr.* 2007 150, 618-22.

[4] Farooqi, S; O'Rahilly, S. Genetics of obesity in humans. *Endocr. Rev.* 2006 27, 710–18.

[5] Feigerlova, E; Diene, G; Conte-Auriol, F. Hyperghrelinemia precedes obesity in Prader-Willi syndrome. *J. Clin. Endocrinol. Metab.* 2008 93, 2800–05.

[6] Cummings, DE ; Clement, K; Purnell, JQ. Elevated plasma ghrelin levels in Prader Willi syndrome. *Nat. Med.* 2002 8, 643–44.

[7] Seo, S; Guo, DF; Bugge, K; Morgan, DA; Rahmouni, K; Sheffi, VC. Requirement of Bardet-Biedl syndrome proteins for leptin receptor signaling. *Hum. Mol. Genet.* 2009 18 1323–31.

[8] Davenport, JR; Watts, AJ; Roper, VC. Disruption of intrafl agellar transport in adult mice leads to obesity and slow-onset cystic kidney disease. *Curr. Biol.* 2007 17, 1586–94.

[9] Han, JC; Liu, QR; Jones, M. Brain-derived neurotrophic factor and obesity in the WAGR syndrome. *N. Engl. J. Med.* 2008 359, 918–27.

[10] Kim, JH; Choi, JH. Pathophysiology and clinical characteristics of hypothalamic obesity in children and adolescents. *Ann. Pediatr Endocrinol. Metab.* 2013 18, 161-167.

[11] Jauch-Chara, K; Ottmans, KM. Obesity – A neuropsychological disease? Systematic review and neuropsychological model. *Progress in Neurobiology* 2014 114, 84–101.

[12] Atlantis, E; Baker, M. Obesity effects on depression: systematic review of epidemiological studies. *Int. J. Obes.* 2008 32, 881–891.
[13] Barry, D; Clarke, M; Petry. Obesity and its relationship to addictions: is overeating a form of addictive behavior? *Am. J. Addict.* 2009 18, 439–451.
[14] Berthoud, HR; Morrison, C. The brain, appetite, and obesity. *Annu. Rev. Psychol.* 2008 59, 55–92.
[15] Gadalla,TM. Association of obesity with mood and anxiety disorders in the adult general population. *Chronic Dis. Can.* 2009 30, 29–36.
[16] Sinha, R; Jastreboff, AM. Stress as a Common Risk Factor for Obesity and Addiction. *Biol. Psychiatry* 2013 73, 827–835.
[17] Mavanji, V; Teske, JA; Billington, CJ; Kotz, CM. Partial sleep deprivation by environmental noise increases food intake and body weight in obesity-resistant rats. *Obesity (Silver Spring)* 2013 21, 1396-405.
[18] Shechter, A; O'Keeffe, M; Roberts, AL; Zammit, GK; RoyChoudhury, A; St-Onge, MP. Alterations in sleep architecture in response to experimental sleep curtailment are associated with signs of positive energy balance. *Am. J. Physiol. Regul. Integr. Comp. Physiol.* 2012 303, 883-9.
[19] Jean-Louis, G; Williams, NJ; Sarpong, D; Pandey, A; Youngstedt, S; Zizi, F. Associations between inadequate sleep and obesity in the US adult population: analysis of the national health interview survey. *BMC Public Health* 2014 14, 290.
[20] Hargens, TA; Kaleth, AS; Edwards, ES; Butner, KL. Association between sleep disorders, obesity, and exercise: a review. *Nat. Sci. Sleep* 2013 5, 27-35.
[21] Liu, J; Zhang, A; Li, L. Sleep duration and overweight/obesity in children: review and implications for pediatric nursing. *J. Special Pediatr Nurs* 2012 17, 193-204.
[22] Hart, CN; Carskadon, MA; Considine, RV; Fava, JL; Lawton, J; Raynor, HA. Changes in children's sleep duration on food intake, weight, and leptin. *Pediatrics* 2013 132, 1473-80.
[23] Beebe, DW; Simon, S; Summer, S; Hemmer, S; Strotman, D; Dolan, LM. Dietary intake following experimentally restricted sleep in adolescents. *Sleep* 2013 36, 827-34.
[24] Cipolla-Neto, J; Amaral, FG; Afeche, SC; Tan, DX; Reiter, RJ. Melatonin, energy metabolism, and obesity: a review. *J. Pineal Res.* 2014 56, 371–381.
[25] Janesick. A; Blumberg, B. Endocrine disrupting chemicals and the developmental programming of adipogenesis and obesity. *Birth Defects Res. Part C Embryo Today Rev.* 2011 93, 34-50.
[26] Zuo, Z; Chen, S; Wu, T; Zhang, J; Su, Y; Chen, Y. Tributyltin causes obesity and hepatic steatosis in male mice. *Environ. Toxicol.* 2011 26, 79-85.
[27] Mackay, H; Patterson, ZR; Khazall, R; Patel, S; Tsirlin, D; Abizaid, A. Organizational effects of perinatal exposure to bisphenol-A and diethylstilbestrol on arcuate nucleus circuitry controlling food intake and energy expenditure in male and female CD-1 mice. *Endocrinology* 2013 154, 1465-75.
[28] Ryan, KK; Haller, AM; Sorrell, JE; Woods, SC; Jandacek, RJ; Seeley, RJ. Perinatal exposure to bisphenol-a and the development of metabolic syndrome in CD-1 mice. *Endocrinology* 2010 151, 2603-12.
[29] Kendig, EL; Buesing, DR; Christie, SM; Cookman, CJ; Gear, RB; Hugo, ER. Estrogen-like disruptive effects of dietary exposure to bisphenol A or 17alpha-ethinyl estradiol in CD1 mice. *Int. J. Toxicol.* 2012 31, 537-50.

[30] Tang-Peronard, JL; Andersen, HR; Jensen, TK; Heitmann, BL. Endocrine-disrupting chemicals and obesity development in humans: a review. *Obes. Rev.* 2011; 12: 622-36.
[31] Reinehr, T. Obesity and thyroid function. Molecular and Cellular Endocrinology 2010 316, 165–171.
[32] Reinehr, T. Thyroid function in the nutritionally obese child and adolescent. *Current Opinion in Pediatrics* 2011 23, 415–420.
[33] Herbts, KL. Rare adipose disorders (RADs) masquerading as obesity. *Acta Pharmacologica Sinica* 2012 33, 155–172.
[34] Garg, A. Lipodystrophies: genetic and acquired body fat disorders. *J. Clin. Endocrinol. Metab.* 2011 96, 3313–25.
[35] Vickers, MH; Gluckman, PD; Coveny, AH; Hofman, PL; Cutfield, WS; Gertler, A. Neonatal leptin treatment reverses developmental programming. *Endocrinology* 2005 146, 4211-6.
[36] Samuelsson, AM; Matthews, PA; Argenton, M; Christie, MR; McConnell, JM; Jansen, EH. Diet-induced obesity in female mice leads to offspring hyperphagia, adiposity, hypertension, and insulin resistance: a novel murine model of developmental programming. *Hypertension* 2008 51, 383-92.
[37] Krasnow, SM; Nguyen, ML; Marks, DL. Increased maternal fat consumption during pregnancy alters body composition in neonatal mice. *Am. J. Physiol. Endocrinol. Metab.* 2011 301, 1243-53.
[38] Kral, JG; Biron, S; Simard, S; Hould, FS; Lebel, S; Marceau, S. Large maternal weight loss from obesity surgery prevents transmission of obesity to children who were followed for 2 to 18 years. *Pediatrics* 2006 118, 1644-9.
[39] Ong, KK; Loos, RJ. Rapid infancy weight gain and subsequent obesity: systematic reviews and hopeful suggestions. *Acta Paediatr* 2006 95, 904-8.
[40] Kiel, DW; Dodson, EA; Artal, R; Boehmer, TK; Leet, TL. Gestational weight gain and pregnancy outcomes in obese women: how much is enough? *Obstetrics Gynecol.* 2007 110, 752-8.
[41] Dabelea, D. The predisposition to obesity and diabetes in off spring of diabetic mothers. *Diabetes Care* 2007 30, 169–74.
[42] Lawlor, DA; Fraser, A; Lindsay, RS. Association of existing diabetes, gestational diabetes and glycosuria in pregnancy with macrosomia and off spring body mass index, waist and fat mass in later childhood: fi ndings from a prospective pregnancy cohort. *Diabetologia* 2010 53, 89–97.
[43] Kral, JG; Biron S; Simard, S. Large maternal weight loss from obesity surgery prevents transmission of obesity to children who were followed for 2 to 18 years. *Pediatrics* 2006 118, 1644–49.
[44] Lawlor, DA ; Timpson, NJ; Harbord, RM. Exploring the developmental overnutrition hypothesis using parental-off spring associations and FTO as an instrumental variable. *PLoS Med.* 2008 5, 33.
[45] Soares, MJ; Murhadi; LL; Kurpad, AV; Chan, WL; Piers, LS. Mechanistic roles for calcium and vitamin D in the regulation of body weight. *Obesity Reviews* 2012 13, 592–605.
[46] Gilbert, J-A; Joanisse, DR; Chaput, J-P. Milk supplementation facilitates appetite control in obese women during weight loss: a randomised, single-blind, placebo-controlled trial. *Br. J. Nutr.* 2011 105, 133–143.

[47] Boon, N; Hul, GBJ; Viguerie, N; Sicard, A; Langin, D; Saris, WHM. Effects of 3 diets with various calcium contents on 24-h energy expenditure, fat oxidation, and adipose tissue message RNA expression of lipid metabolism–related proteins. *Am. J. Clin. Nutr.* 2005 82, 1244–1252.

[48] Lorenzen, JK; Astrup, A. Dairy calcium intake modifies responsiveness of fat metabolism and blood lipids to a high-fat diet. *Br. J. Nutr.* 2011 105, 1823–1831.

[49] Whigham, LD; Israel, BA; Atkinson, RL. Adipogenic potential of multiple human adenoviruses in vivo and in vitro in animals. *Am. J. Physiol. Regul. Integr. Comp. Physiol.* 2006 290, 190-4.

[50] Schilder, RJ; Marden, JH. Metabolic syndrome and obesity in an insect. *Proc. Natl. Acad. Sci. USA* 2006 103, 18805-9.

[51] Fernandez-Real, JM; Ferri, MJ; Vendrell, J; Ricart, W. Burden of infection and fat mass in healthy middle-aged men. *Obesity (Silver Spring)* 2007 15, 245-52.

[52] Yamada, T; Hara, K; Kadowaki, T. Association of adenovirus 36 infection with obesity and metabolic markers in humans: a meta-analysis of observational studies. *PloS ONE* 2012 7, e42031.

[53] Goossens, VJ; de Jage,r SA ; Grauls, GE ; Gielen, M ; Vlietinck, RF ; Derom, CA. Lack of evidence for the role of human adenovirus-36 in obesity in a European cohort. *Obesity (Silver Spring)* 2011 19, 220-1.

[54] Turnbaugh, PJ; Ley, RE; Mahowald, MA; Magrini, V; Mardis, ER; Gordon, JI. An obesity-associated gut microbiome with increased capacity for energy harvest. *Nature* 2006 444, 1027-31.

[55] Everard, A; Lazarevic, V; Derrien, M; Girard, M; Muccioli, GG; Neyrinck, AM. Responses of gut microbiota and glucose and lipid metabolism to prebiotics in genetic obese and diet-induced leptin-resistant mice. *Diabetes* 2011 60, 2775-86.

[56] Buhmann, H; le Roux, CW; Bueter, M. The gut-brain axis in obesity. *Best Practice & Research Clinical Gastroenterology* 2014 28, 559-571.

[57] Moran, CP; Shanahan, F. Gut microbiota and obesity: Role in aetiology and potential therapeutic target. *Best Practice & Research Clinical Gastroenterology* 2014 28, 585-597.

[58] Jessen, AB; Toubro, S; Astrup, A. Effect of chewing gum containing nicotine and caffeine on energy expenditure and substrate utilization in men. *Am. J. Clin. Nutr.* 2003 77, 1442-7.

[59] Filozof, C; Fernandez Pinilla, MC; Fernandez-Cruz A. Smoking cessation and weight gain. *Obes. Rev.* 2004 5, 95-103.

[60] Marti, B; Tuomilehto, J; Korhonen, HJ; Kartovaara, L; Vartiainen, E; Pietinen, P. Smoking and leanness: evidence for change in Finland. *BMJ* 1989 298, 1287-90.

[61] Honjo, K; Siegel, M. Perceived importance of being thin and smoking initiation among young girls. *Tob. Control* 2003 12, 289-95.

[62] Centers for Disease Control and Prevention. Disability and Obesity. Available from, www.cdc.gov/ncbddd/disabilityandhealth/obesity.html; 2012

[63] Melville, CA; Cooper, SA; Morrison, JJ; Allan, LL; Smiley, EE; Williamson, AA. The prevalence and determinants of obesity in adults with intellectual disabilities. *J. Appl. Res. Intellect Disabil.* 2008 21, 425-437.

[64] King, JL; Pomeranz, JL; Merten, JW: Nutrition interventions for people with disabilities: A scoping review. *Disability and Health Journal* 2014 7, 157-163.

[65] Cope, MB; Nagy, TR; Fernandez, JR; Geary, N; Casey, DE; Allison, DB. Antipsychotic drug-induced weight gain: development of an animal model. *Int. J. Obes.* 2005 29, 607-14.

[66] Cooper, GD; Pickavance, LC; Wilding, JP; Harrold, JA; Halford, JC; Goudie, AJ. Effects of olanzapine in male rats: enhanced adiposity in the absence of hyperphagia, weight gain or metabolic abnormalities. *J. Psychopharmacol.* 2007 21, 405-13.

[67] Paulose-Ram, R; Safran, MA; Jonas, BS; Gu, Q; Orwig, D. Trends in psychotropic medication use among U.S. adults. *Pharmacoepidemiol. Drug Saf.* 2007 16, 560-70.

[68] Messerli, FH; Bell, DS; Fonseca V; Katholi, RE; McGill, JB; Phillips, RA. Body weight changes with beta-blocker use: results from GEMINI. *Am. J. Med.* 2007 120, 610-5.

[69] Ratliff, JC; Barber, JA; Palmese, LB; Reutenauer, EL; Tek, C. Association of prescription H1 antihistamine use with obesity: results from the National Health and Nutrition Examination Survey. *Obesity (Silver Spring).* 2010 18, 2398-400.

CONCLUSION

We hope that this book may meet the readers' interest by stimulating a deeper curiosity about overweight problems.

We'd like to give our little contribution to keep the debate and the interest on overweight alive and to contribute to considering overweight as a complex situation.

We'd like to thank all the authors who contributed to carrying out this book: for their precious effort and competence while dealing with such a complex problem like overweight.

We strongly hope to convey to our readers that passion which we always have when dealing with obese and overweight patients.

We'd like to thank our patients too, because they constantly encourage us to go beyond our knowledge.

Finally we'd like to thank the publishers who allowed us to share our experience.

AFFILIATIONS

Bolognesi Antonia
Psychologist, Psychotherapist,
Italian Society for the Study of Eating Disorder (SISDCA).
Rome, Italy
antoniabolognesi@libero.it

Bosello Ottavio, MD
Department of Medicine
University of Verona,
Former President SIO (Italian Society for Obesity)
Verona, Italy
ottavio.bosello@univr.it

Donini Lorenzo M., MD
Experimental Medicine Department
Medical Pathophysiology, Food Science and Endocrinology Section
Food Science and Human Nutrition Research Unit
Sapienza University of Rome
National Council Member,
Italian Society for the Study of Eating Disorder (SISDCA)
Rome, Italy
Lorenzomaria.donini@uniroma1.it

Luxardi Gian Luigi,
Clinical Psychologist,
Chief of Center for Eating Disorders of ASL n.6,
"Friuli Occidentale", Italy
President, Triveneto Section,
Italian Society for the Study of Eating Disorders (SISDCA)
Rome, Italy
gianluigi.luxardi@ass6.sanita.fvg.it

Manzato Emilia
Psychiatrist,
University of Ferrara, Italy
National Council Member,
Italian Society for the Study of Eating Disorder (SISDCA),
Rome, Italy
Emilia.manzato@gmail.com

Marchiol Fiorenza,
Clinical Psychologist,
Center for Eating Disorders of ASL n.6,
"Friuli Occidentale", Italy
Italian Society for the Study of Eating Disorders (SISDCA)
Rome, Italy

Melchionda Nazario, MD
University of Bologna, Italy
President, Italian Society for the Study of Eating Disorder (SISDCA)
Rome, Italy
melchiondauno@gmail.com

Roncarati Eleonora
Dietitian,
Italian Society for the Study of Eating Disorders (SISDCA)
Rome, Italy
Eleonora.roncarati@libero.it

Giulietta Tarrini
Dietista Coordinatrice, Azienda Ospedaliera di Bologna,
Policlinico S.Orsola-Malpighi,
Servizio di Malattie del Metabolismo e Dietetica Clinica, Italy
gtarrini@gmail.com

Vania Andrea, MD
Former President of ECOG (European Childhood Obesity Group)
Department of Paediatrics and Paediatric Neuropsychiatry,
Sapienza University of Rome, Italy
andrea.vania@uniroma1.it

Vanzo Angiola, MD
Department of Prevention, Food Hygiene and Nutrition Service,
ASL 6 Vicenza, Veneto, Italy
angiola.vanzo@ulssvicenza.it

INDEX

B

D

E

F

G

H

I

J

K

L

M

N

O

P

Q

R

S

T

U

V

W

Y